SLEEP DISORDERS AND SLEEP DEPRIVATION

AN UNMET PUBLIC HEALTH PROBLEM

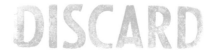

Committee on Sleep Medicine and Research

Board on Health Sciences Policy

Harvey R. Colten and Bruce M. Altevogt, *Editors*

INSTITUTE OF MEDICINE
OF THE NATIONAL ACADEMIES

THE NATIONAL ACADEMIES PRESS
Washington, DC
www.nap.edu

THE NATIONAL ACADEMIES PRESS • 500 Fifth Street, N.W. • Washington, DC 20001

NOTICE: The project that is the subject of this report was approved by the Governing Board of the National Research Council, whose members are drawn from the councils of the National Academy of Sciences, the National Academy of Engineering, and the Institute of Medicine. The members of the committee responsible for the report were chosen for their special competences and with regard for appropriate balance.

This study was supported by contracts between the National Academy of Sciences and the American Academy of Sleep Medicine, the Department of Health and Human Services (contract No. N01-OD-4-2139), the National Sleep Foundation, and the Sleep Research Society. Any opinions, findings, conclusions, or recommendations expressed in this publication are those of the author(s) and do not necessarily reflect the view of the organizations or agencies that provided support for this project.

Library of Congress Cataloging-in-Publication Data

Sleep disorders and sleep deprivation : an unmet public health problem / Committee on Sleep Medicine and Research, Board on Health Sciences Policy ; Harvey R. Colten and Bruce M. Altevogt, editors.
    p. ; cm.
    Includes bibliographical references and index.
    Supported by contracts between the National Academy of Sciences and the American Academy of Sleep Medicine, the Department of Health and Human Services, the National Sleep Foundation, and the Sleep Research Society Contract no. N01-OD-4-2139
    ISBN 0-309-10111-5 (hardback)
    1. Sleep disorders—Social aspects. 2. Sleep deprivation—Social aspects. 3. Sleep—Social aspects. 4. Public health. I. Colten, Harvey R. II. Altevogt, Bruce M. III. Institute of Medicine (U.S.). Committee on Sleep Medicine and Research.
    [DNLM: 1. Sleep Disorders—United States. 2. Health Policy—United States. 3. Sleep Deprivation—United States. WM 188 S63178 2006]
    RC547.S554 2006
    362.196'8498—dc22
                                                                      2006014107

Additional copies of this report are available from the National Academies Press, 500 Fifth Street, N.W., Lockbox 285, Washington, DC 20055; (800) 624-6242 or (202) 334-3313 (in the Washington metropolitan area); Internet, http://www.nap.edu.

For more information about the Institute of Medicine, visit the IOM home page at: www.iom.edu.

"Knowing is not enough; we must apply.
Willing is not enough; we must do."
—Goethe

INSTITUTE OF MEDICINE
OF THE NATIONAL ACADEMIES

Advising the Nation. Improving Health.

THE NATIONAL ACADEMIES
Advisers to the Nation on Science, Engineering, and Medicine

The **National Academy of Sciences** is a private, nonprofit, self-perpetuating society of distinguished scholars engaged in scientific and engineering research, dedicated to the furtherance of science and technology and to their use for the general welfare. Upon the authority of the charter granted to it by the Congress in 1863, the Academy has a mandate that requires it to advise the federal government on scientific and technical matters. Dr. Ralph J. Cicerone is president of the National Academy of Sciences.

The **National Academy of Engineering** was established in 1964, under the charter of the National Academy of Sciences, as a parallel organization of outstanding engineers. It is autonomous in its administration and in the selection of its members, sharing with the National Academy of Sciences the responsibility for advising the federal government. The National Academy of Engineering also sponsors engineering programs aimed at meeting national needs, encourages education and research, and recognizes the superior achievements of engineers. Dr. Wm. A. Wulf is president of the National Academy of Engineering.

The **Institute of Medicine** was established in 1970 by the National Academy of Sciences to secure the services of eminent members of appropriate professions in the examination of policy matters pertaining to the health of the public. The Institute acts under the responsibility given to the National Academy of Sciences by its congressional charter to be an adviser to the federal government and, upon its own initiative, to identify issues of medical care, research, and education. Dr. Harvey V. Fineberg is president of the Institute of Medicine.

The **National Research Council** was organized by the National Academy of Sciences in 1916 to associate the broad community of science and technology with the Academy's purposes of furthering knowledge and advising the federal government. Functioning in accordance with general policies determined by the Academy, the Council has become the principal operating agency of both the National Academy of Sciences and the National Academy of Engineering in providing services to the government, the public, and the scientific and engineering communities. The Council is administered jointly by both Academies and the Institute of Medicine. Dr. Ralph J. Cicerone and Dr. Wm. A. Wulf are chair and vice chair, respectively, of the National Research Council.

www.national-academies.org

Independent Report Reviewers

This report has been reviewed in draft form by individuals chosen for their diverse perspectives and technical expertise, in accordance with procedures approved by the National Research Council's Report Review Committee. The purpose of this independent review is to provide candid and critical comments that will assist the institution in making its published report as sound as possible and to ensure that the report meets institutional standards for objectivity, evidence, and responsiveness to the study charge. The review comments and draft manuscript remain confidential to protect the integrity of the deliberative process. We wish to thank the following individuals for their review of this report:

Ruth Benca, Department of Psychiatry, University of Wisconsin, Madison
Mary A. Carskadon, Sleep Research Laboratory, Brown University
Norman H. Edelman, Health Sciences Center, SUNY Stony Brook University
Stephen L. Hauser, Department of Neurology, University of California, San Francisco
Meir H. Kryger, Sleep Disorders Center, St. Boniface General Hospital Winnipeg, Manitoba, Canada
Lawrence S. Lewin, Executive Consultant, Chevy Chase, Maryland
Thomas Roth, Sleep Center, Henry Ford Hospital, Detroit, Michigan
Joan L. Shaver, College of Nursing, University of Illinois at Chicago
Joseph S. Takahashi, Department of Neurobiology & Physiology, Northwestern University

Terry B. Young, Department of Population Health Sciences, University of Wisconsin

Although the reviewers listed above have provided many constructive comments and suggestions, they were not asked to endorse the conclusions or recommendations, nor did they see the final draft of the report before its release. The review of this report was overseen by **David J. Kupfer,** University of Pittsburgh School of Medicine, and **Floyd E. Bloom,** Professor Emeritus Department of Neuropharmacology, The Scripps Research Institute. Appointed by the National Research Council and Institute of Medicine, they were responsible for making certain that an independent examination of this report was carried out in accordance with institutional procedures and that all review comments were carefully considered. Responsibility for the final content of this report rests entirely with the authoring committee and the institution.

Preface

Sleep has been a subject of intense interest to poets and mystics and is found in folklore since antiquity. Only in the last half a century have scientists and physicians attempted a systematic study of the biology and disorders of sleep. Within the past four decades remarkable advances in the neurophysiology of normal sleep and in circadian biology and the discovery of the genes that regulate these biological rhythms have provided a scientific framework for the elucidation of the etiology, pathogenesis, and potential treatment of sleep disorders. These scientific advances and input from many clinical disciplines such as internal medicine, neurology, nursing, otolaryngology, pediatrics, psychiatry, psychology, and pulmonology have enriched the study and management of sleep pathology. However, the broad intellectual and service requirements for dealing with sleep has created difficulties in coordination and planning of research and clinical services. Recognition of around 90 distinct clinical disorders of sleep has created a platform and need for specialization in the study of sleep (somnology) and sleep pathology. Accordingly, professional societies such as the American Academy of Sleep Medicine, the American Sleep Apnea Association, the National Sleep Foundation, and the Sleep Research Society have been established and the discipline has been recognized by the American Board of Medical Specialties. Moreover, the National Institutes of Health (NIH) formed the National Center on Sleep Disorders Research (NCSDR) to coordinate research in sleep. Although these developments are positive, they do not yet fully address the scope and depth of the public and individual health consequences of sleep deprivation and sleep disorders. For example, more than 50 million Americans suffer a chronic sleep disorder and many others experience disruption of normal daytime activities owing to sleep deprivation. Sadly, the majority of individuals with substantial sleep disorders are not diagnosed and appropriately treated.

In recognition of the limited appreciation of the importance of sleep disorders and sleep deprivation for individuals and the public health, the American Academy of Sleep Medicine, the NCSDR at the NIH, the National Sleep Foundation, and the Sleep Research Society requested that the Institute of Medicine (IOM) do the following:

1. Review and quantify the public health significance of sleep health, sleep loss, and sleep disorders, including assessments of the contribution of sleep disorders to poor health, reduced quality of life, and early mortality, as well as the economic consequences of sleep loss and sleep disorders.

2. Identify gaps in the public health system relating to the understanding, management, and treatment of sleep loss and sleep disorders and assess the adequacy of the current resources and infrastructure for addressing the gaps.

3. Identify barriers to and opportunities for improving and stimulating multi- and interdisciplinary research and education in sleep medicine and biology. Delineate organizational models that will promote and facilitate sleep research in the basic sciences, collaborative research between basic scientists, clinicians, and population scientists in relevant specialties, and education of practitioners and scientists in sleep health, sleep disorders, and sleep research.

4. Develop a comprehensive plan for enhancing sleep medicine and sleep research for improving the public's health.

In response, the IOM appointed a 14-member committee with expertise in pulmonology, cardiology, nursing, neurology, pediatrics, adolescent medicine, psychiatry, epidemiology, public health, otolaryngology, academic and medical administration, and health sciences research. The committee met five times during the course of its work and held two workshops. In addition, the committee received input from relevant federal, private, and nonprofit organizations.

Our findings confirmed the enormous public health burden of sleep disorders and sleep deprivation and the strikingly limited capacity of the health care enterprise to identify and treat the majority of individuals suffering sleep problems.

The direct effects of sleep disorders as well as the comorbidity with other substantial public health problems such as obesity, diabetes, stroke, and depression have a profound economic and social impact. Only minimal estimates of the economic impact of sleep disorders and their derivative consequences are possible because of underrecognition and underreporting.

At a minimum, however, the total direct and indirect cost of sleep disorders and sleep deprivation in the United States is hundreds of billions of dollars. The magnitude of the effect of sleep pathology is shocking even to experts in the field of somnology and sleep medicine. We found that there are too few professionals dedicated to sleep problems to meet the size and importance of the problem and there are too few educational programs that have the potential to increase the workforce of health care practitioners and scientists to meet even current demands. In addition, research that will advance our understanding of sleep pathology and its treatment has been underfunded. We therefore have outlined recommendations to address these shortcomings, in the hope that the burden of sleep disorders and sleep deprivation can be minimized. These recommendations fall into four broad categories: education (public, professional); technology; coordination of research initiatives at the NIH; and organization of research, clinical care, and education in academic health centers.

EDUCATION

The lack of public awareness should prompt a multimedia public education campaign that also targets elementary, middle, and high school students as well as undergraduate college health education programs about the impact of inadequate sleep.

Professional education will be enhanced by integrating the teaching of sleep medicine and biology into medical, nursing, and pharmacology curricula and into residency and specialty fellowships. Strategies to facilitate careers in somnology will be needed to meet the demand for sound science and expert clinical capacity to take care of the health problems related to sleep disorders.

TECHNOLOGY

The cumbersome nature and cost of diagnosis and treatment of sleep disorders and sleep loss will require research to develop and validate the efficacy of advances in diagnostic technologies, including ambulatory monitoring and imaging as well as the development of new therapeutic options for specific sleep disorders.

NATIONAL INSTITUTES OF HEALTH

The NCSDR at the NIH should take a more proactive role in promoting integration of research disciplines pertinent to somnology and sleep disorders, and it should promote training programs that increase the pipeline of highly qualified investigators. Together with other federal agencies, the

NCSDR can support increased public awareness and generation of more reliable prevalence data.

ORGANIZATION OF ACADEMIC HEALTH CENTERS

Within academic health centers new and existing sleep programs should be organized as Interdisciplinary Sleep Programs that encompass the relevant basic and clinical disciplines. The complexity of these programs will vary in accord with the capacity and goals of each center; therefore, we have proposed several different models. Networking among the most complex of these programs will facilitate research progress and accelerate implementation of new clinical strategies with help from the NCSDR.

The committee has been fortunate in having superb support from IOM staff and willing consultants in related fields. Without their help this report could not have been completed. We are most grateful.

Harvey R. Colten, M.D., *Chair*

Acknowledgments

The committee acknowledges with appreciation the individuals who provided information to the committee. These individuals include Richard Allen, Johns Hopkins University School of Medicine; Sonia Ancoli-Israel, University of California, San Diego School of Medicine; Bonnie Austin, AcademyHealth; Donald Bliwise, Emory University; Martha Brewer, American Heart Association; Debra J. Brody, National Center for Health Statistics; Kathleen C. Buckwalter, University of Iowa Center on Aging; Roger Bulger, Association of Academic Health Centers; Daniel Buysse, University of Pittsburgh School of Medicine; Andrea Califano, Columbia University; Sue Ciezadlo, American College of Chest Physicians; Charles A. Czeisler, Harvard University School of Medicine; William Dement, Stanford University School of Medicine; David Dinges, University of Pennsylvania School of Medicine; Darrel Drobnich, National Sleep Foundation; Paul Eggers, National Institute of Diabetes and Digestive and Kidney Diseases; Lawrence Epstein, Sleep HealthCenters; Gary Ewart, American Thoracic Society; David Lewis, SleepMed, Inc; Magda Galindo, American Diabetes Association; Lee Goldman, University of California, San Francisco Medical School; Allan Gordon, American Thoracic Society; Daniel Gottlieb, Boston University School of Medicine; David Gozal, University of Louisville; Meir Kryger, University of Manitoba; James Kiley, National Heart, Lung, and Blood Institute; David J. Kupfer, University of Pittsburgh School of Medicine; Story Landis, National Institute of Neurological Disorders and Stroke; Kathy Lee, University of California, San Francisco; Eugene J. Lengerich, Pennsylvania Cancer Control Consortium; Carole Marcus, The Children's Hospital of Pennsylvania; Jennifer Markkanen, American Academy of Sleep

Medicine; Michael Martin, Center for Scientific Review, National Institutes of Health; William McLeod, Institute of Medicine; John McGrath, National Institute of Child Health & Human Development; Merrill Mitler, National Institute of Neurological Disorders and Stroke; Rosanne Money, American Academy of Sleep Medicine; Hal Moses, Vanderbilt-Ingram Cancer Center; Judith Owens, Brown University Medical School; Barbara Phillips, University of Kentucky College of Medicine; Stuart Quan, University of Arizona; Roger Rosa, National Institute for Occupational Safety and Health; Thomas Roth, Henry Ford Health System of Detroit; Michael Sateia, Dartmouth University; Jerome Siegel, University of California, Los Angeles; John Slater, American Academy of Sleep Medicine; Margaret Snyder, National Institutes of Health; Ed Sondik, The National Center for Health Statistics; Ray Vento, American Lung Association; James Walsh, St. Luke's Hospital; David White, Brigham and Women's Hospital; Steven Wolinsky, Northwestern University; Terry Young, University of Wisconsin.

This study was sponsored by the American Academy of Sleep Medicine, the National Center on Sleep Disorders Research of the National Institutes of Health, the National Sleep Foundation, and the Sleep Research Society. We appreciate their support and especially thank Jerry Barrett, Richard Gelula, Al Golden, Carl Hunt, and Michael Twery for their efforts on behalf of this study.

We appreciate the work of John Fontanesi, University of California, San Diego for his commissioned paper. We also thank Andrew Pope for his guidance and Judy Estep for her expertise in formatting the report for production. Finally, we especially thank Cathy Liverman for all of her thoughtful guidance throughout the project.

Contents

SLEEP DISORDERS AND SLEEP DEPRIVATION

AN UNMET PUBLIC HEALTH PROBLEM

Summary

ABSTRACT   It is estimated that 50 to 70 million Americans chronically suffer from a disorder of sleep and wakefulness, hindering daily functioning and adversely affecting health and longevity. The cumulative long-term effects of sleep deprivation and sleep disorders have been associated with a wide range of deleterious health consequences including an increased risk of hypertension, diabetes, obesity, depression, heart attack, and stroke. The Institute of Medicine (IOM) Committee on Sleep Medicine and Research concluded that although clinical activities and scientific opportunities in the field are expanding, awareness among the general public and health care professionals is low, given the magnitude of the burden. The available human resources and capacity are insufficient to further develop the science and to diagnose and treat individuals with sleep disorders. Therefore, the current situation necessitates a larger and more interdisciplinary workforce. Traditional scientific and medical disciplines need to be attracted into the somnology and sleep medicine field. Renewed and revitalized commitments to the field from the National Institutes of Health (NIH), academic health centers, private foundations, and professional societies are essential to ensure appropriate public and professional awareness, education and training, basic and clinical research, and patient care. Finally, the fragmentation of research and clinical care currently present in most academic institutions requires the creation of accredited interdisciplinary sleep programs in academic institutions.

1

Fitful sleep, restless nights, and hitting the alarm clock button for an additional 10 minutes of sleep are all too familiar manifestations of the interactions of life with one of the frontiers of science and clinical practice—somnology[1] and sleep medicine. It is estimated that 50 to 70 million Americans suffer from a chronic disorder of sleep and wakefulness, hindering daily functioning and adversely affecting health. Hundreds of billions of dollars a year are spent on direct medical costs associated with doctor visits, hospital services, prescriptions, and over-the-counter medications. Almost 20 percent of all serious car crash injuries in the general population are associated with driver sleepiness, independent of alcohol effects. However, given this burden, awareness among the general public and health care professionals is low. In addition, the current clinical and scientific workforce is not sufficient to diagnose and treat individuals with sleep disorders.

Six million individuals suffer moderate to severe obstructive sleep apnea, a disorder characterized by brief periods of recurrent cessation of breathing caused by airway obstruction. Chronic insomnia, which hampers a person's ability to fall or stay asleep, occurs in approximately 30 million Americans. Restless legs syndrome and periodic limb movement disorder are neurological conditions characterized by an irresistible urge to move the legs and nocturnal limb movements; they affect approximately 6 million individuals, making it one of the most common movement disorders.

The cumulative effects of sleep loss and sleep disorders have been associated with a wide range of deleterious health consequences including an increased risk of hypertension, diabetes, obesity, depression, heart attack, and stroke. At the same time, the majority of people with sleep disorders are yet to be diagnosed. Compared to healthy individuals, those suffering from sleep loss and sleep disorders are less productive, have an increased health care utilization, and have an increased likelihood of injury.

In 2003 the NIH National Center on Sleep Disorders Research (NCSDR) published a research plan, which contained a set of research priorities for the field. However, recognizing that continued scientific and clinical advances will require a new coordinated strategy to improve public awareness and strengthen the field of Somnology and Sleep Medicine, the American Academy of Sleep Medicine, the NCSDR at the NIH, the National Sleep Foundation, and the Sleep Research Society requested that the IOM conduct a study that would examine: (1) the public health significance of sleep, sleep loss, and sleep disorders, (2) gaps in the public health system and adequacy

---

[1]Somnology is the branch of science devoted to the study of the physiology of sleep, the behavioral dimensions of sleep, and the consequences of sleep loss and sleep disorders on an individual's and the general population's health, performance, safety, and quality of life. Sleep medicine is the branch of clinical medicine devoted to the diagnosis and treatment of individuals suffering from chronic sleep loss or sleep disorders.

of the current resources and infrastructures for addressing the gaps, (3) barriers and opportunities for improving interdisciplinary research and medical education and training in the area of sleep and sleep medicine, and (4) develop a comprehensive plan for enhancing sleep medicine and sleep research.

In response to the request the IOM appointed a 14-member committee with expertise in academic and medical administration, adolescent medicine, cardiology, epidemiology, geriatrics, health sciences research, neurology, nursing, otolaryngology, pediatrics, psychiatry, and pulmonology. The committee met five times during the course of its work and held two workshops that provided input on: (1) the current public health burden of sleep loss and chronic sleep disorders, and (2) the organization and operation of various types of academic sleep programs.

This committee recognizes that with the continued leadership of the NCSDR and its advisory board a coordinated strategy, described below, is needed to ensure continued advances (Box ES-1). This strategy requires concurrent commitment to the following activities:

- Establish the workforce required to meet the clinical and scientific demands of the field.
- Increase awareness of the burden of sleep loss and sleep disorders among the general public.
- Improve surveillance and monitoring of the public health burden of sleep loss and sleep disorders.
- Expand awareness among health care professionals through education and training.
- Develop and validate new and existing diagnostic and therapeutic technologies.
- Expand accreditation criteria to emphasize treatment, long-term patient care, and chronic disease management strategies.
- Strengthen the national research infrastructure to connect individual investigators, research programs, and research centers.
- Increase the investment in interdisciplinary sleep programs in academic health centers that emphasize long-term clinical care, training, and research.

THE NATIONAL INSTITUTES OF HEALTH LEADERSHIP IN RESEARCH AND TRAINING

To a greater extent than most scientific and medical disciplines, the field of somnology and sleep medicine cuts across many clinical and basic research disciplines, including but not limited to cardiology, dentistry, endocrinology, epidemiology, geriatrics, molecular biology, neurology, neuroscience, nursing, otolaryngology, pediatrics, pharmacology, psychiatry, psychology, and pulmonology. In 2004, there were 331 sleep-related research project grants sponsored by 17 institutes at the NIH. The NIH has two entities to coordinate its sleep-related activities, the Trans-NIH Sleep Research Coordinating Committee and the NCSDR. However, major challenges remain in involving all relevant NIH institutes, centers, and offices; developing a coordinated research and training program; and integrating the efforts of the NCSDR, its advisory board, and the Trans-NIH Sleep Research Coordinating Committee.

Investment in sleep-related research has grown dramatically over the past 10 years; however, the growth in research and training programs have not kept up with the rapid pace of scientific advances. At the same time that the science and magnitude of the problem requires greater investment, NIH funding to sleep-related activities is reaching a plateau. This has partially overlapped the period when the overall NIH budget has plateaued. Consequently, the future outlook for somnology and sleep medicine is unclear. In 2004, for the first time since the NCSRD was established in 1993, there was a decrease in annual NIH expenditures for sleep-related programs, fewer research project grants were funded, and the number of new grants awarded decreased. Over the last three years the NCSDR has only sponsored two programs—one request for applications and one program announcement—a marked reduction since the inception of the NCSDR. This presents an even greater challenge for a field that requires growth in scientific workforce and technology. Thus, there must be incremental growth in this field to meet the public health and economic burden caused by sleep loss and sleep disorders. It is important that research priorities continue to be defined for both short- and long-term goals. To address this problem the committee makes the following recommendation.

Recommendation 8.1 The National Center on Sleep Disorders Research and its advisory board should play a more proactive role in stimulating and coordinating the field.

The National Center on Sleep Disorders and Research (NCSDR) should have adequate staff and resources to ensure its ability to fulfill its mission of coordinating and stimulating training, research, and health information dissemination relevant to somnology and sleep disorders. All relevant institutes with significant sleep portfolios should become members of the Trans-NIH Sleep Research Coordinating Committee. Further, the NCSDR Advisory Board should take a more proactive role in advising the director of the NCSDR. On an annual basis, the NCSDR and its advisory board should:

- Identify specific objectives that address each of the three NCSDR missions and evaluate specific actions taken to accomplish each objective. This assessment should be reported in an annual meeting to the NIH-Trans Sleep Coordinating Committee, the institute directors of its members, and to the director of the NIH.
- Directors of the other federal agencies that fund significant sleep-related activities, such as Department of Defense, Department of Commerce, Department of Education, Department of Labor, and Department of Transportation should report annually on their activities to the NCSDR Advisory Board.
- The NCSDR Advisory Board should annually review the current NIH portfolio of sleep-related grants, as well as requests for applications, and program announcements, assess them for responsiveness to the program plan and identify gaps in research and training.
- The NCSDR Advisory Board should annually recommend new, or modify existing, requests for applications that can be presented to appropriate NIH institutes and other federal agencies including the Centers for Disease Control and Prevention and Department of Defense. Multiple members of the Trans-NIH Sleep Coordinating Committee are encouraged to continue to cosponsor sleep-related grants.

ESTABLISHING A SUFFICIENT WORKFORCE

One of the most pressing needs recognized by this committee is to create an infrastructure capable of developing the workforce required to meet the clinical and scientific demands of the field. This will entail increased investment by the NIH, academia, professional societies, private foundations, and industry. In 2004 there were only 151 researchers who had a clinical sleep-related research project grant (R01), and only 126 investigators focused primarily on basic sleep-related research projects, a decrease from the number of R01 awards in 2003. Further, of the top academic institutions that received the greatest number of grants from the NIH, less then half had career development or training grants in somnology or sleep medicine. Only 54 doctorates were awarded with a focus on somnology or sleep medicine in 2004. This workforce is insufficient given the burden of sleep loss and sleep disorders.

The NIH support of career development awards has decreased. Over the period encompassing 2000 to 2004 there was a decrease in the number of career development awards. Further, since 1997 there have been no new requests for application (RFAs) or program announcements (PAs) for sleep-related fellowship (F), training (T), or career development (K) programs. Given these statistics, creating an infrastructure to develop a workforce capable of meeting the clinical and scientific demand is a challenge for the field. Compared to other fields the current number of clinicians and scientists in the field is not sufficient, given the public health burden of sleep loss and sleep disorders. Further, NIH, academia, and private foundations have not sufficiently supported the development of an adequate workforce. To strengthen the interdisciplinary aspect of the field it is not only important to attract new investigators to the field, but also to expand the number of trained scientists in other relevant disciplines electing to focus on sleep-related research. Therefore, the committee makes the following recommendation designed to improve training and mentoring activities.

Recommendation 7.1: The National Institutes of Health and private foundations should increase investment in interdisciplinary somnology and sleep medicine research training and mentoring activities.

The National Institutes of Health, foundations, and professional societies should utilize and develop further funding mechanisms to attract young investigators into the field of somnology and sleep medicine. As a reflection of the interdisciplinary nature of somnology and sleep medicine, members of the Trans-NIH Sleep Research Coordinating Committee should be encouraged to combine resources to sponsor grants for disciplinary and cross-disciplinary training and mentoring activities (T, F, and K funding mechanisms) of medical students, graduate students, postdoctoral fellows, clinical fellows, and junior faculty.

To implement this recommendation the following should be considered:
- The Trans-NIH Sleep Research Coordinating Committee should establish a somnology and sleep medicine career development program. This program should support trainees for a significant number of years, spanning research training in fellowship and research career development as a faculty member. It should also facilitate midcareer training opportunities (e.g., K21, K24), the Academic Career Award for Education and Curriculum Development program (K07), and research education grants (R25).
- Existing training grants or large research programs in disciplines related to somnology or sleep medicine (e.g., internal medicine, neurology, psychiatry, psychology, otolaryngology, nursing, epidemiology, neuroscience, health services research) should allow for the addition of a sleep medicine trainee. Where pertinent expertise is not available on-site, remote mentoring at other institutions should be encouraged.

PUBLIC AND PROFESSIONAL AWARENESS

A well-coordinated strategy to improve sleep-related health care is required, owing to the public health burden of sleep loss and sleep disorders coupled with the low awareness among the general population, health care professionals, professional societies, and policy makers. Increasing the awareness and improving the diagnosis and treatment of sleep disorders requires a multipronged effort that includes three key components: public education, surveillance and monitoring of the burden of sleep loss and sleep disorders, and training for health professionals. The preeminent goal of these activities is to create and sustain a broad societal commitment to adopting proper sleep habits as a primary tenet of health. Such a commitment will require participation by those individuals and organizations in a position to educate the public at national, state, local, and community levels—including K–12 education, colleges and universities, medical schools, nursing schools, hospitals, community clinics, local health departments, private industry, and entertainment media. This will necessitate simultaneous investment in public education campaigns for all age groups and a sustained effort to integrate sleep-related content into curricula of undergraduate education.

Recommendation 5.1: The National Center on Sleep Disorders Research and the Centers for Disease Control and Prevention should establish a multimedia public education campaign.

The National Center on Sleep Disorders Research—working with the Centers for Disease Control and Prevention, the proposed National Somnology and Sleep Medicine Research Network, private organizations and foundations, entertainment and news media, and private industry—should develop, implement, and evaluate a long-term national multimedia and public awareness campaign directed to targeted segments of the population (e.g., children, their parents, and teachers in preschool and elementary school; adolescents; college students and young adults; middle-aged adults; and elderly people) and specific high-risk populations (e.g., minorities).

Improve Surveillance and Monitoring
of the Public Health Burden

Adequate public health education not only requires informing public and health care practitioners, but also adequate monitoring of the public health burden. The development of adequate surveillance and monitoring systems is important for informing policy makers, health care providers, researchers, and the public about the effectiveness of health care services, programs, rules and regulations, and policies. However, there is currently very little ongoing nationwide surveillance. Thus existing national and state-wide databases should be amended to allow for improved surveillance and monitoring of the burden of sleep loss and sleep disorders in the United States population.

> **Recommendation 5.3:** The Centers for Disease Control and Prevention and National Center on Sleep Disorders Research should support additional surveillance and monitoring of sleep patterns and sleep disorders.

The Centers for Disease Control and Prevention, working with the National Center on Sleep Disorders Research, should support the development and expansion of adequate surveillance and monitoring instruments designed to examine the American population's sleep patterns and the prevalence and health outcomes associated with sleep disorders.

Increasing Awareness Among Health Professionals

Increasing education and training of health care professionals in somnology and sleep medicine will improve the awareness of the associated public health burden and attract a new pool of clinicians and scientists interested in the field. Time devoted to sleep-related material in health and life sciences curricula is inadequate given the magnitude of the morbid effects that sleep disorders have on the most common diseases (e.g. obesity, hypertension, heart attack, and diabetes) and accidents. Focused training about sleep can positively influence the performance of health care providers. In particular, medical, nursing, dentistry, and pharmacy students require greater exposure to the public health burden of sleep loss and sleep disorders. Thus the committee makes the following recommendation to increase sleep-related content in health sciences curricula.

> **Recommendation 5.2:** Academic health centers should integrate the teaching of somnology and sleep medicine into baccalaureate and doctoral health sciences programs, as well as residency and fellowship training and continuing professional development programs.

The subjects of sleep loss and sleep disorders should be included in the curricula of relevant baccalaureate and graduate educational and research programs of all the health sciences. Similarly, postgraduate, residency, and fellowship training programs, as well as continuing professional development programs, must include this content. The curriculum should expose students in the fields of medicine and allied health fields to the etiology, pathophysiology, diagnosis, treatment, prevention, and public health burden of sleep loss and sleep disorders. Relevant accrediting bodies and licensing boards ought to define sleep-related curriculum requirements and expectations for knowledge and competency (e.g., Liaison Committee on Medical Education, Accreditation Council for Graduate Medical Education, American Board of Medical Specialties, the National League for Nursing, the Commission on Collegiate Nursing Education, and the Council on Education for Public Health). Further, a means for credentialing nonphysicians should be maintained by the American Board of Sleep Medicine, or new mechanisms should be developed by relevant organizations.

TECHNOLOGY DEVELOPMENT AND ACCREDITATION

As awareness increases, greater investment in the development and validation of new and existing diagnostic and therapeutic technologies is required to meet the anticipated demand. Today, the capacity needed to serve the population seeking diagnosis and treatment is inadequate. The wait time for a polysomnogram, the procedure used to diagnose sleep disorders, can be up to 10 weeks. Most American communities do not have adequate health care resources to meet the clinical demand; therefore, millions of individuals suffering from sleep disorders remain undiagnosed and untreated. It has been estimated that sleep apnea alone, a diagnosis that necessitates polysomnography to meet current criteria set out by third-party payers, annually requires at least 2,300 polysomnograms per 100,000 population. However, on average, only 425 polysomnograms per 100,000 population are performed each year in the United States, a level far below the need. In fact, 33 states perform fewer than 500 polysomnograms per 100,000 people annually. This shortfall will exacerbate as awareness of the clinical consequences and public health burden of sleep loss and disorders increases, particularly with the aging of the United States population. Given the cumbersome nature and cost of the diagnosis and treatment of sleep disorders and sleep loss and the resultant inequities with regard to access, in order to ensure future quality care the committee recommends greater investment in the development of new and validation of existing diagnostic and therapeutic technologies.

Recommendation 6.1: The National Institutes of Health and the Agency for Healthcare Research and Quality should support the validation and development of existing and new diagnostic and therapeutic technologies.

The National Center on Sleep Disorders Research—working with the Trans-NIH Sleep Research Coordinating Committee, the Agency for Health Care Policy and Research, other federal agencies, and private industry—should support the evaluation and validation of existing diagnostic and therapeutic technologies. Further, development of new technologies such as ambulatory monitoring, biological markers, and imaging techniques should be vigorously supported.

Establish Sleep Laboratories in the NIH Clinical Research Program

The intramural clinical research program at the NIH does not have a sleep laboratory. Consequently, many experimental sleep therapies and the relationship between sleep processes and disease development are not being examined. If there is adequate investment in extramural sleep-related programs, the field can continue to make great strides; therefore, the committee does not support use of limited resources to invest in an intramural somnology and sleep disorders research program. However, because appropriateness of sleep patterns is one of the basic tenets of health, the committee strongly urges the NIH intramural clinical research program to ascertain the need for establishing a sleep study laboratory so that evaluation of sleep may be integrated into ongoing relevant clinical research protocols at NIH.

Recommendation 8.3: The National Institutes of Health should ascertain the need for a transdisciplinary sleep laboratory that would serve as a core resource in its intramural clinical research program.

The Director of the National Institutes of Health Intramural Research Program should ascertain the need for a transdisciplinary sleep laboratory within the intramural clinical research program that would serve as a core resource for the community of intramural clinical investigators across all institutes.

Improved Accreditation Standards Are Required

Sleep disorders are chronic conditions frequently associated with other comorbidities (e.g., cardiovascular disease, depression, diabetes), which often require complex treatments. Despite the importance of early recognition and treatment, the primary focus of most existing sleep centers appears to be on diagnosis, rather than on comprehensive care of sleep loss and sleep disorders as chronic conditions. This narrow focus may largely be the unintended result of compliance with criteria for accreditation of sleep laboratories, which emphasize diagnostic standards and reimbursement, for diagnostic testing. To address this it is recommended that accreditation criteria for sleep centers, in which are imbedded sleep laboratories, be expanded to emphasize treatment, long-term patient care, and management strategies.

Recommendation 9.2: Sleep laboratories should be part of accredited sleep centers, the latter to include long-term strategies for patient care and chronic disease management.

All private and academic sleep laboratories should be under the auspices of accredited sleep centers and include adequate mechanisms to ensure long-term patient care and chronic disease management. Accreditation criteria should expand beyond a primary focus on diagnostic testing to emphasize treatment, long-term patient care, and chronic disease management strategies.

INTERDISCIPLINARY SLEEP PROGRAMS IN ACADEMIC HEALTH CENTERS

Accelerating Scientific Advances

A coordinated and integrated strategy requires bolstering clinical and basic research efforts, catalyzing collaborative research efforts, and attracting the breadth of talented researchers who can provide leadership to advance research and clinical care in sleep loss and sleep disorders. Key to accelerating progress in the treatment of chronic sleep loss and sleep disorders is the development of a coordinated, focused, and centralized network that connects individual investigators, research programs, and research centers; facilitates collaborative projects; encompasses relevant research from diverse fields; and builds on the unique strengths of each research effort to move toward effective therapy, prevention, and treatment. Somnology and Sleep Medicine Research Centers of Excellence would spearhead these translational research efforts and promote collaborations among all sites conducting research relevant to somnology and sleep medicine. Similar to cancer centers, the Somnology and Sleep Medicine Centers of Excellence would act as local, regional, and national resources for the scientific community and the community at large. These centers would provide the interdisciplinary environment that is essential to accelerate the development of therapies for chronic sleep loss and sleep disorders. In addition, these centers would facilitate interactions among basic, clinical, and population-focused scientists. These would not only be research centers, but somnology and sleep medicine centers that emphasize the close association among research, clinical care, and education. The committee further envisions a sustained network for somnology and sleep medicine in the United States that would facilitate public education, career development opportunities, translational research, and implementation of multicenter clinical trials. Although in aggregate, sleep loss and sleep disorders are prevalent, among these are many rare conditions that would benefit from a national data collection system and clinical network.

Despite the limited size of the field, the committee believes that the somnology and sleep medicine field is now sufficiently mature for the establishment of a national somnology and sleep medicine research network. Scientific advances and a number of large academic interdisciplinary sleep programs place the proposed network in position to successfully compete for funding from the National Heart, Lung, and Blood Institute and other members of the Trans-NIH Sleep Research Coordinating Committee.

Recommendation 8.2: The National Institutes of Health should establish a National Somnology and Sleep Medicine Research Network.

The National Center on Sleep Disorders Research in collaboration with the Trans-NIH Sleep Research Coordination Committee should establish a National Somnology and Sleep Medicine Research Network. Type III regional interdisciplinary sleep programs designated by the National Institutes of Health would act as regional centers working with basic research laboratories and sleep cores at NIH-designated clinical translational research centers. It is envisioned that the networks would do the following:
• Coordinate and support the current and future cadre of basic and clinical researchers.
• Train new investigators and fellows.
• Provide core capabilities for basic, clinical, and translational research.
• Support multisite clinical research in children, adolescents, adults, and elderly.

- Create and support virtual networking centers to facilitate the standardization and sharing of data and resources online and enhance collaborations with researchers not working in research centers.
- Create a data coordinating center that includes an Internet-based clearing house for the publication of all data produced in cooperation with the research and clinical network.
- Together with the Agency for Healthcare Research and Quality develop standards for research, outcomes, and clinical practice.
- Work with the Center for Disease Control and Prevention to integrate and support surveillance and population-based research.

Criteria for Interdisciplinary Sleep Programs in Academic Health Centers

Somnology and sleep medicine is an emerging interdisciplinary field that is being forged from several disciplines and clinical specialties. However, the limited investment and organization of sleep programs in academic health centers do not favor interdisciplinary research efforts and continued advances in clinical care. Consequently, the committee recommends a three-tier model for interdisciplinary sleep programs, which lays down the guiding principles for their organization in all academic health centers—progressing from programs that emphasize clinical care and education to programs with a considerable capacity for research, advanced training, and public education (Table S-1). It is the belief of the committee that, if these components and guiding principles are followed, interdisciplinary sleep programs can thrive, whether as free-standing departments or as programs within an existing department, division, or unit.

Status as a Type I interdisciplinary sleep program is achievable by many academic health centers nationwide; it primarily focuses on clinical care. This type should highlight the importance of increasing awareness among health care professionals by offering educational programs for medical students and residents in primary care. The Type I interdisciplinary sleep program is a single accredited center that emphasizes a comprehensive diagnosis and treatment program.

A Type II interdisciplinary sleep program includes the characteristics of a Type I program but in addition is designed to provide optimal education, training, and research in somnology and sleep medicine for scientists and physicians, including an accredited sleep fellowship program for physicians. A Type III regional interdisciplinary sleep program includes the characteristics of Type I and II programs; however, this type of program would act as a regional coordinator for the proposed National Somnology and Sleep

Medicine Research Network for education, training, mentoring, clinical care, research, and clinical trials.

Recommendation 9.1: New and existing sleep programs in academic health centers should meet the criteria of a Type I, II, or III interdisciplinary sleep program.

New and existing sleep programs should at a minimum conform to the criteria of a Type I clinical interdisciplinary sleep program. Academic medical centers with a commitment to interdisciplinary training are encouraged to train sleep scientists and fellows in sleep medicine, which would require at least a Type II training and research interdisciplinary sleep program. Research-intensive medical centers should aspire to become Type III regional interdisciplinary sleep programs and coordinators of the National Somnology and Sleep Medicine Research Network. The American Academy of Sleep Medicine should develop accreditation criteria for sleep programs specific to academic health centers.

PRIORITIES TO ADVANCE SOMNOLOGY AND SLEEP MEDICINE

The field is particularly well suited to interdisciplinary and translational strategies. NIH's Roadmap identified a number of initiatives that aim to foster the development of interdisciplinary research and training. The growth of this field fits in with the framework of the Roadmap and thus could serve as a prototypical program for these new cross-institute initiatives.

Recognizing the current fiscal restraints at the NIH and the prerequisite requirements for the field, the committee recommends the following prioritized strategy. Of primary importance is

- improving awareness among the general public and health care professionals,
- increasing investment in interdisciplinary somnology and sleep medicine research training and mentoring activities,
- validating and developing new and existing technologies for diagnosis and treatment.

Transforming academic health centers is also an important part of the strategy. Although many health centers have the components to establish interdisciplinary sleep programs, many do not, and it will take time and energy to develop successful programs. Therefore, it is important that academia and accrediting bodies begin facilitating this transformation.

Finally, although there are only a limited number of academic institutions that currently have the capacity to be a Type III regional interdisciplinary sleep program, this should not delay the establishment of the research network. Initially the network could consist of a limited number of programs. The network would benefit greatly from cultural, ethnic, and environmental diversity. Therefore, a long-range goal should be to have 8 to 10 geographically distributed Type III regional interdisciplinary sleep programs. In this report the committee does not recommend any research priorities. It is the committee's belief that the strategies outlined in the report will generate the appropriate mechanisms for generating a research agenda for the future of somnology and sleep medicine.

TABLE S-1 Guidelines for Interdisciplinary Type I, II, and III Academic Sleep Programs

Attribute	Type I (clinical)	Type II (clinical, training, research)	Type III (regionalized comprehensive centers)
Structure and Composition			
Clinical specialties represented:[a]			
Internal medicine and relevant subspecialties	x	x	x
Neurology	x	x	x
Psychiatry and subdisciplines	x	x	x
Otolaryngology	x	x	x
Pediatrics and subspecialties (as necessary may be separate program)	x	x	x
Nursing	x	x	x
Psychology		x	x
Dentistry			x
Medical director certification in sleep medicine (American Board of Medical Specialties or American Board of Sleep Medicine)[b]	x	x	x
Consultant services from specialties not represented	x	x	x
Sleep specialists provide consultant services	x	x	x
Single accredited clinical sleep center	x	x	x
Comprehensive program for diagnosis and treatment of individuals	x	x	x

continued

TABLE S-1 continued

Attribute	Type I (clinical)	Type II (clinical, training, research)	Type III (regionalized comprehensive centers)
Training Program			
Training program for health care professionals and/or researchers	x	x	x
Medical school training and education	x	x	x
Education for residents in primary care	x	x	x
Residents in neurology, psychiatry, otolaryngology, and fellows in pulmonary medicine rotate through sleep program		x	x
Accredited fellowship program for physicians		x	x
Research training for clinical fellows		x	x
NIH-sponsored training grants for graduate and postgraduate researchers		x	x
Research Program			
Research areas of emphasis:[c]			
Neuroscience		x	x
Epidemiology/public health		x	x
Pharmacology			x
Basic *or* clinical research program		x	
Basic *and* clinical research program			x
Member of proposed national somnology and sleep medicine research and clinical network	x[d]	x	x
Regional coordinator for:			
Core facilities for basic research			x
Multisite clinical trials			x
Core facilities for clinical research			x
Mentoring of sleep fellows			x
Public education			x
Data coordinating site			x

[a]This list is not meant to be exclusive or exhaustive and should be modified as relevant specialties and training programs emerge.

[b]Currently this is American Board of Sleep Medicine. It is anticipated that in 2007 the examination would be supplanted by the American Board of Medical Specialties.

[c]This list is not meant to be exclusive or exhaustive. Other research areas could be involved (e.g., genetics, systems neurobiology, and bioengineering).

[d]Type I programs would be responsible for generating and submitting data to the national data registry established by the proposed National Somnology and Sleep Medicine Research and Clinical Network.

BOX S-1
Summary of Committee's Recommendations to Address
and Remedy the Unmet Public Health Need

The following is a summary of the committee's recommendations. Complete text of each recommendation can be found in the corresponding chapters.

NATIONAL INSTITUTES OF HEALTH LEADERSHIP IN RESEARCH AND TRAINING

The National Center on Sleep Disorders Research and its advisory board should play a more proactive role in stimulating and coordinating the field. (Recommendation 8.1)

The National Institutes of Health and private foundations must increase investment in interdisciplinary somnology and sleep medicine research training and mentoring activities. (Recommendation 7.1)

The National Institutes of Health should ascertain the need for a transdisciplinary sleep laboratory that would serve as a core resource in its intramural clinical research program. (Recommendation 8.3)

PUBLIC AND PROFESSIONAL AWARENESS

The National Center on Sleep Disorders Research and the Centers for Disease Control and Prevention should establish a multimedia public education campaign. (Recommendation 5.1)

Academic health centers should integrate the teaching of somnology and sleep medicine into baccalaureate and doctoral health sciences programs, as well as residency and fellowship training and continuing professional development programs. (Recommendation 5.2)

SURVIELLANCE AND MONITORING

The Centers for Disease Control and Prevention and National Center on Sleep Disorders Research should support additional surveillance and monitoring of sleep patterns and sleep disorders. (Recommendation 5.3)

continued

BOX S-1 continued

TECHNOLOGY DEVELOPMENT

The National Institutes of Health and the Agency for Healthcare Research and Quality should support the validation and development of existing and new diagnostic and therapeutic technologies. (Recommendation 6.1)

INTERDISCIPLINARY SLEEP PROGRAMS IN ACADEMIC HEALTH CENTERS

New and existing sleep programs in academic health centers should conform to meet the criteria of a type I, II, or III interdisciplinary sleep program. (Recommendation 9.1)
   Type I clinical interdisciplinary sleep program
   Type II clinical, research, and training interdisciplinary sleep program
   Type III regional comprehensive sleep program

It is recommended that the National Institutes of Health establish a national somnology and sleep medicine research network. (Recommendation 8.2)

Sleep laboratories should be part of accredited sleep centers, which include long-term strategies for patient care and chronic disease management. (Recommendation 9.2)

NOTE: For ease of reference, the committee's recommendations are numbered according to the chapter of the main text in which they appear followed by the order in which they appear in the chapter.

1

Introduction

"Sleep that knits up the ravelled sleave of care, The death of each day's life, sore labour's bath, Balm of hurt minds, great Nature's second course, Chief nourisher in life's feast."
Shakespeare, Macbeth

CHAPTER SUMMARY *The public health burden of chronic sleep loss and sleep disorders is immense. Although clinical activities and scientific opportunities in the field are expanding, awareness among the general public and health care professionals is low, given the burden. The available workforce of health care providers is not sufficient to diagnose and treat individuals with sleep disorders. Therefore, the current situation necessitates a larger and more interdisciplinary workforce to meet health care demands as well as advance the field's knowledge base. Further, there is a need to develop and reorganize public health and academic sleep programs to facilitate and improve the efficiency and effectiveness in public awareness, training, research, diagnosis, and treatment of sleep loss and sleep disorders. Finally, the fragmentation of research and clinical care currently present in most academic institutions requires the creation of accredited interdisciplinary sleep programs in academic institutions. The success of existing comprehensive academic Somnology and Sleep Medicine Programs offers evidence of the value of interdisciplinary approaches to patient care, education, research training, faculty development, and science. An interdisciplinary approach requires the coordinated and integrated effort of not only the major medical fields involved in sleep clinical care (internal medicine and its relevant subspecialties, pediatrics, neurology, psychiatry, psychology, and otolaryngology) but also other disciplines such as neuroscience, dentistry, nursing, and pharmacology.*

MAGNITUDE AND COST OF THE PROBLEM

Fitful sleep, restless nights, hitting the alarm clock button for an additional 10 minutes of sleep—all are all too familiar manifestations of the interactions of life with one of the frontiers of science and clinical practice—somnology[1] and sleep medicine. It is estimated that 50 to 70 million Americans suffer from a chronic disorder of sleep and wakefulness (NHLBI, 2003), hindering daily functioning and adversely affecting health. The current capacity of America's health system is not sufficient to diagnose and treat all individuals with sleep disorders. Further, awareness among health care professionals and the general public is low considering the size of the problem. Among those individuals with sleep disorders are 3 to 4 million individuals with moderate to severe obstructive sleep apnea (Young et al., 1993), a disorder characterized by brief periods of recurrent cessation of breathing caused by airway obstruction with morbid or fatal consequences. Chronic insomnia, which hampers a person's ability to fall asleep, is observed in approximately 10 percent of the American population (Ford and Kamerow, 1989; Simon and VonKorff, 1997; Roth and Ancoli-Israel, 1999). Restless legs syndrome and periodic limb movement disorder are neurological conditions characterized by nocturnal limb movements and an irresistible urge to move the legs. These conditions affect approximately 5 percent of the general population (Lavigne and Montplaisir, 1994; Rothdach et al., 2000; NSF, 2000; Montplaisir et al., 2005), making it one of the most common movement disorders (Montplaisir et al., 2005).

The negative public health consequences of sleep loss and sleep-related disorders are enormous. Some of the most devastating human and environmental health disasters have been partially attributed to fatigue-related performance failures,[2] sleep loss, and night shift work-related performance failures, including the tragedy at the Union Carbide chemical plant in Bhopal, India; the nuclear reactor meltdowns at Three Mile Island and Chernobyl; and the grounding of the Exxon *Valdez* oil tanker (NCSDR, 1994; Moss and Sills, 1981; United States Senate Committee on Energy and National Resources, 1986; USNRC, 1987; Dinges et al., 1989). Each of these incidents not only cost millions of dollars but also had a disastrous impact on the environment and the health of local communities.

---

[1]Somnology is the branch of science devoted to the study of the physiology of sleep, the behavioral dimensions of sleep, and the consequences of sleep loss and sleep disorders on an individual's and the general population's health, performance, safety, and quality of life. Sleep medicine is the branch of clinical medicine devoted to the diagnosis and treatment of individuals suffering from chronic sleep loss or sleep disorders.

[2]A significant portion of fatigue, but not all, is caused by chronic sleep loss and/or sleep disorders.

Over the past century, the average amount of time that Americans sleep has decreased by around 20 percent (NCSDR, 1994). Further, 1 out of every 5 workers in industrialized countries (well over 20 million Americans [OTA, 1991]) perform shift-work, which requires them to work at night and attempt to sleep during the daytime hours (AASM, 2005). These reversed sleep patterns cause maladjustment of circadian rhythms that often lead to sleep disruption. Americans are working more hours or multiple jobs and spending more time watching television and using the Internet, resulting in later sleep times and less sleep.

The cumulative long-term effects of sleep loss and sleep disorders have been associated with a wide range of deleterious health consequences, including an increased risk of hypertension, diabetes, obesity, heart attack, and stroke. In addition, sleep loss and sleep disorders have a significant economic impact. Billions of dollars a year are spent on direct medical costs associated with doctor visits, hospital services, prescriptions, and over-the-counter medications (NCSDR, 1994). Compared to healthy individuals, individuals with chronic sleep loss are less productive, have health care needs greater than the norm, and have an increased likelihood of injury; for example, it is estimated that there are 110,000 sleep-related injuries and 5,000 fatalities each year in motor vehicle crashes involving commercial trucks (CNTS, 1996).

HISTORICAL BACKGROUND

For centuries, sleep and dreams have long been topics of immense interest; however, the modern scientific study of sleep began relatively recently. In 1937 an electroencephalograph was used for the first time to observe the electrical activity in the brain during nonrapid eye movement sleep (Loomis et al., 1937). This opened the field to further advances. Rapid eye movement (REM) was discovered in 1953 by Kleitman and colleagues, and its correlation with dreams was a major step forward in understanding sleep physiology (Aserinsky and Kleitman, 1953). The culmination of this work came in 1957 when Dement and Kleitman defined the stages of sleep (see Chapter 2 of this report) (Dement and Kleitman, 1957). Since the 1950s a convergence of findings from many fields (e.g., neurology, pulmonology, neuroscience, psychiatry, otolaryngology, anatomy, and physiology) have led to a greater understanding of sleep as a basic universal biological process that affects the functioning of many organ systems (Shepard et al., 2005). In 1989, a seminal study demonstrated that rats that were subjected to total sleep deprivation developed skin lesions, experienced weight loss in spite of increased food intake, developed bacterial infections, and died within 2 to 3 weeks (Rechtschaffen et al., 1989). Researchers in sleep and circadian biology continue to work toward a greater understanding of the etiology and pathophysiology of sleep disorders. The field is maturing into an interdisciplinary field in which integration and coordination across the traditional medical specialties, other health care providers (e.g. nurses, dentists), and between basic and clinical science is vital.

GROWTH OF SOMNOLOGY AND SLEEP MEDICINE

The maturation of the study of sleep and the field of Somnology and Sleep Medicine (Box 1-1) has seen the establishment of many organizations devoted to promoting public awareness, ensuring quality care for individuals who suffer from chronic sleep loss and sleep disorders, and supporting education and research endeavors. In addition to the National Center on Sleep Disorders Research (NCSDR) at the National Institutes of Health (NIH), professional societies and foundations have been established, including the American Academy of Sleep Medicine, the Sleep Research Society, the American Sleep Apnea Association, the Restless Legs Syndrome Foundation, and the National Sleep Foundation

The field of somnology and sleep medicine has been marked by a number of milestones over the last 35 years. Sleep laboratories dedicated to the evaluation and management of sleep disorders have been established. In 1970, sleep disorders were evaluated at only a handful of sleep laboratories in the world. In 2001, there were close to 1,300 sleep laboratories in the United States (Tachibana et al., 2005). Membership in the American Academy of Sleep Medicine and the Sleep Research Society and participation at the annual meeting of the American Professional Sleep Societies has continued to increase. In 2005 sleep medicine was recognized as a medical subspecialty by the Accreditation Council for Graduate Medical Education and the American Board of Medical Specialties.

CHALLENGES IN ADVANCING THE STUDY
OF SLEEP DISORDERS

Coordinating Research and Research Funding

Integrating and coordinating the efforts of the many relevant institutes and centers at the NIH presents many challenges related to funding and advancing somnology research. For example, it has recently been recognized that restless legs syndrome (National Institute of Neurological Disorders and Stroke) and sleep apnea (National Heart, Lung, and Blood Institute) may be a major cause of attention deficit hyperactivity disorder (National Institute of Child Health and Human Development, National Institute of Mental Health) and other behavioral problems (Chervin et al., 2002). The National Institute on Aging is interested in the increase in sleep

---

BOX 1-1
Defining Somnology and Sleep Medicine

Throughout information gathering workshops and discussions the Committee on Sleep Medicine and Research heard the field and practice of somnology and sleep medicine referred to in many different terms: *sleep, sleep medicine, sleep disorders research, sleep research and medicine,* and the *study of sleep.* These terms and others fail to describe the full extent of the study and practice of somnology and sleep medicine. In response to this and the emergence of the clinical and research field, this committee believes that an enhanced vocabulary would be helpful to describe the study of sleep and circadian rhythms. Therefore, throughout this report the committee will use the terms *somnology* and *sleep medicine.*

Somnology: Somnology is the branch of science devoted to the study of the physiology of sleep, the behavioral dimensions of sleep, and the consequences of sleep loss and sleep disorders on an individual's and the general population's health, performance, safety, and quality of life.

Sleep medicine: Sleep medicine is a branch of clinical medicine devoted to the diagnosis and treatment of individuals suffering from chronic sleep loss or sleep disorders.

---

and wake disruption during senescence. Insomnia is typically treated using behavioral therapy techniques (Office of Behavioral and Social Sciences Research) and is often comorbid with depression, eating disorders, and other mental disorders (National Institute of Mental Health). Drugs of abuse, including alcohol and stimulants (National Institute on Drug Abuse, National Institute on Alcohol Abuse and Alcoholism), have major effects on sleep and are often used to treat underlying sleep problems such as insomnia or narcolepsy. Sleep apnea research and therapy cuts across a number of disciplines, including nursing (National Institute of Nursing Research), dentistry and otolaryngology (National Institute of Dental and Craniofacial Research), surgery, neurology (National Institute of Neurological Disorders and Stroke), cardiology, and pulmonary medicine (National Heart, Lung, and Blood Institute). At the basic research level, somnology research often involves multiple disciplines such as genetics (National Human Genome Research Institute), environmental sciences (National Institute of Environmental Health Sciences), epidemiology, immunology (National Institute of Allergy and Infectious Diseases), endocrinology (National Institute of Diabetes and Digestive and Kidney Diseases), neurosciences (National

Institute of Neurological Disorders and Stroke, National Institute of Mental Health, National Eye Institute), and otolaryngology (National Institute on Deafness and Other Communication Disorders).

Trans-NIH Sleep Research Coordinating Committee

To facilitate an interchange of information on somnology research the Trans-NIH Sleep Research Coordinating Committee was formed in 1986. The coordinating committee consists of representatives from 13 NIH institutes and centers and meets quarterly to discuss current sleep-related activities in the NIH and to develop new programs.

National Center on Sleep Disorders Research

In 1993 the National Heart, Lung, and Blood Institute established the NCSDR. As described in the congressional language, the mission of the NCSDR is the "conduct and support of biomedical and related research and research training, the dissemination of health information, and the conduct of other programs with respect to various sleep disorders, the basic understanding of sleep, biological and circadian rhythm research, chronobiology, and other sleep related research"[3] (see Appendix D).

The function of the NCSDR and the Trans-NIH Sleep Research Coordinating Committee are intertwined. The director of the NCSDR serves as Chair of the Coordinating Committee. Further, the NCSDR is responsible for coordinating the information collected by individual institutions for the Coordinating Committee's annual report; including sleep related activities, initiatives, and funding of sleep-related activities.

NIH funding for somnology research has increased by more than 150 percent since the NCSDR became fully operational in 1996, reaching a total of $196.2 million (0.07 percent of the NIH budget) in fiscal year 2004 (NHLBI, 2003). However, this growth occurred during the same period that the overall budget to the NIH doubled, and currently NIH funding for sleep-related activities is reaching a plateau. In 2004, for the first time since the NCSDR was established, there was a decrease in annual NIH expenditures for sleep-related projects; there were fewer research project grants funded in 2004, and the number of new grants awarded also decreased (see Appendix G). Consequently, the future outlook for somnology and sleep medicine is unclear. This presents an even greater challenge for a field that requires growth in its scientific workforce and technology.

---

[3]National Institutes of Health Revitalization Act of 1993. Pub. L. No. 103-43 (1993).

Increasing the Numbers of Trained Researchers and Clinicians

New investigators and clinicians knowledgeable about sleep-related research and clinical care are needed. The growth of the discipline in terms of clinical volume has not been reflected in a corresponding increase in the number of clinical and basic sleep researchers. In the spring of 2005 there were 781 American members of the Sleep Research Society, a number representing the majority of individuals performing sleep-related research. There are only 253 principal investigators who work on sleep-related research. There are 151 researchers involved primarily in clinical sleep research, and 126 focus primarily on basic research projects. In 2004, of the top 30 academic institutions that received the greatest number of grants from the NIH, less than half had career development and training awards in somnology and sleep medicine, and only 17 had NIH-sponsored fellowships that were sleep related. Between the years 2000 and 2004, the NIH increased its support of sleep-related training and fellowship grants; however, during this same period there was a decrease in the number of career development awards. Over the same period, the number of academic institutions receiving sleep-related career development awards also decreased. Therefore, creating an infrastructure to develop a workforce capable of meeting the clinical and scientific demand remains a major challenge.

Time devoted in medical school curriculum to sleep medicine is limited. The percentage of medical schools that include sleep disorders in their curriculums has risen modestly from 54 percent in 1978 (Orr et al., 1980) to 63 percent in 1993, but the time devoted averages only 2.11 hours (Rosen et al., 1998). Similar analysis has not recently been performed, but there is no evidence to suggest that medical schools are placing increased emphasis on sleep-related content in their curriculums. Clearly, the educational effort is still inadequate given the magnitude of the morbid effects that sleep loss and sleep disorders have on the most common diseases (e.g., obesity, hypertension, heart attack, and diabetes). In response to this perceived shortcoming in sleep education, the National Heart, Lung, and Blood Institute supported a series of grants (K07 funding mechanism) to develop model medical school curricula. This resulted in the establishment of MEDSleep, a collection of over 75 sleep education tools and products (AASM, 2005). Although this program generated a large number of resources, it is unclear how many of them have been used and implemented. Despite these advances, physician education regarding the recognition, diagnosis, management, and treatment of sleep disorders is still inadequate (Strohl et al., 2003; Owens, 2005).

To strengthen the interdisciplinary aspects of the field it is important to attract new investigators to the field and expand the number of trained somnology scientists in other relevant and related disciplines. These areas include, but are not limited to, biology and health informatics, health service research, nursing, epidemiology and genetic epidemiology, clinical trials, functional imaging, genetics, pathology, neurosciences, and molecular biology.

Distribution of Resources and Technology Development

Today, the capacity needed to serve the population seeking diagnosis and treatment is inadequate. Analysis commissioned on behalf of the committee indicated that in many health care systems and communities, the waiting time for a polysomnogram, the procedure used to diagnose many sleep disorders, may be as much as 10 weeks (see Chapter 9). This shortfall will worsen as awareness of the clinical consequences and public health burden of sleep disorders increases. A substantial investment is needed to enlarge the clinical and research workforce and improve the technology for diagnosis and treatment. Ambulatory diagnostic technologies currently available need to be validated. Further, there is a need for improved treatments for individuals with chronic sleep loss and sleep disorders. For example, the most common treatment for sleep apnea, continuous positive airway pressure therapy, which requires an individual to wear a mask over the face while sleeping, has a low rate of compliance, between 45 to 70 percent (Kribbs et al., 1993).

There are approximately 1,300 sleep laboratories in the United States, 39 percent of which are accredited by the American Academy of Sleep Medicine (Tachibana et al., 2005). However, millions of individuals suffering from sleep disorders remain undiagnosed and untreated (Young et al., 1997; Kapur et al., 2002). The utilization and capacity of sleep laboratories is not distributed based on the prevalence of sleep disorders (Tachibana et al., 2005). Apart from creating new sleep centers and laboratories, developing and validating reliable portable diagnostic technologies is required to meet the demand that will arise from greater awareness among the general public (see Chapter 6).

SOMNOLOGY AND SLEEP MEDICINE RESEARCH IN ACADEMIC INSTITUTIONS

The division of a university and medical school into academic departments is based upon distinct clinical and graduate training programs. Many of the most promising new lines of academic research and the most effective clinical services depend on strong, interdisciplinary programs that emerge from the knowledge base of the more traditional disciplines (CFAT, 2001). Unfortunately, the organization of academic disciplines among the schools and colleges does not effectively support existing interdisciplinary programs or those that could be created (Ehrenberg and Epifantseva, 2001; Thursby and Thursby, 2002).

Somnology and Sleep Medicine Is an Interdisciplinary Field

The field of Somnology and Sleep Medicine is an emerging interdisciplinary field that is being forged from several existing sciences and medical specialties. However, the current organization of academic health centers houses clinicians and scientists in discrete departments that do not favor interdisciplinary research efforts. Although the scientific enterprise of the field requires interdisciplinary strategies, the clinical service of patients is multidisciplinary and requires linkages to other medical specialties.

As described in the National Academy of Sciences (2004) report *Facilitating Interdisciplinary Research:*

> **Interdisciplinary** research is a mode of research performed by teams or individuals that integrates information, data, techniques, tools, perspectives, concepts, and/or theories from two or more disciplines or bodies of specialized knowledge to advance fundamental understanding or to solve problems whose solutions are beyond the scope of a single discipline or field of research practice (Figure 1-1A).

> **Multidisciplinary** research is taken to mean research that involves more than a single discipline in which each discipline makes a separate contribution. Investigators may share facilities and research approaches while working separately on distinct aspects of a problem (Figure 1-1B) (NAS, 2004).

There are a wide range of programs in Somnology and Sleep Medicine. Some are solely clinical in nature; others are clinical programs that include training of physicians and some research. There are also a limited number of comprehensive programs that emphasize clinical care education and training, as well as basic and clinical research. With few exceptions most programs continue to be not integrated and embedded in medical departments. This organization has many adverse implications for the field; including:

- Clinical training in sleep loss and sleep disorders is often limited to those in the department where the program is housed to the exclusion of others.
- The absence of interdisciplinary clinical teams hinders patient care.
- A limited sense of identity with, or focus on the field, and an absence of an established career path for faculty makes it difficult to attract new students, researchers, and clinicians into the field.

A) Interdisciplinary

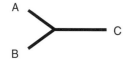

Joined together to work on a common question or problem. Interaction may forge a new research field or discipline.

B) Multidisciplinary

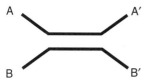

Disciplines joined together to work on a common question or problem, split apart when work is complete, having likely gained new knowledge, insight, strategies from other disciplines.

FIGURE 1-1 Interdisciplinary and multidisciplinary research.
SOURCE: National Academy of Sciences, 2004.

- Research or clinical funds generated from sleep-related activities are not generally reinvested to enhance sleep programs.
- Collaboration can be more difficult because researchers and clinicians are geographically dispersed.

Sleep Loss and Sleep Disorders Require Long-Term Patient Care and Chronic Disease Management

Sleep disorders are chronic conditions necessitating complex treatments. They are frequently comorbid with other sleep disorders and other conditions (e.g., cardiovascular disease, depression, or diabetes), which, by themselves, are complex to treat. Despite the importance of early recognition and treatment, the primary focus of most existing sleep centers is on diagnosis, rather than on comprehensive care of sleep loss and sleep disorders as chronic conditions. The narrow focus of sleep centers may largely be the unintended result of accreditation criteria, which emphasize diagnostic standards and reimbursement for the diagnostic testing (see Chapter 9).

SCOPE AND ORGANIZATION OF THIS REPORT

Increased public education and greater awareness of the burden of sleep loss and sleep disorders as well as scientific advances have poised the field of somnology and sleep medicine for great strides. In 2003 the NCSDR published a set of research priorities for the field. However, advances will require an organized strategy to increase and coordinate efforts in training and educating the public, researchers, and clinicians, as well as improved infrastructure and funding for this endeavor.

Recognizing the need to develop a new coordinated strategy to improve public awareness and strengthen the field of Somnology and Sleep Medicine, the NCSDR at the NIH, along with the American Academy of Sleep Medicine, the National Sleep Foundation, and the Sleep Research Society, requested that the Institute of Medicine (IOM) conduct a study that would examine: (1) the public health significance of sleep, sleep loss, and sleep disorders, (2) gaps in the public health system and adequacy of the current resources and infrastructures for addressing the gaps, (3) barriers and opportunities for improving interdisciplinary research and medical education and training in the area of sleep and sleep medicine, and (4) develop a comprehensive plan for enhancing sleep medicine and sleep research (Box 1-2).

The IOM appointed a 14-member committee with expertise in academic and medical administration, adolescent medicine, cardiology, epidemiology, geriatrics, health sciences research, neurology, nursing, otolaryngology, pediatrics, psychiatry, and pulmonology. The committee met five times during the course of its work and held two workshops that provided input on the current public health burden of sleep loss and chronic sleep disorders and the organization and operation of various types of academic sleep programs.

Chapter 2 of this report describes the basic biology and physiology of sleep and circadian rhythms. Chapter 3 introduces the primary sleep disorders and their associated health burdens, and Chapter 4 describes their impact on an individual's performance and associated economic impact. Chapter 5 provides an overview of the barriers to providing optimal patient care, including the lack of public and professional education. Chapter 6 highlights the need for greater capacity to diagnose and treat individuals with sleep loss and sleep disorders. In Chapter 7, the committee examines the education and training programs for students, scientists, and health care professionals. Chapter 8 discusses the current investment by the NIH and the NCSDR and the potential role of a national somnology and sleep medicine research network for advancing therapeutic interventions for sleep loss and sleep disorders. Chapter 9 highlights the infrastructure of the field and proposes recommendations for developing academic programs in somnology and sleep medicine.

BOX 1-2
Statement of Task

The Institute of Medicine will convene an ad hoc committee of experts in public health, academic and medical administration, and health sciences research to identify (1) the public health significance of sleep, sleep loss, and sleep disorders; (2) barriers and opportunities for improving interdisciplinary research and medical education and training in the area of sleep and sleep medicine; and (3) strategies for developing increased support for sleep medicine and sleep research in academic health centers.

The committee will:

1. Review and quantify the public health significance of sleep health, sleep loss, and sleep disorders based on current knowledge. This task will include assessments of (a) the contribution of sleep disorders to poor health, reduced quality of life, and early mortality; and (b) the economic consequences of sleep loss and sleep disorders, including lost wages and productivity. Target populations will be segmented as children, adults, and the elderly.

2. Identify gaps in the public health system relating to the understanding, management, and treatment of sleep loss and sleep disorders, and assess the adequacy of the current resources and infrastructures for addressing the gaps. The committee, however, will not be responsible for making any budgetary recommendations.

3. Identify barriers to and opportunities for improving and stimulating multidisciplinary research, education, and training in sleep medicine. Delineate fiscal and academic organizational models that promote and facilitate (a) sleep research in the basic sciences; (b) cooperative research efforts between basic science disciplines and clinical practice specialties; and (c) multidisciplinary efforts in education and training of practitioners in sleep health, sleep disorders, and sleep research.

4. Develop a comprehensive plan for enhancing sleep medicine and sleep research, as appropriate, for improving the public's health. This will include interdisciplinary initiatives for research, medical education, training, clinical practice, and health policy.

REFERENCES

AASM (American Academy of Sleep Medicine). 2005. *Medsleep*. [Online]. Available: http://www.aasmnet.org/Medsleep_Home.aspx [accessed December 17, 2005].

Aserinsky E, Kleitman N. 1953. Regularly occurring periods of eye motility, and concomitant phenomena, during sleep. *Science* 118(3062):273–274.

CFAT (Carnegie Foundation for the Advancement of Teaching). 2001. *The Carnegie Classification of Institutions of Higher Education*. Princeton, NJ: Carnegie Foundation for the Advancement of Teaching.

Chervin RD, Hedger Archbold K, Dillon JE, Pituch KJ, Panahi P, Dahl RE, Guilleminault C. 2002. Associations between symptoms of inattention, hyperactivity, restless legs, and periodic leg movements. *Sleep* 25(2):213–218.

CNTS (Center for National Truck Statistics). 1996. *Truck and Bus Accident Factbook—1994*. UMTRI-96-40. Washington, DC: Federal Highway Administration Office of Motor Carriers.

Dement W, Kleitman N. 1957. Cyclic variations in EEG during sleep and their relation to eye movements, body motility, and dreaming. *Electroencephalography and Clinical Neurophysiology Supplement* 9(4):673–690.

Dinges DF, Graeber RC, Carskadon MA, Czeisler CA, Dement WC. 1989. Attending to inattention. *Science* 245(4916):342.

Ehrenberg RG, Epifantseva J. 2001. Has the growth of science crowded out other things at universities? *Change* 26:46–52.

Ford DE, Kamerow DB. 1989. Epidemiologic study of sleep disturbances and psychiatric disorders. An opportunity for prevention? *Journal of the American Medical Association* 262(11):1479–1484.

Kapur V, Strohl KP, Redline S, Iber C, O'Connor G, Nieto J. 2002. Underdiagnosis of sleep apnea syndrome in U.S. communities. *Sleep and Breathing* 6(2):49–54.

Kribbs NB, Pack AI, Kline LR, Smith PL, Schwartz AR, Schubert NM, Redline S, Henry JN, Getsy JE, Dinges DF. 1993. Objective measurement of patterns of nasal CPAP use by patients with obstructive sleep apnea. *American Review of Respiratory Disease* 147(4):887–895.

Lavigne GJ, Montplaisir JY. 1994. Restless legs syndrome and sleep bruxism: Prevalence and association among Canadians. *Sleep* 17(8):739–743.

Loomis AL, Harvey EN, Hobart GA. 1937. Cerebral states during sleep as studied by human brain potentials. *Journal of Experimental Psychology* 21:127–144.

Montplaisir J, Allen RP, Walters AD, Lerini-Strambi L. 2005. Restless legs syndrome and periodic limb movements during sleep. In: Kryger MH, Roth T, Dement WC, eds. *Principles and Practice of Sleep Medicine*. 4th ed. Philadelphia: Elsevier/Saunders. Pp. 839–852.

Moss TH, Sills DL, 1981. *The Three Mile Island Nuclear Accident: Lessons and Implications*. New York: New York Academy of Sciences.

NAS (National Academy of Sciences). 2004. *Facilitating Interdisciplinary Research*. Washington, DC: The National Academies Press.

NCSDR (National Commission on Sleep Disorders Research). 1994. *Wake Up America: A National Sleep Alert. Volume II: Working Group Reports*. 331-355/30683. Washington, DC: Government Printing Office.

NHLBI (National Heart, Lung, and Blood Institute). 2003. *National Sleep Disorders Research Plan, 2003*. Bethesda, MD: National Institutes of Health.

NSF (National Sleep Foundation). 2000. *2000 Omnibus Sleep in America Poll.* [Online]. Available: http://www.sleepfoundation.org/publications/2001poll.html [accessed May 25, 2005].

Orr WC, Stahl ML, Dement WC, Reddington D. 1980. Physician education in sleep disorders. *Journal of Medical Education* 55(4):367–369.

OTA (Office of Technology Assessment). 1991. *Biological Rhythms: Implications for the worker.* OTA-BA-463. Washington, DC: Government Printing Office.

Owens J. 2005. Introduction to special section: NIH Sleep Academic Award program. *Sleep Medicine* 6(1):45–46.

Rechtschaffen A, Bergmann BM, Everson CA, Kushida CA, Gilliland MA. 1989. Sleep deprivation in the rat: X. Integration and discussion of the findings. *Sleep* 12(1):68–87.

Rosen R, Mahowald M, Chesson A, Doghramji K, Goldberg R, Moline M, Millman R, Zammit G , Mark B, Dement W. 1998. The Taskforce 2000 Survey on Medical Education in Sleep and Sleep Disorders. *Sleep* 21(3):235–238.

Roth T, Ancoli-Israel S. 1999. Daytime consequences and correlates of insomnia in the United States: Results of the 1991 National Sleep Foundation survey. II. *Sleep* 22(suppl 2):S354–S358.

Rothdach AJ, Trenkwalder C, Haberstock J, Keil U, Berger K. 2000. Prevalence and risk factors of RLS in an elderly population: The MEMO study. Memory and morbidity in Augsburg elderly. *Neurology* 54(5):1064–1068.

Shepard JJW, Buysse DJ, Chesson JAL, Dement WC, Goldberg R, Guilleminault C, Harris CD, Iber C, Mignot E, Mitler MM, Moore KE, Phillips BA, Quan SF, Rosenberg RS, Roth T, Schmidt HS, Silber MS, Walsh JK, White DP. 2005. History of the development of sleep medicine in the United States. *Journal of Clinical Sleep Medicine* 1(1):61–82.

Simon GE, VonKorff M. 1997. Prevalence, burden, and treatment of insomnia in primary care. *American Journal of Psychiatry* 154(10):1417–1423.

Strohl KP, Veasey S, Harding S, Skatrud J, Berger HA, Papp KK, Dunagan D, Guilleminault C. 2003. Competency-based goals for sleep and chronobiology in undergraduate medical education. *Sleep* 26(3):333–336.

Tachibana N, Ayas TA, White DP. 2005. A quantitative assessment of sleep laboratory activity in the United States. *Journal of Clinical Sleep Medicine* 1(1):23–26.

Thursby JG, Thursby TM. 2002. Who is selling the ivory tower? Sources of growth in university licensing. *Management Science* 48(1):90–104.

United States Senate Committee on Energy and Natural Resources. 1986. *The Chernobyl Accident.* Washington, DC: Government Printing Office.

USNRC (United States Nuclear Regulatory Commission). 1987. *Report on the Accident at the Chernobyl Nuclear Power Station.* NU-REG 1250. Washington, DC: Government Printing Office.

Young T, Palta M, Dempsey J, Skatrud J, Weber S, Badr S. 1993. The occurrence of sleep-disordered breathing among middle-aged adults. *New England Journal of Medicine* 328(17):1230–1235.

Young T, Evans L, Finn L, Palta M. 1997. Estimation of the clinically diagnosed proportion of sleep apnea syndrome in middle-aged men and women. *Sleep* 20(9):705–706.

2

Sleep Physiology

CHAPTER SUMMARY   *This chapter provides a brief overview of sleep physiology and how sleep patterns change over an individual's life span. Humans spend about one-third of their lives asleep. There are two types of sleep, non-rapid eye movement (NREM) sleep and rapid eye movement (REM) sleep. NREM sleep is divided into stages 1, 2, 3, and 4, representing a continuum of relative depth. Each has unique characteristics including variations in brain wave patterns, eye movements, and muscle tone. Circadian rhythms, the daily rhythms in physiology and behavior, regulate the sleep-wake cycle. In addition, the sleep-wake system is thought to be regulated by the interplay of two major processes, one that promotes sleep and one that maintains wakefulness.*

Humans spend about one-third of their lives asleep, yet most individuals know little about sleep. Although its function remains to be fully elucidated, sleep is a universal need of all higher life forms including humans, absence of which has serious physiological consequences. This chapter provides an overview of basic sleep physiology and describes the characteristics of REM and NREM sleep. Sleep and circadian-generating systems are also reviewed. The chapter ends with a discussion about how sleep patterns change over an individual's life span.

SLEEP ARCHITECTURE

Sleep architecture refers to the basic structural organization of normal sleep. There are two types of sleep, non-rapid eye-movement (NREM) sleep and rapid eye-movement (REM) sleep. NREM sleep is divided into stages 1, 2, 3, and 4, representing a continuum of relative depth. Each has unique characteristics including variations in brain wave patterns, eye movements, and muscle tone. Sleep cycles and stages were uncovered with the use of electroencephalographic (EEG) recordings that trace the electrical patterns of brain activity (Loomis et al., 1937; Dement and Kleitman, 1957a).

Two Types of Sleep

Over the course of a period of sleep, NREM and REM sleep alternate cyclically (Figure 2-1). The function of alternations between these two types of sleep is not yet understood, but irregular cycling and/or absent sleep stages are associated with sleep disorders (Zepelin et al., 2005). For example, instead of entering sleep through NREM, as is typical, individuals

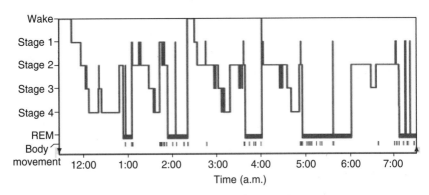

FIGURE 2-1 Progression of sleep states across a single night in young adult.
SOURCE: Carskadon and Dement (2005).

with narcolepsy enter sleep directly into REM sleep (Carskadon and Rechtschaffen, 2005).

NREM and REM Sleep Cycles

A sleep episode begins with a short period of NREM stage 1 progressing through stage 2, followed by stages 3 and 4 and finally to REM. However, individuals do not remain in REM sleep the remainder of the night but, rather, cycle between stages of NREM and REM throughout the night (Figure 2-1). NREM sleep constitutes about 75 to 80 percent of total time spent in sleep, and REM sleep constitutes the remaining 20 to 25 percent. The average length of the first NREM-REM sleep cycle is 70 to 100 minutes. The second, and later, cycles are longer lasting—approximately 90 to 120 minutes (Carskadon and Dement, 2005). In normal adults, REM sleep increases as the night progresses and is longest in the last one-third of the sleep episode. As the sleep episode progresses, stage 2 begins to account for the majority of NREM sleep, and stages 3 and 4 may sometimes altogether disappear.

Four Stages of NREM Sleep

The four stages of NREM sleep are each associated with distinct brain activity and physiology. Figure 2-2 shows the EEG patterns characteristic of the four NREM stages. Other instruments are used to track characteristic changes in eye movement and muscle tone.

Stage 1 Sleep

NREM stage 1 sleep serves a transitional role in sleep-stage cycling. Aside from newborns and those with narcolepsy and other specific neurological disorders, the average individual's sleep episode begins in NREM stage 1. This stage usually lasts 1 to 7 minutes in the initial cycle, constituting 2 to 5 percent of total sleep, and is easily interrupted by a disruptive noise. Brain activity on the EEG in stage 1 transitions from wakefulness (marked by rhythmic alpha waves) to low-voltage, mixed-frequency waves. Alpha waves are associated with a wakeful relaxation state and are characterized by a frequency of 8 to 13 cycles per second (Carskadon and Dement, 2005).

Stage 2 Sleep

Stage 2 sleep lasts approximately 10 to 25 minutes in the initial cycle and lengthens with each successive cycle, eventually constituting between 45 to 55 percent of the total sleep episode. An individual in stage 2 sleep

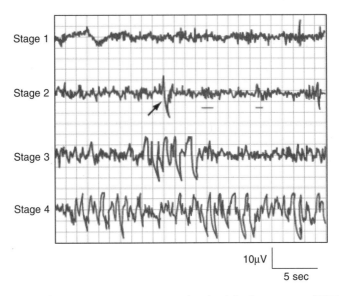

FIGURE 2-2 Characteristic EEG activity of each of the four stages of NREM sleep. NOTE: In stage 2, the arrow indicates a K-complex, and the underlining shows two sleep spindles.
SOURCE: Carskadon and Dement (2005).

requires more intense stimuli than in stage 1 to awaken. Brain activity on an EEG shows relatively low-voltage, mixed-frequency activity characterized by the presence of sleep spindles and K-complexes (Figure 2-2). It is hypothesized that sleep spindles are important for memory consolidation. Individuals who learn a new task have a significantly higher density of sleep spindles than those in a control group (Gais et al., 2002).

Stages 3 and 4, Slow-Wave Sleep

Sleep stages 3 and 4 are collectively referred to as slow-wave sleep (SWS), most of which occurs during the first third of the night. Each has distinguishing characteristics. Stage 3 lasts only a few minutes and constitutes about 3 to 8 percent of sleep. The EEG shows increased high-voltage, slow-wave activity (Figure 2-2).

The last NREM stage is stage 4, which lasts approximately 20 to 40 minutes in the first cycle and makes up about 10 to 15 percent of sleep. The arousal threshold is highest for all NREM stages in stage 4. This stage is characterized by increased amounts of high-voltage, slow-wave activity on the EEG (Carskadon and Dement, 2005).

REM Sleep

REM sleep is defined by the presence of desynchronized (low-voltage, mixed-frequency) brain wave activity, muscle atonia, and bursts of rapid eye movements (Carskadon and Dement, 2005). "Sawtooth" wave forms, theta activity (3 to 7 counts per second), and slow alpha activity also characterize REM sleep. During the initial cycle, the REM period may last only 1 to 5 minutes; however, it becomes progressively prolonged as the sleep episode progresses (Carskadon and Dement, 2005). There are numerous physiological differences between NREM and REM sleep (Table 2-1).

TABLE 2-1 Physiological Changes During NREM and REM Sleep

Physiological Process	NREM	REM
Brain activity	Decreases from wakefulness	Increases in motor and sensory areas, while other areas are similar to NREM
Heart rate	Slows from wakefulness	Increases and varies compared to NREM
Blood pressure	Decreases from wakefulness	Increases (up to 30 percent) and varies from NREM
Sympathetic nerve activity	Decreases from wakefulness	Increases significantly from wakefulness
Muscle tone	Similar to wakefulness	Absent
Blood flow to brain	Decreases from wakefulness	Increases from NREM, depending on brain region
Respiration	Decreases from wakefulness	Increases and varies from NREM, but may show brief stoppages; coughing suppressed
Airway resistance	Increases from wakefulness	Increases and varies from wakefulness
Body temperature	Is regulated at lower set point than wakefulness; shivering initiated at lower temperature than during wakefulness	Is not regulated; no shivering or sweating; temperature drifts toward that of the local environment
Sexual arousal	Occurs infrequently	Greater than NREM

SOURCES: NHLBI (2003), Somers et al. (1993), Madsen et al. (1991b).

Dreaming is most often associated with REM sleep. Loss of muscle tone and reflexes likely serves an important function because it prevents an individual from "acting out" their dreams or nightmares while sleeping (see Chapter 3) (Bader et al., 2003). Approximately 80 percent of vivid dream recall results after arousal from this stage of sleep (Dement and Kleitman, 1957b). REM sleep may also be important for memory consolidation (Crick and Mitchison, 1983; Smith and Lapp, 1991).

Physiology During Sleep

In addition to the physiological changes listed in Table 2-1, there are other body system changes that occur during sleep. Generally, these changes are well tolerated in healthy individuals, but they may compromise the sometimes fragile balance of individuals with vulnerable systems, such as those with cardiovascular diseases (Parker and Dunbar, 2005). Physiological changes also occur in the following systems:

• Cardiovascular: Changes in blood pressure and heart rate occur during sleep and are primarily determined by autonomic nervous system activity. For instance, brief increases in blood pressure and heart rate occur with K-complexes, arousals, and large body movements (Lugaresi et al., 1978; Catcheside et al., 2002; Blasi et al., 2003; Tank et al., 2003). Further, there is an increased risk of myocardial infarction in the morning due to the sharp increases in heart rate and blood pressure that accompany awakening (Floras et al., 1978; Mulcahy et al., 1993).

• Sympathetic-nerve activity: Sympathetic-nerve activity decreases as NREM sleep deepens; however, there is a burst of sympathetic-nerve activity during NREM sleep due to the brief increase in blood pressure and heart rate that follows K-complexes. Compared to wakefulness, there is a rise in activity during REM sleep (Somers et al., 1993).

• Respiratory: Ventilation and respiratory flow change during sleep and become increasingly faster and more erratic, specifically during REM sleep (Krieger, 2000; Simon et al., 2002). Ventilation data during REM sleep are somewhat unclear, but they suggest that hypoventilation (deficient ventilation of the lungs that results in reduction in the oxygen content or increase in the carbon dioxide content of the blood or both) occurs in a similar way as during NREM sleep (NLM, 2006). Several factors contribute to hypoventilation during NREM, and possibly REM, sleep such as reduced pharyngeal muscle tone (Krieger, 2000; Simon et al., 2002). Further, during REM sleep, there is reduced rib cage movement and increased upper airway resistance due to the loss of tone in the intercostals and upper airway muscles (Parker and Dunbar, 2005). More generally, ventilation and respiratory flow show less effective adaptive responses during sleep. The cough reflex, which normally reacts to irritants in the airway, is suppressed during REM and NREM sleep. The hypoxic ventilatory response is also lower in NREM sleep than during wakefulness and decreases further during REM sleep. Similarly, the arousal response to respiratory resistance (for example, resistance in breathing in or out) is lowest in stage 3 and stage 4 sleep (Douglas, 2005).

• Cerebral blood flow: NREM sleep is associated with significant reductions in blood flow and metabolism, while total blood flow and metabolism in REM sleep is comparable to wakefulness (Madsen et al., 1991b). However, metabolism and blood flow increase in certain brain regions during REM sleep, compared to wakefulness, such as the limbic system (which is involved with emotions), and visual association areas (Madsen et al., 1991a).

• Renal: There is a decreased excretion of sodium, potassium, chloride, and calcium during sleep that allows for more concentrated and reduced urine flow. The changes that occur during sleep in renal function are complex and include changes in renal blood flow, glomerular filtration, hormone secretion, and sympathetic neural stimulation (Cianci et al., 1991; Van Cauter, 2000; Buxton et al., 2002).

• Endocrine: Endocrine functions such as growth hormone, thyroid hormone, and melatonin secretion are influenced by sleep. Growth hormone secretion typically takes place during the first few hours after sleep onset and generally occurs during SWS, while thyroid hormone secretion takes place in the late evening. Melatonin, which induces sleepiness, likely by reducing an alerting effect from the suprachiasmatic nucleus, is influenced by the light-dark cycle and is suppressed by light (Parker and Dunbar, 2005).

SLEEP-WAKE REGULATION

The Two-Process Model

The sleep-wake system is thought to be regulated by the interplay of two major processes, one that promotes sleep (process S) and one that maintains wakefulness (process C) (Gillette and Abbott, 2005). Process S is the homeostatic drive for sleep. The need for sleep (process S) accumulates across the day, peaks just before bedtime at night and dissipates throughout the night.

Process C is wake promoting and is regulated by the circadian system. Process C builds across the day, serving to counteract process S and promote wakefulness and alertness. However, this wake-promoting system begins to decline at bedtime, serving to enhance sleep consolidation as the need for sleep dissipates across the night (Gillette and Abbott, 2005). With an adequate night's rest, the homeostatic drive for sleep is reduced, the circadian waking drive begins to increase, and the cycle starts over. In the absence of process C, total sleep time remains the same, but it is randomly distributed over the day and night; therefore, process C also works to consolidate sleep and wake into fairly distinct episodes (Gillette and Abbott, 2005). Importantly, through synchronization of the circadian system, process C assists in keeping sleep-wakefulness cycles coordinated with environmental light-dark cycles.

Sleep-Generating Systems in the Brainstem

Sleep process S is regulated by neurons that shut down the arousal systems, thus allowing the brain to fall asleep. Many of these neurons are found in the preoptic area of the hypothalamus (Figure 2-3A). These neurons, containing molecules that inhibit neuronal communication, turn off the arousal systems during sleep. Loss of these nerve cells causes profound insomnia (Saper et al., 2005a,c). Inputs from other regions of the brain also greatly influence the sleep system. These include inputs from the lower brainstem that relay information about the state of the body (e.g., a full stomach is conducive to falling asleep), as well as from emotional and cognitive areas of the forebrain. In addition, as described further in the next section, there are inputs from the circadian system that allow the wake-sleep system to synchronize with the external day-night cycle, but also to override this cycle when it is necessitated by environmental needs.

The sleep-generating system also includes neurons in the pons that intermittently switch from NREM to REM sleep over the course of the night. These neurons send outputs to the lower brainstem and spinal cord that cause muscle atonia, REMs, and chaotic autonomic activity that characterize REM sleep. Other outputs are sent to the forebrain, including activation of the cholinergic pathways to the thalamus to activate the EEG.

Wake-Generating Systems in the Brainstem

Wakefulness is generated by an ascending arousal system from the brainstem that activates forebrain structures to maintain wakefulness (Figure 2-3B). This idea, originally put forward by Morruzzi and Magoun (1949), has more recently been refined (Jones, 2005a; Saper et al., 2005c). The main source for the ascending arousal influence includes two major pathways that originate in the upper brainstem. The first pathway, which takes origin from cholinergic neurons in the upper pons, activates parts of the thalamus that are responsible for maintaining transmission of sensory information to the cerebral cortex. The second pathway, which originates in cell groups in the upper brainstem that contain the monoamine neurotransmitters (norepinephrine, serotonin, dopamine, and histamine),

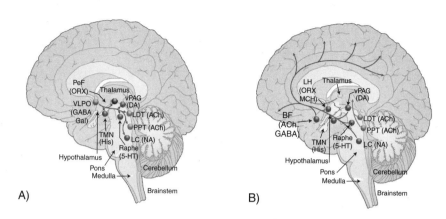

FIGURE 2-3 Sleep-generating (A) and wake-generating (B) systems in the brain.
NOTE: Cholinergic (ACh) cell groups; basal forebrain (BF); dopamine (DA);
gamma-aminobutyric acid (GABA); galanin (Gal); histamine (His); serotonin (5-HT);
locus coeruleus (LC); laterodorsal tegmental nuclei (LDT); lateral hypothalamus
(LH); melanin-concentrating hormone (MCH); noradrenaline (NA); orexin (ORX);
perifornical (PeF); the pedunculopontine (PPT); tuberomammillary nucleus (TMN);
ventrolateral preoptic nucleus (VLPO); ventral periaqueductal gray (vPAG).
SOURCE: Saper et al. (2005c).

enters the hypothalamus, rather than the thalamus, where it picks up
inputs from nerve cells that contain peptides (orexin or hypocretin and
melanin-concentrating hormone). These inputs then traverse the basal forebrain, where they pick up additional inputs from cells containing acetyl-
choline and gamma-aminobutyric acid. Ultimately, all of these inputs
enter the cerebral cortex, where they diffusely activate the nerve cells
and prepare them for the interpretation and analysis of incoming sensory
information.

CIRCADIAN RHYTHMS, THE 24-HOUR CLOCK

Circadian rhythms refer, collectively, to the daily rhythms in physiology
and behavior. They control the sleep-wake cycle, modulate physical activity
and food consumption, and over the course of the day regulate body temperature, heart rate, muscle tone, and hormone secretion. The rhythms are
generated by neural structures in the hypothalamus that function as a biological clock (Dunlap et al., 2004). Animals and plants possess endogenous clocks
to organize daily behavioral and physiological rhythms in accord with the
external day-night cycle (Bunning, 1964). The basis for these clocks is believed
to be a series of molecular pathways involving "clock" genes that are
expressed in a nearly 24-hour rhythm (Vitaterna et al., 2005).

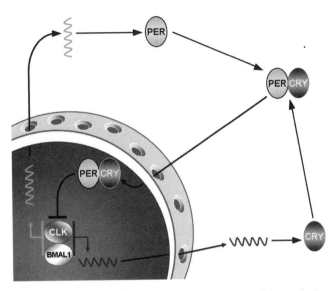

FIGURE 2-4 Molecular mechanisms underlying the activity of the circadian clock. NOTE: The activation and deactivation of *Period* and *Cryptochrome* protein production is the basis of a negative-feedback loop that controls the ~24-hour cycle time of circadian clocks. Thus, the ability of the *Period* and *Cryptochrome* proteins to modulate their own production allows the system to self-regulate.

In mammals, two proteins, Clock and Bmal1, bind together and move into the nucleus of the cell, where they bind to specific sites in the DNA that activate specific genes (Figure 2-4). Among the genes that they activate are *Period* and *Cryptochrome*. The products of these genes also move back into the nucleus, where they disrupt the binding of Clock and Bmal1 to the DNA, thus inhibiting their own synthesis. This results in a rising and falling pattern of expression of the *Period* and *Cryptochrome* gene products with a periodicity that is very close to 24 hours.

Many other genes are also regulated by Clock and Bmal1, and these genes cycle in this way in many tissues in the body, giving rise to daily patterns of activity. These rhythmically expressed genes contribute to many aspects of cellular function, including glucose and lipid metabolism, signal transduction, secretion, oxidative metabolism, and many others, suggesting the importance of the circadian system in many central aspects of life.

The Suprachiasmatic Nucleus

The suprachiasmatic nucleus (SCN) is responsible for regulating circadian rhythms in all organs. It receives direct inputs from a class of nerve cells in the retina that act as brightness detectors, which can reset the clock genes in the SCN on a daily basis. The SCN then transmits to the rest of the brain and body signals that bring all of the daily cycles in synchrony with the external day-night cycle.

The main influence of the SCN on sleep is due to a series of relays through the dorsomedial nucleus of the hypothalamus, which signals to the wake-sleep systems to coordinate their activity with the day-night cycles. The SCN also coordinates cycles of feeding, locomotor activity, and hormones, such as corticosteroids (Chou et al., 2003). Under some conditions (e.g., limited food availability) when there are changes in the external temperature, or even under conditions of behavioral stress (e.g., the need to avoid a predator), animals must shift their daily cycles to survive. In such circumstances, the dorsomedial nucleus may shift to a new daily cycle, which can be completely out of phase with the SCN and the light-dark cycle, and its signals also shift the daily cycles of sleep, activity, feeding, and corticosteroid hormone secretion (Saper et al., 2005b,c).

Another major output of the SCN is to a pathway that controls the secretion of melatonin, a hormone produced by the pineal gland. Melatonin, which is mainly secreted at night, acts to further consolidate the circadian rhythms but has only limited effects directly on sleep.

Sleep and Thermoregulation

Body temperature regulation is subject to circadian system influence. An individual's body temperature is higher during the day than at night (Figure 2-5). At night there is a gradual decline in body temperature, a decrease in heat production (called the falling phase of the body temperature rhythm), and an increase in heat loss, all which promote sleep onset and maintenance, as well as EEG slow-wave activity. Conversely, there is a gradual increase in body temperature several hours before waking. The brain sends signals to other parts of the body that increase heat production and conservation in order to disrupt sleep and promote waking (Szymusiak, 2005).

SLEEP PATTERNS CHANGE WITH AGE

Sleep architecture changes continuously and considerably with age. From infancy to adulthood, there are marked changes in how sleep is initiated and maintained, the percentage of time spent in each stage of sleep, and overall sleep efficiency (i.e., how successfully sleep is initiated and maintained). A general trend is that sleep efficiency declines with age (Figure 2-6). Although the consequences of decreased sleep efficiency are relatively well documented, the reasons are complex and poorly understood. Exami-

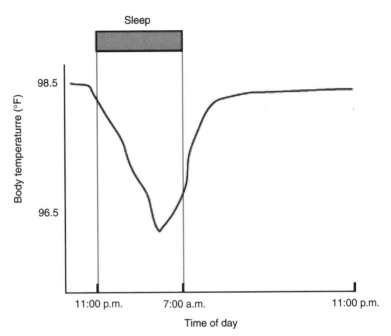

FIGURE 2-5 Body temperature in relation to time of day.
SOURCE: NHBLI (2003).

nation of sleep characteristics by age, however, allows a closer understanding of the function of sleep for human development and successful aging.

Newborns and Infants

At birth, sleep timing is distributed evenly across day and night for the first few weeks, with no regular rhythm or concentration of sleeping and waking. Newborns sleep about 16 to 18 hours per day; however, it is discontinuous with the longest continuous sleep episode lasting only 2.5 to 4 hours (Adair and Bauchner, 1993; Roffwarg et al., 1966). Newborns have three types of sleep: quiet sleep (similar to NREM), active sleep (analogous to REM), and indeterminate sleep (Davis et al., 2004). Sleep onset occurs through REM, not NREM, and each sleep episode consists of only one or two cycles (Jenni and Carskadon, 2000; Davis et al., 2004). This distinctive sleep architecture occurs mostly because circadian rhythms have not yet been fully entrained (Davis et al., 2004).

Circadian rhythms begin to arise around 2 to 3 months of age, leading to sleep consolidation that manifests in greater durations of wakefulness

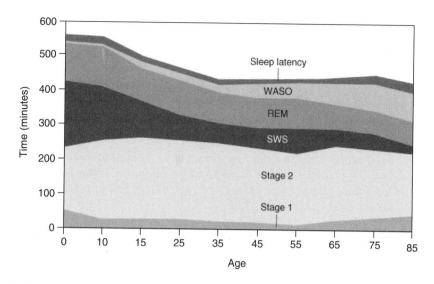

FIGURE 2-6 Changes in sleep with age.
NOTE: Time (in minutes) for sleep latency, amount of time spent awake after initially falling asleep (WASO), rapid eye movement (REM), non-rapid eye movement (NREM), stages 1, 2, and slow-wave sleep (SWS).
SOURCE: Carskadon and Rechtschaffen (2005).

during the day and longer periods of sleep at night (Sheldon, 2002). Circadian rhythm development in the first 3 months includes: emergence of the 24-hour core body temperature cycle (1 month of age); progression of nocturnal sleeping (2 months of age); and cycling of melatonin and cortisol hormones in a circadian rhythm (3 months of age) (Jenni and Carskadon, 2000).

Sleep cycles also change because of the emergence of the circadian rhythm and a greater responsiveness to social cues (such as breast-feeding and bedtime routines). By 3 months of age, sleep cycles become more regular: sleep onset now begins with NREM, REM sleep decreases and shifts to the later part of the sleep cycle, and the total NREM and REM sleep cycle is typically 50 minutes (Anders et al., 1995; Jenni and Carskadon, 2000). By 6 months of age, total sleep time reduces slightly and the longest continuous sleep episode lengthens to approximately 6 hours (Anders et al., 1995; Jenni and Carskadon, 2000). As sleep cycles mature, the typical muscle paralysis of REM sleep replaces the propensity for movement in what was called "active sleep" as a newborn. By 12 months old, the infant typically sleeps 14 to 15 hours per day with the majority of sleep consolidated in the evening and during one to two naps during the day (Anders et al., 1995).

Young Children

There are a limited number of studies that address normal sleep architecture in young children; however, one trend that appears to be consistent is that sleep amounts decrease as a child gets older. The reduction cannot be attributed solely to physiologic requirements, because cultural environments and social changes also influence changing sleep characteristics in young children. Total sleep time decreases by 2 hours from age 2 to age 5 (13 hours to 11) (Roffward et al., 1966). Socially, the decrease in time asleep may be a result of decreased daytime napping, as most children discontinue napping between 3 and 5 years old (Jenni and Carskadon, 2000). Other social and cultural factors that begin to influence sleep include how, with whom, and where children sleep and the introduction of school time routines (Jenni and O'Connor, 2005).

Physiologically, it has been suggested that by the time children enter school (typically 6 years old) they begin to manifest circadian sleep phase preferences—a tendency to be a "night owl" or "morning bird" (Jenni and Carskadon, 2000). Older children, however, are significantly more likely to experience challenges in initiating and maintaining sleep than younger children. In addition, older children are more likely to have nightmares, which usually disrupt sleep, making it discontinuous (Beltramini and Hertzig, 1983). One study found that children appear to have longer REM sleep latencies than adolescents and consequently spend a greater percentage of sleep time in stages 3 and 4 (Gaudreau et al., 2001).

Adolescents

A complex and bidirectional relationship exists between pubertal development and sleep. Studies underscore the importance of using pubertal stage, rather than chronologic age as the metric in understanding sleep, as has been found for other physiologic parameters in the second decade of life. It has been determined that adolescents require 9 to 10 hours of sleep each night (Carskadon et al., 1993; Mercer et al., 1998), though few adolescents obtain adequate sleep. In the United States, the average total sleep time in a sample of eighth-grade students was found to be 7.9 hours (Wolfson et al., 2003). Over a quarter of high school and college students were found to be sleep deprived (Wolfson and Carskadon, 1998).

SWS and sleep latency time progressively declines with advancing pubertal development (Carskadon et al., 1980); however, time spent in stage 2 increases (Carskadon, 1982). These changes are likely in part due to pubertal and hormonal changes that accompany the onset of puberty (Karacan et al., 1975). For instance, at midpuberty, there is significantly greater daytime sleepiness than at earlier stages of puberty. Afternoon sleepiness is greater than that in late afternoon and evening in more mature adolescents than in younger subjects. With increasing age, the total time spent sleeping decreases, as does REM sleep. However, if bedtime is fixed, the duration of REM sleep remains constant (Carskadon, 1982; Carskadon et al., 1983).

Adults

Sleep architecture continues to change with age across adulthood. Two major attributes of age-related sleep changes are earlier wake time and reduced sleep consolidation (Dijk et al., 2000). A hallmark change with age is a tendency toward earlier bedtimes and wake times. Older adults (approximately ages 65 to 75) typically awaken 1.33 hours earlier, and go to bed 1.07 hours earlier, than younger adults (approximately ages 20 to 30) (Duffy et al., 1998). There are no conclusive studies that demonstrate why older adults experience earlier wake times, despite decreased sleep efficiency, but one hypothesis may be an advanced circadian pacemaker that accompanies age (Dijk et al., 2000). It is unclear if this is due to older adults experiencing an increased sensitivity to light (Dijk et al., 2000; Ancoli-Israel, 2005). Nonetheless, the consequences of an advanced circadian rhythm are a 1-hour advance in body temperature increase in the early morning and misaligned melatonin and cortisol secretion rhythms with the circadian clock (Dijk et al., 2000).

Younger adults may experience brief awakenings, but they are usually minor and occur close to an REM sleep transition; thus, sleep remains relatively consolidated. Arousal occurring mostly from REM sleep in young adults suggests that there is a protective mechanism to keep from awakening during NREM sleep; however, this protective effect appears to also decline with age (Dijk, 1998). As an individual ages (between the ages of 20 to 60), SWS declines at a rate of about 2 percent per decade (Figure 2-6) (Dijk et al., 1989; Astrom and Trojaborg, 1992; Landolt et al., 1996; Ancoli-Israel, 2005). Because arousal thresholds are typically highest during SWS, and because SWS declines with age, older adults experience more frequent awakenings during a sleep episode. Another important variable may be an age-related reduction both in homeostatic sleep pressure and circadian pacemaker effectiveness during the night (Dijk et al., 2000).

Gender Differences

Although there have been few systematic studies, there appear to be gender-based differences in sleep and circadian rhythms. Available evidence is strongest in adults; however, gender differences have also been observed in infancy (Bach et al., 2000; Moss and Robson, 1970; Hoppenbrouwers et al., 1989), childhood (Meijer et al., 2000; Sadeh et al., 2000; Acebo et al., 1996), and adolescence (Giannotti et al., 2002; Laberge et al., 2001). In adults, men spend greater time in stage 1 sleep (Bixler et al., 1984) and experience more awakenings (Kobayashi et al., 1998). Although women maintain SWS longer than men, they complain more often of difficulty falling asleep and midsleep awakenings. In contrast, men are more likely to complain of daytime sleepiness (Ancoli-Israel, 2000).

In women, the menstrual cycle may influence sleep-wake activity; however, methodological challenges have limited the number of conclusive findings (Metcalf, 1983; Leibenluft et al., 1994). There have been a number of studies that suggest that women's sleep patterns are greatly affected during pregnancy and the postpartum period (Karacan et al., 1968; Hertz et al., 1992; Lee and Zaffke, 1999; Driver and Shapiro, 1992). For example, women often experience considerable daytime sleepiness during pregnancy and during the first few postpartum months, and as will be discussed in greater detail in Chapter 3, they are also at a higher risk of developing restless legs syndrome (Goodman et al., 1998; Lee et al., 2001).

Elderly People

Problematic sleep has adverse effects on all individuals, regardless of age; however, older people typically show an increase in disturbed sleep that can create a negative impact on their quality of life, mood, and alertness (Ancoli-Israel, 2005; Bliwise, 2005). Elderly individuals sleep 36 percent less than children at age 5 (Figure 2-6). Although the ability to sleep becomes more difficult, the need to sleep does not decrease with age (Ancoli-Israel, 2005). Difficulty in initiating and maintaining sleep is cited in 43 percent of the elderly (Foley et al., 1995), although these problems are more commonly among adults suffering from depression, respiratory symptoms, and physical disability, among others (Ancoli-Israel, 2005). However, declining sleep efficiency and quality has also been observed in healthy older people (Dijk et al., 2000).

Changes in sleep patterns affect males and females differently. The progressive decrease in SWS is one of the most prominent changes with aging; however, it appears to preferentially affect men. The gender difference is unclear, but it has been suggested that older women have "better-preserved" SWS than men (Reynolds et al., 1985). Women ages 70 and older spend around 15 to 20 percent of total sleep time in stages 3 and 4; men of the same age spend only around 5 percent of total sleep time in stages 3 and 4 (Redline et al., 2004). Another gender contrast is that older women go to bed and wake up earlier than older men, which suggests that body temperature rhythms are phase-advanced in elderly women (Campbell et al., 1989;

Moe et al., 1991; Monk et al., 1995). However, both men and women have increased stage 1 and decreased REM sleep.

Older people also experience a decrease in melatonin levels, which may be due to the gradual deterioration of the hypothalamic nuclei that drive circadian rhythms (Ancoli-Israel, 2005). The inability to maintain long sleep episodes and bouts of wakefulness may reflect, in addition to other medical factors, a continuously decreasing sleep homeostasis (Dijk et al., 2000; Bliwise, 2005). Other prominent factors are the continuous increase in sleep latency and nighttime awakenings and inconsistency of external cues such as light exposure (which tends to be low), irregular meal times, nocturia, and decreased mobility leading to a reduction in exercise (Dijk et al., 2000; Ancoli-Israel, 2005; Bliwise, 2005).

REFERENCES

Acebo C, Millman RP, Rosenberg C, Cavallo A, Carskadon MA. 1996. Sleep, breathing, and cephalometrics in older children and young adults. Part I: Normative values. *Chest* 109(3):664–672.

Adair RH, Bauchner H. 1993. Sleep problems in childhood. *Current Problems in Pediatrics* 23(4):142,147–170.

Ancoli-Israel S. 2000. Insomnia in the elderly: A review for the primary care practitioner. *Sleep: Supplement* 23(1): S23–S30, discussion S36–S38.

Ancoli-Israel S. 2005. Normal human sleep at different ages: Sleep in older adults. In: Sleep Research Society, eds. *SRS Basics of Sleep Guide.* Westchester, IL: Sleep Research Society. Pp. 21–26.

Anders TF, Sadeh A, Appareddy V. 1995. Normal sleep in neonates and children. In: Ferber RKM, ed. *Principles and Practice of Sleep Medicine in the Child.* Philadelphia: Saunders. Pp. 7–18.

Astrom C, Trojaborg W. 1992. Relationship of age to power spectrum analysis of EEG during sleep. *Journal of Clinical Neurophysiology* 9(3):424–430.

Bach V, Telliez F, Leke A, Libert JP. 2000. Gender-related sleep differences in neonates in thermoneutral and cool environments. *Journal of Sleep Research* 9(3):249–254.

Bader G, Gillberg C, Johnson M, Kadesjö B, Rasmussen P. 2003. Activity and sleep in children with ADHD. *Sleep* 26:A136.

Beltramini AU, Hertzig ME. 1983. Sleep and bedtime behavior in preschool-aged children. *Pediatrics* 71(2):153–158.

Bixler EO, Kales A, Jacoby JA, Soldatos CR, Vela-Bueno A. 1984. Nocturnal sleep and wakefulness: Effects of age and sex in normal sleepers. International *Journal of Neuroscience* 23(1):33–42.

Blasi A, Jo J, Valladares E, Morgan BJ, Skatrud JB, Khoo MC. 2003. Cardiovascular variability after arousal from sleep: Time-varying spectral analysis. *Journal of Applied Physiology* 95(4):1394–1404.

Bliwise D. 2005. Normal aging. In: Kryger MH, Roth T, Dement WC, eds. *Principles and Practice of Sleep Medicine.* 4th ed. Philadelphia: Saunders. Pp. 24–38.

Bunning E. 1964. *The Physiological Clock.* Berlin, Germany: Springer-Verlag.

Buxton OM, Spiegel K, Van Cauter E. 2002. Modulation of endocrine function and metabolism by sleep and sleep loss. In: Lee-Chiong TL, Sateia MJ, Carskadon MA, eds. *Sleep Medicine.* Philadelphia: Hanley & Belfus. Pp. 59–69.

Campbell SS, Gillin JC, Kripke DF, Erikson P, Clopton P. 1989. Gender differences in the circadian temperature rhythms of healthy elderly subjects: Relationships to sleep quality. *Sleep* 12(6):529–536.

Carskadon MA. 1982. The second decade. Guilleminault C, ed. *Sleeping and Waking Disorders: Indications and Techniques.* Menlo Park, CA: Addison-Wesley. Pp. 99–125.

Carskadon M, Dement W. 2005. Normal human sleep: An overview. In: Kryger MH, Roth T, Dement WC, eds. *Principles and Practice of Sleep Medicine.* 4th ed. Philadelphia: Elsevier Saunders. Pp. 13–23.

Carskadon MA, Rechtschaffen A. 2005. Monitoring and staging human sleep. In: Kryger MH, Roth TT, Dement WC, eds. *Principles and Practice of Sleep Medicine.* 4th ed. Philadelphia: Elsevier Saunders. Pp. 1359–1377.

Carskadon MA, Harvey K, Duke P, Anders TF, Litt IF, Dement WC. 1980. Pubertal changes in daytime sleepiness. *Sleep* 2(4):453–460.

Carskadon MA, Orav EJ, Dement WC. 1983. Evolution of sleep and daytime sleepiness in adolescents. In: Guilleminault CLE, ed. *Sleep/Wake Disorders: Natural History, Epidemiology, and Long-Term Evolution.* New York: Raven Press. Pp. 201–216.

Carskadon MA, Vieira C, Acebo C. 1993. Association between puberty and delayed phase preference. *Sleep* 16(3):258–262.

Catcheside PG, Chiong SC, Mercer J, Saunders NA, McEvoy RD. 2002. Noninvasive cardiovascular markers of acoustically induced arousal from non-rapid-eye-movement sleep. *Sleep* 25(7):797–804.

Chou TC, Scammell TE, Gooley JJ, Gaus SE, Saper CB, Lu J. 2003. Critical role of dorsomedial hypothalamic nucleus in a wide range of behavioral circadian rhythms. *Journal of Neuroscience* 23(33):10691–10702.

Cianci T, Zoccoli G, Lenzi P, Franzini C. 1991. Loss of integrative control of peripheral circulation during desynchronized sleep. *American Journal of Physiology* 261(2 Pt 2): R373–R377.

Crick F, Mitchison G. 1983. The function of dream sleep. *Nature* 304(5922):111–114.

Davis KF, Parker KP, Montgomery GL. 2004. Sleep in infants and young children: Part one: Normal sleep. *Journal of Pediatric Health Care* 18(2):65–71.

Dement W, Kleitman N. 1957a. Cyclic variations in EEG during sleep and their relation to eye movements, body motility, and dreaming. *Electroencephalography and Clinical Neurophysiology: Supplement* 9(4):673–690.

Dement T, Kleitman N. 1957b. The relation of eye movements during sleep to dream activity: An objective method for the study of dreaming. *Journal of Experimental Psychology* 53(5):339–346.

Dijk DCC. 1998. REM sleep as a gate to wakefulness during forced desynchrony in young and older people [abstract]. *Sleep* 21(3):S298.

Dijk DJ, Beersma DG, van den Hoofdakker RH. 1989. All night spectral analysis of EEG sleep in young adult and middle-aged male subjects. *Neurobiology of Aging* 10(6):677–682.

Dijk DJ, Duffy JF, Czeisler CA. 2000. Contribution of circadian physiology and sleep homeostasis to age-related changes in human sleep. *Chronobiology International* 17(3): 285–311.

Douglas, NJ. 2005. Respiratory physiology: Control of ventilation. In: Kryger MH, Roth T, Dement WC, eds. *Principles and Practice of Sleep Medicine.* 4th ed. Philadelphia: Elsevier Saunders. Pp. 224–229.

Driver HS, Shapiro CM. 1992. A longitudinal study of sleep stages in young women during pregnancy and postpartum. *Sleep* 15(5):449–453.

Duffy JF, Dijk DJ, Klerman EB, Czeisler CA. 1998. Later endogenous circadian temperature nadir relative to an earlier wake time in older people. *American Journal of Physiology* 275(5 Pt 2):R1478–R1487.

Dunlap JC, Loros JJ, DeCoursey PJ. 2004. *Chronobiology: Biological Timekeeping.* Sunderland, MA: Sinauer Associates.

Floras JS, Jones JV, Johnston JA, Brooks DE, Hassan MO, Sleight P. 1978. Arousal and the circadian rhythm of blood pressure. *Clinical Science and Molecular Medicine Supplement* 55(4):395s–397s.

Foley DJ, Monjan AA, Brown SL, Simonsick EM, Wallace RB, Blazer DG. 1995. Sleep complaints among elderly persons: An epidemiologic study of three communities. *Sleep* 18(6):425–432.

Gais S, Molle M, Helms K, Born J. 2002. Learning-dependent increases in sleep spindle density. *Journal of Neuroscience* 22(15):6830–6834.

Gaudreau H, Carrier J, Montplaisir J. 2001. Age-related modifications of NREM sleep EEG: From childhood to middle age. *Journal of Sleep Research* 10(3):165–172.

Giannotti F, Cortesi F, Sebastiani T, Ottaviano S. 2002. Circadian preference, sleep and daytime behaviour in adolescence. *Journal of Sleep Research* 11(3):191–199.

Gillette M, Abbott S. 2005. Fundamentals of the circadian system. In: Sleep Research Society, eds. *SRS Basics of Sleep Guide.* Westchester, IL: Sleep Research Society. Pp. 131–138.

Goodman JD, Brodie C, Ayida GA. 1988. Restless leg syndrome in pregnancy. *British Medical Journal* 297(6656):1101–1102.

Hertz G, Fast A, Feinsilver SH, Albertario CL, Schulman H, Fein AM. 1992. Sleep in normal late pregnancy. *Sleep* 15(3):246–251.

Hoppenbrouwers T, Hodgman J, Arakawa K, Sterman MB. 1989. Polysomnographic sleep and waking states are similar in subsequent siblings of SIDS and control infants during the first six months of life. *Sleep* 12(3):265–276.

Jenni OG, Carskadon MA. 2000. Normal human sleep at different ages: Infants to adolescents. In: Sleep Research Society, eds. *SRS Basics of Sleep Guide.* Westchester, IL: Sleep Research Society. Pp. 11–19.

Jenni OG, O'Connor BB. 2005. Children's sleep: An interplay between culture and biology. *Pediatrics* 115(1 Suppl):204–216.

Jones BE. 2005. Basic mechanisms of sleep-wake states. In: Kryger MH, Roth T, Dement WC, eds. *Principles and Practice of Sleep Medicine.* 4th ed. Philadelphia: Elsevier/Saunders. Pp. 136–153.

Karacan IH, Agnew H, Williams RL, Webb W, Ross J. 1968. Characteristics of sleep patterns during late pregnancy and postpartum periods. *American Journal of Obstetrics and Gynecology* 297(6656):1101–1102.

Karacan I, Anch M, Thornby JI, Okawa M, Williams RL. 1975. Longitudinal sleep patterns during pubertal growth: Four-year follow up. *Pediatrics Research* 9(11):842–846.

Kobayashi R, Kohsaka M, Fukuda N, Honma H, Sakakibara S, Koyama, T. 1998. Gender differences in the sleep of middle-aged individuals. *Psychiatry and Clinical Neurosciences* 52(2):186–187.

Krieger J. 2000. Respiratory physiology: Breathing in normal subjects. In: Kryger M, Roth T, Dement WC, eds. *Principles and Practice of Sleep Medicine.* 4th ed. Philadelphia: Elsevier Saunders. Pp. 229–241.

Laberge L, Petit D, Simard C, Vitaro F, Tremblay RE, Montplaisir J. 2001. Development of sleep patterns in early adolescence. *Journal of Sleep Research* 10(1):59–67.

Landolt HP, Dijk DJ, Achermann P, Borbely AA. 1996. Effect of age on the sleep EEG: Slow-wave activity and spindle frequency activity in young and middle-aged men. *Brain Research* 738(2):205–212.

Lee KA, Zaffke ME. 1999. Longitudinal changes in fatigue and energy during pregnancy and the postpartum period. *Journal of Obstetric, Gynecologic, and Neonatal Nursing* 28(2):183–191.

Lee KA, Zaffke ME, Baratte-Beebe K. 2001. Restless legs syndrome and sleep disturbance during pregnancy: The role of folate and iron. *Journal of Women's Health and Gender-based Medicine* 10(4):335–341.

Leibenluft E, Fiero PL, Rubinow DR. 1994. Effects of the menstrual cycle on dependent variables in mood disorder research. *Archives of General Psychiatry* 51(10):761–781.

Loomis AL, Harvey EN, Hobart GA. 1937. Cerebral states during sleep as studied by human brain potentials. *Journal of Experimental Psychology* 21(2):127–144.

Lugaresi E, Coccagna G, Cirignotta F, Farneti P, Gallassi R, Di Donato G, Verucchi P. 1978. Breathing during sleep in man in normal and pathological conditions. *Advances in Experimental Medicine and Biology* 99:35–45.

Madsen PL, Holm S, Vorstrup S, Friberg L, Lassen NA, Wildschiodtz G. 1991a. Human regional cerebral blood flow during rapid-eye-movement sleep. *Journal of Cerebral Blood Flow Metabolism* 11(3):502–507.

Madsen PL, Schmidt JF, Wildschiodtz G, Friberg L, Holm S, Vorstrup S, Lassen N A. 1991b. Cerebral O_2 metabolism and cerebral blood flow in humans during deep and rapid-eye-movement sleep. *Journal of Applied Physiology* 70(6):2597–2601.

Meijer AM, Habekothe HT, Van Den Wittenboer GL. 2000. Time in bed, quality of sleep and school functioning of children. *Journal of Sleep Research* 9(2):145–153.

Mercer PW, Merritt SL, Cowell JM. 1998. Differences in reported sleep need among adolescents. *Journal of Adolescent Health* 23(5):259–263.

Metcalf MG. 1983. Incidence of ovulation from the menarche to the menopause: Observations of 622 New Zealand women. *The New Zealand Medical Journal* 96(738): 645–648.

Moe KE, Prinz PN, Vitiello MV, Marks AL, Larsen LH. 1991. Healthy elderly women and men have different entrained circadian temperature rhythms. *Journal of the American Geriatrics Society* 39(4):383–387.

Monk TH, Buysse DJ, Reynolds CF III, Kupfer DJ, Houck PR. 1995. Circadian temperature rhythms of older people. *Experimental Gerontology* 30(5):455–474.

Morruzzi G, Magoun HW. 1949. Brain stem reticular formation and activation of the EEG. *Electroencephalography and Clinical Neurophysiology* 1:455–473.

Moss HA, Robson KS. 1970. The relation between the amount of time infants spend at various states and the development of visual behavior. *Child Development* 41(2):509–517.

Mulcahy D, Wright C, Sparrow J, Cunningham D, Curcher D, Purcell H, Fox K. 1993. Heart rate and blood pressure consequences of an afternoon SIESTA (Snooze-Induced Excitation of Sympathetic Triggered Activity). *American Journal of Cardiology* 71(7):611–614.

NHLBI (National Heart, Lung, and Blood Institute). 2003. *Sleep, Sleep Disorders, and Biological Rhythms: NIH Curriculum Supplement Series, Grades 9-12.* Colorado Springs, CO: Biological Sciences Curriculum Study.

NLM (National Library of Medicine), NIH (National Institutes of Health). *Medline Plus Online Medical Dictionary.* [Online]. Available: http://www.nlm.nih.gov/medlineplus/mplusdictionary.html [accessed February 6, 2006].

Parker KP, Dunbar SB. 2005. Cardiac nursing. In: Woods SL, Froelicher ESS, Motzer SU, Bridges E, eds. *Sleep.* 5th ed. Philadelphia: Lippincott Williams and Wilkins. Pp. 197–219.

Redline S, Kirchner HL, Quan SF, Gottlieb DJ, Kapur V, Newman A. 2004. The effects of age, sex, ethnicity, and sleep-disordered breathing on sleep architecture. *Archives of Internal Medicine* 164(4):406–418.

Reynolds CF III, Kupfer DJ, Taska LS, Hoch CC, Sewitch DE, Spiker DG. 1985. Sleep of healthy seniors: A revisit. *Sleep* 8(1):20–29.

Roffward HP, Muzio JN, Dement WC. 1966. Ontogenetic development of the human sleep-dream cycle. *Science* 152(3722):604–619.

Sadeh A, Raviv A, Gruber R. 2000. Sleep patterns and sleep disruptions in school-age children. *Developmental Psychology* 36(3):291–301.

Saper CB, Cano G, Scammell TE. 2005a. Homeostatic, circadian, and emotional regulation of sleep. *Journal of Comparitive Neurology* 493(1):92–98.

Saper CB, Lu J, Chou TC, Gooley J. 2005b. The hypothalamic integrator for circadian rhythms. *Trends in Neuroscience* 28(3):152–157.

Saper CB, Scammell TE, Lu J. 2005c. Hypothalamic regulation of sleep and circadian rhythms. *Nature* 437(7063):1257–1263.

Sheldon SH. 2002. Sleep in infants and children. In: Lee-Choing TK, Sateia MJ, Carskadon MA, eds. *Sleep Medicine*. Philadelphia: Hanley and Belfus. Pp. 99–103.

Simon PM, Landry SH, Leifer JC. 2002. Respiratory control during sleep. In: Lee-Chiong TK, Sateia MJ, Carskadon MA, eds. *Sleep Medicine*. Philadelphia: Hanley and Belfus. Pp. 41–51.

Smith C, Lapp L. 1991. Increases in number of REMS and REM density in humans following an intensive learning period. *Sleep* 14(4):325–330.

Somers V, Dyken M, Mark A, Abboud F. 1993. Sympathetic-nerve activity during sleep in normal subjects. *New England Journal of Medicine* 328(5):303–307.

Szymusiak R. 2005. Thermoregulation and sleep. In: Sleep Research Society, eds. *SRS Basics of Sleep Guide*. Westchester, IL: Sleep Research Society. Pp. 119–126.

Tank J, Diedrich A, Hale N, Niaz FE, Furlan R, Robertson RM, Mosqueda-Garcia R. 2003. Relationship between blood pressure, sleep K-complexes, and muscle sympathetic nerve activity in humans. *American Journal of Physiology. Regulatory, Integrative and Comparative Physiology* 285(1):R208–R214.

Van Cauter E. 2000. Endocrine physiology. In: Kryger MH, Roth T, Dement WC, eds. *Principles and Practice of Sleep Medicine*. Philadelphia: Elsevier/Saunders. Pp. 266–278.

Vitaterna M, Pinto L, Turek F. 2005. Molecular genetic basis for mammalian circadian rhythms. In: Kryger MH, Roth T, Dement WC, eds. *Principles and Practice of Sleep Medicine*. 4th ed. Philadelphia: Elsevier/Saunders. Pp. 363–374.

Wolfson AR, Carskadon MA. 1998. Sleep schedules and daytime functioning in adolescents. *Child Development* 69(4):875–887.

Wolfson AR, Carskadon MA, Acebo C, Seifer R, Fallone G, Labyak SE, Martin JL. 2003. Evidence for the validity of a sleep habits survey for adolescents. *Sleep* 26(2):213–216.

Zepelin H, Siegel JM, Tobler I. 2005. Mammalian sleep. In: Kryger MH, Roth T, Dement WC, eds. *Principles and Practice of Sleep Medicine*. 4th ed. Philadelphia: Elsevier/Saunders. Pp. 91–100.

3

Extent and Health Consequences of Chronic Sleep Loss and Sleep Disorders

CHAPTER SUMMARY *It is estimated that 50 to 70 million Americans chronically suffer from a disorder of sleep and wakefulness, hindering daily functioning and adversely affecting health and longevity. There around 90 distinct sleep disorders; most are marked by one of these symptoms: excessive daytime sleepiness, difficulty initiating or maintaining sleep, and abnormal events occurring during sleep. The cumulative long-term effects of sleep loss and sleep disorders have been associated with a wide range of deleterious health consequences including an increased risk of hypertension, diabetes, obesity, depression, heart attack, and stroke. After decades of research, the case can be confidently made that sleep loss and sleep disorders have profound and widespread effects on human health. This chapter focuses on manifestations and prevalence, etiology and risk factors, and comorbidities of the most common sleep conditions, including sleep loss, sleep-disordered breathing, insomnia, narcolepsy, restless legs syndrome, parasomnias, sleep-related psychiatric disorders, sleep-related neurological disorders, sleep-related medical disorders, and circadian rhythm sleep disorders.*

Sleep loss and sleep disorders are among the most common yet frequently overlooked and readily treatable health problems. It is estimated that 50 to 70 million Americans chronically suffer from a disorder of sleep and wakefulness, hindering daily functioning and adversely affecting health and longevity (NHLBI, 2003). Questions about sleep are seldom asked by physicians (Namen et al., 1999, 2001). For example, about 80 to 90 percent of adults with clinically significant sleep-disordered breathing remain undiagnosed (Young et al., 1997b). Failure to recognize sleep problems not only precludes diagnosis and treatment—it also precludes the possibility of preventing their grave public health consequences.

The public health consequences of sleep loss and sleep-related disorders are far from benign. The most visible consequences are errors in judgment contributing to disastrous events such as the space shuttle *Challenger* (Walsh et al., 2005). Less visible consequences of sleep conditions are far more prevalent, and they take a toll on nearly every key indicator of public health: mortality, morbidity, performance, accidents and injuries, functioning and quality of life, family well-being, and health care utilization. Some of these consequences, such as automobile crashes, occur acutely within hours (or minutes) of the sleep disorder, and thus are relatively easy to link to sleep problems. Others—for example, obesity and hypertension—develop more insidiously over months and years of chronic sleep problems. After decades of research, the case can be confidently made that sleep loss and sleep disorders have profound and widespread effects on human health.

Although there are around 90 distinct sleep disorders, according to the International Classification of Sleep Disorders (AASM, 2005), most are marked by one of these symptoms: excessive daytime sleepiness, difficulty initiating or maintaining sleep, or abnormal movements, behaviors, and sensations occurring during sleep. The cumulative effects of sleep loss and sleep disorders have been associated with a wide range of deleterious health consequences including an increased risk of hypertension, diabetes, obesity, depression, heart attack, and stroke.

This chapter focuses on the most common sleep conditions, including sleep loss, sleep-disordered breathing, insomnia, narcolepsy, restless legs syndrome (RLS), parasomnias, sleep-related psychiatric disorders, sleep-related neurological disorders, sleep-related medical disorders, and circadian rhythm sleep disorders. The manifestations and prevalence, etiology and risk factors, and comorbidities for each condition are briefly described. There is a large body of data on these disorders, in part because they encompass the most frequently cited sleep disorders or they carry the greatest public health burden. As such, the committee chose to focus primarily on these disorders.

SLEEP LOSS

Manifestations and Prevalence

Sleep loss generally, in adults, refers to sleep of shorter duration than the average basal need of 7 to 8 hours per night. The main symptom of sleep loss is excessive daytime sleepiness, but other symptoms include depressed mood and poor memory or concentration (Dinges et al., 2005). Chronic sleep loss, while neither a formal syndrome nor a disorder, has serious consequences for health, performance, and safety, as described in Chapter 4.

Sleep loss is a highly prevalent problem that continues to worsen in frequency as individuals grow older. Recent studies find that at least 18 percent of adults report receiving insufficient sleep (Liu et al., 2000; Kapur et al., 2002; Strine and Chapman, 2005). Historically, there have been a limited number of nationally representative surveys that provide reliable data on sleep patterns in the population. The National Health Interview Survey (NHIS), run by the Centers for Disease Control and Prevention (CDC) (see Chapter 5), included the following question in the 1977, 1985, 1990 cycles: "On average how many hours of sleep do you get a night (24-hour period)?" The same question was added to the core NHIS questionnaire in 2004. Based on these data, it has been estimated that the percentage of men and women who sleep less than 6 hours has increased significantly over the last 20 years (Figure 3-1) (CDC, 2005). More than 35 years ago, adults reported sleeping 7.7 hours per night (Tune, 1968).

Adolescents also frequently report receiving insufficient sleep. Contrary to public perceptions, adolescents need as much sleep as preteens. A large survey of over 3,000 adolescents in Rhode Island found that only 15 percent reported sleeping 8.5 or more hours on school nights, and 26 percent reported sleeping 6.5 hours or less (Wolfson and Carskadon, 1998). The optimal sleep duration for adolescents, about 9 hours per night, is based on research about alertness, sleep-wake cycles, hormones, and circadian rhythms (Carskadon et al., 2004). Among adolescents, extensive television viewing and growing social, recreational, and academic demands contribute to sleep loss or sleep problems (Wolfson and Carskadon, 1998; Johnson et al., 2004).

Etiology and Risk Factors

The causes of sleep loss are multifactoral. They fall under two major, somewhat overlapping categories: lifestyle/occupational (e.g., shift work,[1]

---

[1] The term "shift work" is defined by regular employment outside of the normal day work hours of 7:00 a.m. to 6:00 p.m.

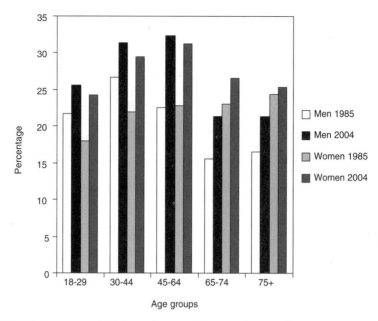

FIGURE 3-1 Percent of adults in the United States who usually slept 6 hours or less a night.
SOURCE: CDC (2005).

prolonged working hours, jet lag, irregular sleep schedules[2]), and sleep disorders (e.g., insomnia, sleep-disordered breathing, RLS, narcolepsy, and circadian rhythm disorders). Unfortunately, available epidemiological data are not sufficient to determine the extent to which sleep loss is caused by pathology versus behavioral components. The increase in sleep loss is driven largely by broad societal changes, including greater reliance on longer work hours, shift work, and greater access to television and the Internet. About 20 percent of workers are engaged in some kind of shift work (Monk, 2005), of whom there is a growing number of night shift workers suffering chronic sleep loss and disruption of circadian rhythms (Harma et al., 1998; Drake et al., 2004). One indication of the growing trend is the number of adults departing for work between midnight and 5:30 a.m.; that number has grown, over a 10-year period, by 24 percent (United States Census Bureau, 1990). A greater prevalence of insomnia also may contribute to the rise in sleep loss, but probably to a lesser extent than do occupational or lifestyle

---

[2]Irregular sleep schedules frequently include significant disparities between sleep on weekdays and weekends, which contribute to shifts in sleep phase and sleep problems.

changes. Adults are sleeping less to get more work accomplished and are staying up later to watch television or use the Internet (NSF, 2005b).

Sleep Loss Affects Health

In the past 10 or more years, research has overturned the dogma that sleep loss has no health effects, apart from daytime sleepiness. The studies discussed in this section suggest that sleep loss (less than 7 hours per night) may have wide-ranging effects on the cardiovascular, endocrine, immune, and nervous systems, including the following:

- Obesity in adults and children
- Diabetes and impaired glucose tolerance
- Cardiovascular disease and hypertension
- Anxiety symptoms
- Depressed mood
- Alcohol use

Many of the studies find graded associations, insofar as the greater the degree of sleep deprivation, the greater the apparent adverse effect (although the difference may not reach statistical significance). Another common finding is the relationship that adverse effects occur with either short or long sleep duration, as compared to a sleep time of 7 to 8 hours. This type of association is often described as a U-shaped relationship. It should be noted, however, that the majority of these studies are observational in nature, and thus definite causal inferences cannot be made. The associations observed in some studies might be subject to different types of biases, such as temporal (or "reverse causality") bias, whereby sleep loss might be a *manifestation* or a *symptom* of the disease in question. The latter is most likely in cross-sectional studies but could also affect associations observed in cohort studies, particularly when they are relatively short term and/or when the disease under investigation has a long preclinical phase. In the discussion that follows, and wherever possible, potential physiological mechanisms behind epidemiological associations and that support the plausibility of a true causal relationship are noted.

Sleep Loss Is Associated with Obesity

When a person sleeps less than 7 hours a night there is a dose-response relationship between sleep loss and obesity: the shorter the sleep, the greater the obesity, as typically measured by body mass index (BMI)—weight in kilograms divided by height in meters squared. Although most studies were cross-sectional, one prospective study was a 13-year cohort study of nearly

500 adults. By age 27, individuals with short sleep duration (less than 6 hours) were 7.5 times more likely to have a higher body mass index, after controlling for confounding factors such as family history, levels of physical activity, and demographic factors (Hasler et al., 2004). Another study, a large population-based study of more than 1,000 adults, found a U-shaped relationship between sleep duration, measured by polysomnography, and BMI (Figure 3-2). Adults who slept 7.7 hours had the lowest BMI; those with shorter and longer sleep duration had progressively higher BMI. The U-shaped association also applies to other health outcomes, such as heart attacks. The impact of sleep loss diminishes with age. The study also sought to investigate physiological mechanisms behind the relationship between sleep duration and BMI. Measuring two appetite-related hormones, the study found that sleep insufficiency increased appetite. Sleep insufficiency was associated with lower levels of leptin, a hormone produced by an adipose tissue hormone that suppresses appetite, and higher levels of ghrelin, a peptide that stimulates appetite (Taheri et al., 2004). Another study—a small randomized, cross-over clinical trial—also found that sleep restriction was associated with lower leptin and higher ghrelin levels (Spiegel et al., 2004). The findings suggest that a hormonally mediated increase in appetite may help to explain why short sleep is related to obesity. Several mediating mechanisms have been proposed, including effects of sleep deprivation on

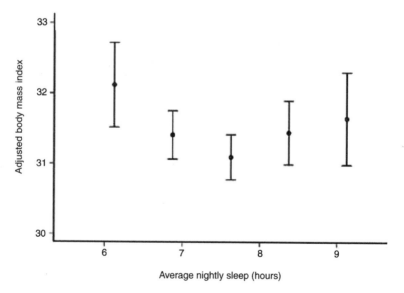

FIGURE 3-2 Curvilinear relationship between BMI and average nightly sleep. SOURCE: Taheri et al. (2004).

the sympathetic nervous system and/or hypothalamic hormones (Spiegel et al., 2004), which also influence appetite.

Obesity also contributes to obstructive sleep apnea (OSA). This most likely occurs through fat deposition in airways, causing them to narrow. This point is inferred from studies finding that large neck size is a better predictor of OSA than is BMI (Katz et al., 1990) and the finding that central obesity (obesity around the waist) is a better predictor of OSA than total obesity (Grunstein, 2005b). The relationship has been found in well-designed epidemiological studies of young children (Locard et al., 1992; Sekine et al., 2002; von Kries et al., 2002) and adults (Vioque et al., 2000; Kripke et al., 2002; Gupta et al., 2002; Taheri et al., 2004; Hasler et al., 2004).

Taken as a whole, the body of evidence suggests that the serious public health problem of obesity may continue to grow as sleep loss trends continue to worsen. It also suggests that addressing obesity will likely benefit sleep disorders, and treating sleep deprivation and sleep disorders may benefit individuals with obesity (Taheri et al., 2004).

Sleep Loss Is Associated with Diabetes and Impaired Glucose Tolerance

Two large epidemiological studies and one experimental study found an association between sleep loss and diabetes, or impaired glucose tolerance. Impaired glucose tolerance, which is a precursor to diabetes, is manifested by glucose levels rising higher than normal and for a longer period after an intravenous dose of glucose. In the Sleep Heart Health Study, which is a community-based cohort, adults (middle-aged and older) who reported 5 hours of sleep or less were 2.5 times more likely to have diabetes, compared with those who slept 7 to 8 hours per night (Figure 3-3, [Gottlieb et al., 2005]). Those reporting 6 hours per night were about 1.7 times more likely to have diabetes. Both groups were also more likely to display impaired glucose tolerance. Adults with sleep times of 9 hours or more also showed these effects, a finding consistent with the Nurses Health Study. Adjustment for waist girth, a measure of obesity, did not alter the significance of the findings, suggesting that the diabetes effect was independent of obesity.

The relationship between shorter sleep times and impaired glucose tolerance is also supported by an experimental study in which 11 healthy male volunteers were restricted to 4 hours of sleep for a total of six nights (Spiegel et al., 1999). Even after this relatively short period of time, the study found that sleep loss, compared with a fully rested state, led to impaired glucose tolerance. The effect resolved after restoring sleep to normal. Glucose clearance was 40 percent slower with sleep loss than with sleep recovery. Further, mice that have a mutation in a gene that regulates

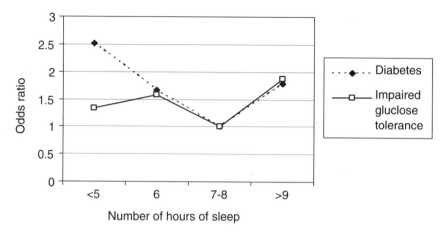

FIGURE 3-3 Sleep duration impacts prevalence of diabetes.
NOTE: Data were adjusted for age, sex, race, waist girth, caffeine, alcohol, smoking, and apnea-hypopnea index.
SOURCE: Gottlieb et al. (2005).

circadian rhythms have metabolic disorders (Turek et al., 2005). The association between sleep loss and diabetes or impaired glucose tolerance may mediate the relationship between sleep loss and cardiovascular morbidity and mortality, as discussed below.

Sleep Loss Is Associated with Cardiovascular Morbidity

Sleep loss and sleep complaints are associated with heart attacks (myocardial infarction) and perhaps stroke, according to several large epidemiological studies (Eaker et al., 1992; Qureshi et al., 1997; Schwartz et al., 1998; Newman et al., 2000; Ayas et al., 2003; Yaggi et al., 2005; Bradley et al., 2005; Caples et al., 2005) and one case-control study (Liu et al., 2002). One of these studies, of incident cases of heart attacks in the Nurses Health Study, was discussed earlier because it also found increased incidence of diabetes (Ayas et al., 2003). The cohort had no coronary heart disease at baseline. Ten years later, in 1996, the likelihood of nonfatal and fatal heart attack was modestly increased for both short and long sleep duration. Five hours of sleep or less was associated with a 45 percent increase in risk (odds ratio [OR] = 1.45, 95% confidence interval [CI], 1.10–1.92), after adjusting for age, BMI, smoking, and snoring. Similarly elevated risks were also found for sleeping 9 hours or more. The effects were independent of a history of hypertension or diabetes because additional adjustment for these conditions yielded slightly lower, but still significantly elevated, relative risks.

Several potential mechanisms could explain the link between sleep loss and cardiovascular events, including blood pressure increases, sympathetic hyperactivity, or impaired glucose tolerance. Experimental data, showing that acute sleep loss (3.6 hours sleep) for one night results in increased blood pressure in healthy young males, may provide a biological mechanism for the observed associations between sleep loss and cardiovascular disease (Tochikubo et al., 1996; Meier-Ewert et al., 2004).

Sleep Loss, Mood, Anxiety, and Alcohol Use

Sleep loss is associated with adverse effects on mood and behavior. Adults with chronic sleep loss report excess mental distress, depressive symptoms, anxiety, and alcohol use (Baldwin and Daugherty, 2004; Strine and Chapman, 2005; Hasler et al., 2005). A meta-analysis of 19 original articles found that partial sleep deprivation alters mood to an even greater extent that it does cognitive or motor functions (Pilcher and Huffcutt, 1996).

Several studies of adolescents, including one with more than 3,000 high school students, found that inadequate sleep is associated with higher levels of depressed mood, anxiety, behavior problems, alcohol use (Carskadon, 1990; Morrison et al., 1992; Wolfson and Carskadon, 1998), and attempted suicide (Liu, 2004). Nevertheless, it is not clear from cross-sectional studies whether sleep influences mood or anxiety level, or vice versa. On the other hand, a large, 3-year longitudinal study of more than 2,200 middle school students (ages 11 to 14) found that self-reported sleep loss was associated with more depressive symptoms and lower self-esteem over time (Fredriksen et al., 2004). The study measured sleep loss using a single question about sleep duration on school nights and measured depressive symptoms and self-esteem by the Children's Depressive Inventory and the Self-Esteem Questionnaire, respectively. Therefore, although this study suggests an association, the evidence is still limited.

Sleep Loss and Disease Mortality

Sleep loss is also associated with increased age-specific mortality, according to three large, population-based, prospective studies (Kripke et al., 2002; Tamakoshi et al., 2004; Patel et al., 2004). The studies were of large cohorts, ranging from 83,000 to 1.1 million people. In three studies, respondents were surveyed about their sleep duration, and then they were followed for periods ranging from 6 to 14 years. Deaths in short or long sleepers were compared with those who slept 7 hours (the reference group), after adjusting for numerous health and demographic factors. Sleeping 5 hours or less increased mortality risk, from all causes, by roughly 15 percent. The largest American study, depicted in Figure 3-4, graphically illustrates what has been found in all three studies: a U-shaped curve, showing that progressively shorter or longer sleep duration is associated with greater mortality. Other epidemiological studies suggest that sleep-loss-related mortality is largely from acute heart attacks (Ayas et al., 2003). Potential pathophysiological mechanisms accounting for the relationship, while poorly understood, have become the focus of growing interest and are discussed later in this chapter.

Management and Treatment

Management and treatment of sleep loss are rarely addressed by clinicians, despite the large toll on society (Chapters 4, 5, and 7). There are no formal treatment guidelines in primary or specialty care for dealing with sleep loss (Dinges et al., 1999). The most effective treatment for sleep loss is to sleep longer or take a short nap lasting no more than 2 hours (Veasey et al., 2002), and to have a better understanding of proper sleep habits. Catching up on sleep on the weekends—a popular remedy for sleep loss—does not return individuals to baseline functioning (Szymczak et al., 1993; Dinges et al., 1997; Klerman and Dijk, 2005; Murdey et al., 2005). If extended work hours or shift work cannot be avoided, specific behavioral tips to stay alert are available (NSF, 2005c), as are such wake-promoting

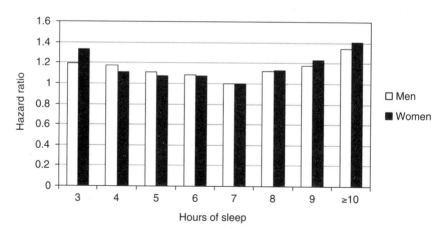

FIGURE 3-4 Shorter or longer sleep duration is associated with greater mortality. NOTE: Hazard ratio is an individual's relative risk of dying compared to the general population, based upon average number of hours of sleep per night. SOURCE: Kripke et al. (2002).

medications as caffeine, modafinil, and sympathomimetic medications (direct and indirect acting), including pemoline and methylphenidate (Mitler and O'Malley, 2005). In a randomized clinical trial caffeine and modafinil showed similar benefits for performance and alertness (Wesensten et al., 2002). Modafinil is the only FDA-approved drug for shift work sleep disorder, although it is not approved for sleep loss. Behavioral approaches developed for insomnia also may be useful for sleep loss, but no formal studies have been undertaken expressly for sleep loss. Furthermore, there have been no large-scale clinical trials examining the safety and efficacy of modafinil, or other drugs, in children and adolescents.

SLEEP-DISORDERED BREATHING

Manifestations and Prevalence

Sleep-disordered breathing refers to a spectrum of disorders that feature breathing pauses during sleep. The most common disorder is characterized by obstructive apneas and hypopneas (White, 2005), where repeated episodes of collapse (apneas) or partial collapse of the pharyngeal airway occur, usually a result of obstruction by soft tissue in the rear of the throat. Snoring, which is produced by vibrations of the soft tissues, is a good marker for OSA (Netzer, et al., 2003). Apneas or hypopneas (a reduction without cessation in airflow or effort) typically result in abrupt and intermittent reduction in blood oxygen saturation, which leads to sleep arousal, often accompanied by loud snorts or gasps as breathing resumes. Episodic interruptions of breathing also frequently cause cortical and brainstem arousals, interrupting sleep continuity, reducing sleep time, and causing increased sympathetic nervous system activation. These broad systemic effects on gas exchange and nervous system activation may lead to a range of systemic effects that affect vascular tone, levels of inflammatory mediators, and hormonal changes. As discussed in the following sections, these in turn may contribute to the development of hypertension, coronary artery disease, congestive heart failure, arrhythmias, stroke, glucose intolerance, and diabetes.

The defining symptom of sleep-disordered breathing is excessive daytime sleepiness. The symptom is likely influenced by sleep fragmentation tied to recurrent arousals that occur in response to breathing pauses. Other symptoms of fragmented sleep include decreased concentration and mood changes. The diagnosis of OSA requires detection, by polysomnography, of at least five or more apneas or hypopneas per hour of sleep (Thorpy, 2005). This rate is expressed as an index, the apnea-hypopnea index (or respiratory disturbance index), which is the average hourly number of apneas plus hypopneas.

OSA is found in at least 4 percent of men and 2 percent of women in the middle-aged workforce, according to the first major United States population-based study of the condition conducted about 15 years ago (Young et al., 1993). Those prevalence figures are based on a cutoff apnea-hypopnea index of 5 or higher, plus a requirement for daytime sleepiness. The prevalence is higher, 9 percent of women and 24 percent of men, with the same apnea-hypopnea index cutoff (Box 3-1), but without the daytime sleepiness requirement. In view of the epidemic increase of obesity (an important determinant of OSA) in recent years, these numbers might underestimate the current prevalence. However, other more recent population-based studies support these prevalence figures (Bixler et al., 1998, 2001).

OSA prevalence appears to increase with age. Adults 65 to 90 years of age had a threefold higher prevalence rate than middle-aged adults (Ancoli-Israel et al., 1991), while the prevalence in children has been reported to be around 2 percent (Ali et al., 1993; Rosen et al., 2003), with higher estimates occurring in ethnic minorities (Gislason and Benediktsdottir, 1995; Redline et al., 1999; Rosen et al., 2003). Underdiagnosis of OSA is common, with between 10 and 20 percent of OSA being diagnosed in adults (Young et al., 1997b). Less than 1 percent of older adults in primary care are referred for polysomnography (Haponik, 1992), although these numbers might have increased in recent years due to increased awareness of the disease. Similarly, children's OSA often goes undiagnosed too, partly because the implications of snoring are not often recognized by pediatricians. Although OSA can occur in children of any age, it is most common at preschool ages, a time coincident with tonsils and adenoids being largest relative to the underlying airway (Jeans et al., 1981).

Obstructive Sleep Apnea Causes Hypertension

OSA causes chronic elevation in daytime blood pressure (Young et al., 2002a; Young and Javaheri, 2005). The strongest evidence for a rise in systemic hypertension comes from several large, well-designed epidemiological studies, both cross-sectional (Young et al., 1997a; Nieto et al., 2000; Bixler et al., 2000; Duran et al., 2001) and prospective (Peppard et al., 2000). The Wisconsin Sleep Cohort study, a prospective study, tracked adults with sleep-disordered breathing for at least 4 years to determine new onset hypertension and other outcomes. The hypertensive effect was independent of obesity, age, gender, and other confounding factors. Controlling for obesity is especially important because it is a risk factor for hypertension as well as for OSA.

A causal association between OSA and hypertension is supported by evidence of a dose-response relationship; the higher the apnea-hypopnea index, the greater the increase in blood pressure (Peppard et al., 2000; Nieto

---

BOX 3-1
Definitions Impact Disease Prevalence Estimates

The metric used most commonly to define obstructive sleep apnea and to quantify its severity is the apnea-hypopnea index, derived by identifying and manually counting each respiratory disturbance (apnea and hypopnea) with subsequent division of the sum by the number of hours slept. Technology for measuring changes in airflow and ventilatory effort has evolved rapidly, with laboratories varying in the implementation of specific sensors and scoring approaches for identifying respiratory events. Variation in event identification has been particularly great for hypopneas (Moser et al., 1994), which requires identification of more subtle changes in airflow than do apneas, and often requires visualization of corroborative changes in oxygen desaturation or evidence of a cortical arousal. Variation in the sensors used to detect breathing changes, the amplitude criteria (from discernible to greater than 50 percent) applied to identify any given reductions in breathing signals as hypopneas, and different uses of corroborative data (associated desaturation and arousal) to discriminate "normal" from "hypopneic" breaths have all contributed to marked laboratory differences in events scored for clinical or research purposes. Likewise, there has been variation in the choice of threshold values for the apnea-hypopnea index considered to define the disease state. An analysis of over 5,000 records from the Sleep Heart Health Study underscores the potential variability introduced by varying either hypopnea definitions or threshold values. This analysis showed that the magnitude of the median apnea-hypopnea index varied 10-fold (i.e., 29.3 when the apnea-hypopnea index was based on events identified on the basis of flow or volume amplitude criteria alone to 2.0 for an apnea-hypopnea index that required an associated 5 percent desaturation with events) (Redline et al., 2000). Using any given definition but varying the threshold to define disease also resulted in marked differences in the percentage of subjects classified as diseased. For example, using an apnea-hypopnea index cutoff value of greater than 15 and an apnea-hypopnea index definition requiring a 5 percent level of desaturation resulted in a prevalence estimate of 10.8 percent. In contrast, almost the entire cohort was identified to be "affected" when sleep-disordered breathing was defined using an apnea-hypopnea index threshold of 5 and when all hypopneas were scored regardless of associated corroborative physiological changes. These data and others have identified the critical need for standardization. As such, at least three efforts led by professional organizations have attempted to develop standards. The latest efforts by the American Academy of Sleep Medicine (2005) have attempted to apply evidence-based guidelines to the recommendations. Unfortunately, the lack of prospective studies that allow various definitions to be compared relative to predictive ability have limited these initiatives, resulting in some recommendations reflecting consensus or expert opinion that may change as further research is developed.

et al., 2000). Both the Wisconsin Sleep Cohort study and the Sleep Heart Health Study showed dose-response relationships. The Sleep Heart Health Study is a community-based multicenter study of more than 6,000 middle-aged and older adults whose apnea-hypopnea index was measured by polysomnography. The likelihood of hypertension was greater at higher apnea-hypopnea index levels. Case-control studies reveal that approximately 30 percent of patients diagnosed with essential hypertension (hypertension in which the underlying cause cannot be determined) turn out to have sleep apnea (Partinen and Hublin, 2005). Further, evidence from pediatric studies indicate elevations in systemic blood pressure during both wakefulness and sleep in children with sleep apnea (Amin et al., 2004), with additional evidence of left ventricular wall changes by echocardiography.

The causal nature of the relationship between OSA and hypertension is reinforced by randomized controlled clinical trials showing that the most effective treatment for OSA, continuous positive airway pressure (CPAP) therapy, can reduce blood pressure levels. Although findings have been mixed in other studies, a critical review article that evaluated each study's methodology and results concluded that the trials show convincing decreases in blood pressure in those patients with severe OSA. The benefit is greatest in patients with severe OSA, determined by objective (polysomnography) and subjective (daytime sleepiness) criteria. The review also concluded that there was a lack of benefit in patients who had no daytime sleepiness (Robinson et al., 2004b). However, each of these studies was relatively small (less than 150 individuals), and findings can be considered only tentative.

How does OSA cause sustained hypertension? During the night, the apneas and hypopneas of OSA cause a transient rise in blood pressure (30 mm Hg or more) and increased activity of the sympathetic nervous system (Figure 3-5). Over time, the transient changes become more sustained and are detectable during the daytime, including evidence of sympathetic overactivity (Narkiewicz and Somers, 2003). Studies have found that people with OSA (versus those with similar blood pressure, but no OSA) have faster heart rates, blunted heart rate variability, and increased blood pressure variability—all of which are markers of heightened cardiovascular risk (Caples et al., 2005). The precise pathophysiological steps from transient vascular changes to systemic hypertension are far from clear but may involve oxidative stress, upregulation of vasoactive substances (Caples et al., 2005), and endothelial dysfunction (Faulx et al., 2004; Nieto et al., 2004; Young and Javaheri, 2005).

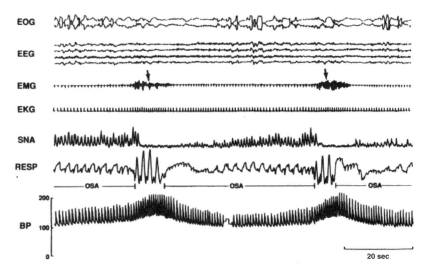

FIGURE 3-5 REM sleep recordings for an individual with OSA. NOTE: During even the lowest phase, blood pressure during REM was higher than in the awake state. Electrooculogram (EOG), electroencephalogram (EEG), electromyogram (EMG), electrocardiogram (EKG), sympathetic nerve activity (SNA), respiration (RESP), blood pressure (BP). SOURCE: Somers et al. (1995).

Obstructive Sleep Apnea Is Associated with Cardiovascular Disease and Stroke

Epidemiological studies reveal an association between OSA and cardiovascular disease, including arrhythmias (Guilleminault et al., 1983); coronary artery disease (Andreas et al., 1996) and specifically, myocardial infarction (Hung et al., 1990; D'Alessandro et al., 1990; Mooe et al., 1996a,b; Marin et al., 2005); and congestive heart failure (Javaheri et al., 1998). Most case-control studies detecting a relationship with myocardial infarction found adjusted odds ratios of around 4 (Young et al., 2002a,b). The large, cross-sectional Sleep Heart Health Study of nearly 6,500 (Shahar et al., 2001) found that participants in the highest apnea-hypopnea index quartile (index greater than 11) were 42 percent more likely to self-report cardiovascular disease (coronary heart disease, heart failure, or stroke) than those in the lowest quartile (adjusted OR = 1.42, 95% CI, 1.13–1.78). The adjusted OR for stroke was 1.58 (95% CI, 1.02–2.46). A higher probability of stroke associated with OSA is also supported by other studies (Bassetti and Aldrich, 1999; Parra et al., 2000; Yaggi et al., 2005; Bradley et al., 2005). In the Sleep Heart Health Study, apnea-hypopnea index was determined by polysomnography, and adjustments were made for a variety of confounding factors, including hypertension. That the hypertension adjustment did not eliminate the effect suggests that hypertension is not the exclusive means by which OSA may lead to cardiovascular disease. A limitation of cross-sectional and case-control analyses is that cause and effect cannot be determined: heart disease may have resulted in OSA or vice versa. However, an observational cohort study of 1,022 individuals, where 68 percent of individuals had OSA (apnea-hypopnea index of 5 or higher), showed that OSA syndrome significantly increased the risk of stroke or death from any cause, and the increase is independent of other risk factors, including hypertension (Yaggi et al., 2005). Other studies have confirmed the risk of OSA syndrome with stroke or death from any cause (Ayas et al., 2003; Gami et al., 2005). Furthermore, other large prospective studies also have shown an association between snoring—a marker for OSA—and incidence of cardiovascular diseases (Jennum et al., 1995; Hu et al., 2000), providing temporal associations in support of OSA playing a causal role in the development of heart diseases. As will be discussed in the next section, OSA is associated with glucose intolerance and diabetes, both of which are independent risk factors for cardiovascular disease.

Studies of the benefits of CPAP further support an association between cardiovascular disease and OSA. Marin and colleagues (2005), in a large, observational study of 10 years' duration, found that patients with untreated severe OSA (apnea-hypopnea index greater than 30), relative to those receiving CPAP treatment, with similar apnea-hypopnea index severity, had a higher incidence of fatal and nonfatal cardiovascular events. The events included myocardial infarction, stroke, and coronary artery bypass surgery. The untreated patients had refused CPAP but were followed regularly. A second study found an increased mortality rate from cardiovascular disease in individuals who did not maintain CPAP treatment over a 5-year follow-up period (Doherty et al., 2005). However, the number of new cases of cardiovascular disease was independent of CPAP treatment compliance. Although observational evidence of this type is not conclusive proof, because it may be subject to confounding by indication and other biases, it still lends weight to the strength of the association.

Most studies finding elevated cardiovascular disease risk have been conducted in adults. Whether or not children with sleep-disordered breathing are at risk for cardiovascular effects is not known. Children with OSA, as noted previously, do experience changes in blood pressure profiles, heart rate variability, and ventricular wall changes as measured by echocardiography (Marcus et al., 1998; Amin et al., 2005). The paucity of longitudinal data on OSA in children, in whom levels of OSA may vary during growth and development and in whom responses to therapies such as tonsillectomy may be variable (Morton et al., 2001), limits the ability to speculate on the long-term cardiovascular effects of untreated sleep-disordered breathing in children. Nonetheless, evidence that as many as 20 to 25 percent of children may have persistent OSA even after tonsillectomy underscores the potential importance of OSA as an early childhood risk factor for later cardiovascular diseases (Amin et al., 2005; Larkin et al., 2005).

Obstructive Sleep Apnea Is Associated with Impaired Glucose Tolerance and Diabetes

OSA is associated with impaired glucose tolerance and insulin resistance, according data from several studies (Ip et al., 2002; Punjabi et al., 2002), including the Sleep Heart Health Study (Punjabi et al., 2004). Those outcomes were more prevalent in those with the highest apnea-hypopnea index. The study also found a relationship between sleep-related hypoxemia and glucose intolerance, which has implications for understanding mechanisms behind the OSA-glucose intolerance link (see below). The Sleep Heart Health Study, as noted earlier, was a large, cross-sectional, community-based study that used polysomnography to identify OSA. The analyses adjusted for obesity (BMI and waist circumference), self-reported sleep duration, and other confounding factors. The findings suggest that OSA contributes to the onset of diabetes through the development of glucose intolerance and insulin resistance, which are established pathophysiological processes in diabetes (Martin et al., 1992).

Of studies that have examined diabetes as an outcome measure, the largest was the prospective Nurses' Health Study. The study found that, after 10 years of follow-up, occasional snoring (versus nonsnoring) was associated with an elevated risk of new onset diabetes in women, and the risk was even greater for regular snoring (Al-Delaimy et al., 2002). Regular or habitual snoring is an indicator of OSA.

The relationship between OSA and metabolic changes that may lead to diabetes is reinforced by studies of the benefits of CPAP. CPAP alleviates glucose intolerance in the short term and long term (Brooks et al., 1994; Harsch et al., 2004). In a separate study of people with type 2 diabetes as well as OSA, CPAP improved glycemic control (Babu et al., 2005). Recent data also indicate that diabetics with OSA have poorer control of glucose levels, with improvement following treatment of OSA with CPAP (Babu et al., 2005).

The mechanisms by which OSA disrupts glucose metabolism are not established. Drawing on human studies and animal models, the biochemical cascade begins with intermittent hypoxia and recurrent sleep arousals (sleep fragmentation). These events stimulate the sympathetic nervous system, hypothalamic-pituitary-adrenal axis, and adipocytes (Punjabi and Beamer, 2005). Their activation, in turn, leads to release of catecholamines, cortisol, and inflammatory cytokines and other vasoactive intermediates, which may mediate the development of glucose intolerance, insulin resistance, and, ultimately, type 2 diabetes. Because diabetes is also a risk factor for cardiovascular disease, the interrelationships may partly explain why OSA predisposes to cardiovascular disease (Punjabi and Beamer, 2005).

Obstructive Sleep Apnea May Contribute to Obesity

Up to 40 percent of people who are morbidly obese have OSA (Vgontzas et al., 1994). This finding may reflect the role of obesity as a well-established risk factor for the development of OSA. It may also reflect obesity as a *consequence* of OSA, although the evidence is not yet conclusive (Grunstein, 2005b). Patients with newly diagnosed OSA, compared with controls matched for BMI and percent body fat, show recent weight gain (Phillips et al., 1999). Data from the Wisconsin Sleep Cohort also show that individuals with OSA have reduced levels of physical activity; OSA-related sleepiness may contribute to changes in activity and energy expenditure, and thus contribute to weight gain. OSA-related hormonal changes may also contribute to obesity. In general, patients with OSA have higher levels of leptin, the appetite-suppressing hormone (Phillips et al., 2000; Palmer et al., 2004; Patel et al., 2004) than controls. However, their morning levels are relatively lower than evening levels (Patel et al., 2004). Thus, either via leptin resistance (where high levels of leptin are present, but tissues are poorly responsive to leptin's action) or because of disturbances in diurnal variability in leptin, individuals with OSA may be predisposed to lower effective levels of appetite suppressing hormones. Although CPAP reduces leptin levels, it is not known whether such effects relate to differences in the effectiveness of leptin's actions (Chin et al., 2003). Furthermore, obesity also affects the severity of OSA. Significant weight loss in adolescents who underwent gastric bypass surgery (mean, 58 kg) was associated with a dramatic reduction of OSA severity (Kalra et al., 2005).

Etiology and Risk Factors

In simplest terms, OSA is caused by narrowing or collapse of the airway as a result of anatomical and physiological abnormalities in pharyngeal structures. Apnea episodes cause hypoxemia (insufficient oxygen in the blood) and hypercapnia (high concentration of blood carbon dioxide). The episodes also increase the output of the sympathetic nervous system (Narkiewicz and Somers, 2003), the effect of which is to restore pharyngeal muscle tone and reopen the airway. Although increased sympathetic activity is beneficial for restoring normal breathing and oxygen intake over the short term, it has long-term deleterious effects on vascular tone and blood pressure, among other effects (Caples et al., 2005). These early events—which are mediated by a variety of chemoreceptors in the carotid body and brainstem—trigger pathophysiological changes that occur not only during the obstructive apneas, but also extend into wakeful states during the day. For example, during daytime wakefulness, people with OSA have higher sympathetic activity (Somers, et al., 1995) and heightened chemoreflex sensitivity, which in turn generates an increased ventilatory response (Narkiewicz et al., 1999). The full pathophysiology of OSA remains somewhat elusive, although research is piecing together the relationships between OSA and a range of the previously described long-term health effects. The etiology of central sleep apnea, although also not well understood, is hypothesized to result from instability of respiratory control centers (White, 2005).

There are a number of risk factors for OSA, including:

• Obesity, male gender, and increasing age (Table 3-1) (Young et al., 1993). It is unclear how incidence changes with older age; some data suggest that snoring and OSA may decline after age 65 years (Young et al., 1993); however, other studies show very high prevalence rates of OSA in elderly individuals (Bliwise et al., 1988; Ancoli-Israel et al., 1993; Foley et al., 2003). The pathophysiological roles of these risk factors are not well understood, although evidence suggests that fat deposition in the upper airways, which is more likely in males, contributes to the physical narrow-

TABLE 3-1 Risk Factors for Obstructive Sleep Apnea

Risk Factor	Reference
Obesity and BMI greater than 25 kg/m^2	Grunstein et al., 1993
Male gender	Strohl and Redline, 1996; Kapsimalis and Kryger, 2002; Shepertycky et al., 2005
Familial association	Guilleminault et al., 1995; Pillar and Lavie, 1995; Redline et al., 1995; Buxbaum et al., 2002
Alcohol consumption	Taasan et al., 1981
Cranial facial structure High and narrow hard palate, elongated soft palate, small chin, and abnormal overjet	Ferguson et al., 1995
Enlargement of the tonsils	Behlfelt, 1990
Lesions of the autonomic nervous system	Mondini and Guilleminault, 1985; Rosen et al., 2003
Race: African Americans, Mexican Americans, Pacific Islanders, and East Asians	Schmidt-Nowara et al., 1990; Redline et al., 1997; Li et al., 2000

ing that causes OSA (Robinson et al., 2004a). Menopause also increases the risk of OSA (Bixler et al., 2001; Young et al., 2003), possibly through lower levels of progestational hormones that influence the respiratory system through changes in body fat distribution (Vgontzas and Kales, 1999). However, recent studies suggest that there may be a referral bias that results in a lower apparent rate of sleep apnea in females than in males (Kapsimalis and Kryger, 2002; Shepertycky et al., 2005). Epidemiological evidence suggests that hormone replacement therapy lessens the risk of OSA (Shahar et al., 2003). In children, the main risk factor for OSA is tonsillar hypertrophy, although OSA may also occur in children with congenital and neuromuscular disorders and in children who were born prematurely (Rosen et al., 2003). Asthma, a common childhood respiratory illness, is also associated with OSA in children (Sulit et al., 2005).

- In adolescents, risk factors may be more similar to those seen in adults and include obesity (Redline et al., 1999). Being a minority is a risk factor for both increased prevalence and severity of sleep-disordered breathing in both children and adults (Rosen et al., 1992; Ancoli-Israel et al., 1995; Rosen et al., 2003). The prevalence of sleep-disordered breathing in the United States is approximately three times higher in middle-aged members of minority groups compared to non-Hispanic whites (Kripke et al., 1997). African American children are at increased risk, even after adjusting for obesity or respiratory problems (Redline et al., 1999; Rosen et al., 2003). Familial and probably genetic factors strongly contribute to OSA (Buxbaum et al., 2002; Palmer LJ et al., 2003; Palmer et al., 2004).

- Patients with cardiovascular disease and diabetes are also at higher risk for developing both OSA and central sleep apnea (Sin et al., 1999).

- Patients with impaired baroreflexes (e.g., patients with hypertension or heart failure and premature infants) may be especially susceptible to excessive autonomic responses to chemoreflex stimulation during periods of apnea. In these patient groups, bradyarrhythmias, hypoxia, hypoperfusion, and sympathetic activation during apnea may predispose to sudden death (Somers et al., 1988; 1992).

Sleep-Disordered Breathing May Affect Mortality

Limited evidence suggests that sleep-disordered breathing may affect an individual's mortality (Young et al., 2002a,b; Lavie et al., 2005). Studies of patients at sleep clinics tend to show an association between sleep apnea and mortality (He et al., 1988), but several well-designed, population-based studies failed to find an association (Ancoli-Israel et al., 1996; Lindberg et al., 1998; Kripke et al., 2002), except in one subgroup of patients below age 60 with both snoring and excessive daytime sleepiness. The subgroup experienced twice the risk of mortality (Lindberg et al., 1998). A recent observational study of a large cohort of sleep apnea patients (n = 403), snorers, and healthy controls who had been followed for an average of 10 years, found a threefold higher risk of fatal cardiovascular events with severe OSA (Marin et al., 2005). An observational follow-up study of the long-term effects of CPAP therapy on mortality found that compared to individuals that began receiving CPAP therapy for at least 5 years (n = 107), individuals that were untreated with CPAP (n = 61) were more likely to die from cardiovascular disease (14.8 percent versus 1.9 percent, log rank test, P = .009) (Yaggi et al., 2005; Doherty et al., 2005).

Treatment

In adults, OSA is most effectively treated with CPAP and weight loss (Strollo et al., 2005; Grunstein, 2005a). Evidence of CPAP's efficacy for alleviating daytime sleepiness comes from randomized controlled trials and meta-analysis (Patel et al., 2003). The problem is that many patients are noncompliant with CPAP (see Chapter 6). Other options, although less effective, include a variety of dental appliances (Ferguson and Lowe, 2005) or surgery (e.g., uvulopalatopharyngoplasty) (Powell et al., 2005). In children, the first-line treatment for most cases of OSA is adenotonsillectomy, according to clinical practice guidelines developed by the American Academy of Pediatrics (Marcus et al., 2002). Children who are not good candidates for this procedure can benefit from CPAP. Central apnea treatment is tailored to the cause of the ventilatory instability. Commonly used treatments include oxygen, CPAP, and acetazolamide, a drug that acts as a respiratory stimulant (White, 2005).

INSOMNIA

Manifestations and Prevalence

Insomnia is the most commonly reported sleep problem (Ohayon, 2002). It is a highly prevalent disorder that often goes unrecognized and untreated despite its adverse impact on health and quality of life (Benca, 2005a) (see also Chapter 4). Insomnia is defined by having difficulty falling asleep, maintaining sleep, or by short sleep duration, despite adequate opportunity for a full night's sleep. Other insomnia symptoms include daytime consequences, such as tiredness, lack of energy, difficulty concentrating, and/or irritability (Simon and VonKorff, 1997). The diagnostic criteria for primary insomnia include:

• Difficulty initiating or maintaining sleep or nonrestorative sleep.

• Causing clinically significant distress or impairment in social, occupational, or other important areas of functioning.
• Not occurring exclusively during the course of another sleep disorder.
• Not due to the direct physiological effects of a substance or a medical condition (APA, 1994).

Insomnia symptoms are remarkably common, affecting at least 10 percent of adults in the United States (Ford and Kamerow, 1989; Ohayon et al., 1997; Simon and VonKorff, 1997; Roth and Ancoli-Israel, 1999). Prevalence is higher among women and older individuals (Mellinger et al., 1985; Ford and Kamerow, 1989; Foley et al., 1995). Severe insomnia tends to be chronic, with about 85 percent of patients continuing to report the same symptoms and impairment months or years after diagnosis (Hohagen et al., 1993; Katz and McHorney, 1998). The comorbidity of sleep disorders with psychiatric disorders is covered later in this chapter.

Etiology and Risk Factors

The precise causes of insomnia are poorly understood but, in general terms, involve a combination of biological, psychological, and social factors. Insomnia is conceptualized as a state of hyperarousal (Perlis et al., 2005). Stress is thought to play a leading role in activating the hypothalamic-pituitary axis and setting the stage for chronic insomnia. A key study showed that adults with insomnia, compared with normal sleepers, have higher levels, over a 24-hr period, of cortisol and adrenocorticotropic hormone (ACTH), which are hormones released by the hypothalamic-pituitary-adrenal axis after stress exposure (Vgontzas et al., 2001). The 24-hour pattern of cortisol and ACTH secretion is different, however, from that in individuals who are chronically stressed. Cognitive factors, such as worry, rumination, and fear of sleeplessness, perpetuate the problem through behavioral conditioning. Other perpetuating factors include light exposure and unstable sleep schedules (Partinen and Hublin, 2005).

Insomnia patients often attribute their difficulty sleeping to an overactive brain. Several lines of evidence, from preclinical to sleep neuroimaging studies in insomnia patients, suggest that there are multiple neural systems arranged hierarchically in the central nervous system that contribute to arousal as well as insomnia complaints. Disturbances in these systems may differ according to the nature of insomnia. Structures that regulate sleep and wakefulness, for example the brainstem, hypothalamus and basal forebrain, are abnormally overactive during sleep in primary insomnia patients (Nofzinger et al., 2004b). In addition, limbic and paralimbic structures that regulate basic emotions and instinctual behaviors such as the amygdala, hippocampus, ventromedial prefrontal cortex and anterior cingulate cortex have been shown to be abnormally active during sleep in individuals with primary insomnia and secondary insomnias related to depression (Nofzinger et al., 2004a, 2005). Abnormal activity in neocortical structures that control executive function and are responsible for modulating behavior related to basic arousal and emotions has been observed in individuals with insomnias associated with depression (Nofzinger et al., 2004a, 2005).

The two main risk factors of insomnia are older age and female gender (Edinger and Means, 2005). One large, population-based study found that insomnia was nearly twice as common in women than men, although reporting bias cannot be ruled out as a contributing factor (Ford and Kamerow, 1989). The reason behind the apparent higher prevalence in women is not understood. Other risk factors for insomnia include family history of insomnia (Dauvilliers et al., 2005), stressful life styles, medical and psychiatric disorders, and shift work (Edinger and Means, 2005). Although adolescent age is not viewed a risk factor, insomnia has rarely been studied in this age group.

Treatment

Insomnia is treatable with a variety of behavioral and pharmacological therapies, which may be used alone or in combination. While the therapies currently available to treat insomnia may provide benefit, the 2005 NIH State of the Science Conference on the Manifestations and Management of Chronic Insomnia concluded that more research and randomized clinical trials are needed to further verify their efficacy, particularly for long-term illness management and prevention of complications like depression (NIH, 2005). Behavioral therapies appear as effective as pharmacological therapies (Smith et al., 2002), and they may have more enduring effects after cessation (McClusky et al., 1991; Hauri, 1997). Behavioral therapies, according to a task force review of 48 clinical trials, benefit about 70 to 80 percent of patients for at least 6 months after completion of treatment (Morin et al., 1999; Morin, 2005). The therapies are of several main types (Table 3-2). The major problem with current behavioral therapies is not their efficacy; rather it is lack of clinician awareness of their efficacy and lack of providers sufficiently trained and skilled in their use. Other problems are their cost and patient adherence (Benca, 2005a). A specific strategy to improve an individual's sleep quality is by promoting proper sleep hygiene (Kleitman, 1987; Harvey, 2000).

The most efficacious pharmacological therapies for insomnia are hypnotic agents of two general types, benzodiazepine or nonbenzodiazepine hypnotics (Nowell et al., 1997). Nonbenzodiazepine hypnotics are advantageous because they generally have shorter half-lives, thus producing fewer impairments the next day, but the trade-off is that they may not be as effective at

TABLE 3-2 Psychological and Behavioral Treatments for Insomnia

Therapy	Description
Stimulus control therapy	A set of instructions designed to reassociate the bed/bedroom with sleep and to reestablish a consistent sleep-wake schedule: Go to bed only when sleepy; get out of bed when unable to sleep; use the bed/bedroom for sleep only (e.g., no reading, watching TV); arise at the same time every morning; no napping.
Sleep restriction therapy	A method to curtail time in bed to the actual sleep time, thereby creating mild sleep deprivation, which results in more consolidated and more efficient sleep.
Relaxation training	Clinical procedures aimed at reducing somatic tension (e.g., progressive muscle relaxation, autogenic training) or intrusive thoughts (e.g., imagery training, meditation) interfering with sleep.
Cognitive therapy	Psychotherapeutic method aimed at changing faulty beliefs and attitudes about sleep, insomnia, and the next-day consequences. Other cognitive strategies are used to control intrusive thoughts at bedtime and prevent excessive monitoring of the daytime consequences of insomnia.
Sleep hygiene education	General guidelines about health practices (e.g., diet, exercise, substance use) and environmental factors (e.g., light, noise, temperature) that may promote or interfere with sleep.

SOURCE: Morin (2005).

maintaining sleep throughout the night (Morin, 2005; Benca, 2005a). It is still unclear whether hypnotics lead to dependence. It is suggested that they should not be taken for more than 10 days in a row; however, recent studies suggest that hypnotics do not always lead to dependence (Hajak et al., 2003; Walsh et al., 2005; Benca, 2005a). There have been no large-scale trials examining the safety and efficacy of hypnotics in children and adolescents. Other pharmacological classes used for insomnia include sedating antidepressants, antihistamines, and antipsychotics, but their efficacy and safety for treating insomnia have not been thoroughly studied (Walsh et al., 2005).

SLEEP AND PSYCHIATRIC DISORDERS

Manifestations and Prevalence

Sleep disturbances are common features of psychiatric disorders. The most frequent types of sleep disturbances are insomnia, excessive daytime sleepiness (hypersomnia), and parasomnia. Sleep disturbances are so commonly seen as symptoms of certain psychiatric disorders that they are listed as diagnostic criteria under DSM-IV (APA, 1994). For example, insomnia is a symptom used with others to diagnose major depression. The comorbidity, or coexistence, of a full-blown sleep disorder (particularly insomnia and hypersomnia) with a psychiatric disorder is also common. Forty percent of those diagnosed with insomnia, in a population-based study, also have a psychiatric disorder (Ford and Kamerow, 1989). Among those diagnosed with hypersomnia, the prevalence of a psychiatric disorder is somewhat higher—46.5 percent.

The reasons behind the comorbidity of sleep and psychiatric disorders are not well understood. Comorbidity might be due to one disorder being a risk factor or cause of the other; they might both be manifestations of the same or overlapping physiological disturbance; one might be a consequence of the other. In some cases, the sleep disturbance can be both cause and consequence. In generalized anxiety disorder, for example, the symptoms of fatigue and irritability used to diagnose it are often the result of a sleep disturbance, which itself is also a diagnostic symptom.

Adolescents with major depressive disorders report higher rates of sleep problems and, conversely, those with sleep difficulties report increased negative mood or mood regulation (Ryan et al., 1987). In addition, sleep-onset abnormalities during adolescence have been associated with an increased risk of depression in later life (Rao et al., 1996).

The best studied and most prevalent comorbidity is insomnia with major depression. Insomnia as a symptom of depression is highly common. On the basis of longitudinal studies, insomnia is now established as a risk factor for major depression. Not all people with insomnia have a depression diagnosis; however, studies have found that 15 to 20 percent of people diagnosed with insomnia have major depression (Ford and Kamerow, 1989; Breslau et al., 1996).

Depressed individuals have certain abnormalities detected by polysomnography. One is shorter rapid eye movement (REM) latency (a shorter period of time elapsing from onset of sleep to onset of REM sleep), an effect that persists even after treatment for depression. Other abnormalities include shortened initial REM period, increased REM density, and slow-wave deficits (Benca, 2005a). Shorter REM latency and slow-wave sleep (SWS) deficits tend to run in families; these abnormalities are also found in first-degree relatives of people with major depression, but who are unaffected by depression (Giles et al., 1998). A variety of polysomnographic abnormalities have been found with other psychiatric disorders (Benca, 2005a).

Etiology and Risk Factors

The etiological basis for the comorbidity of sleep disorders and psychiatric disorders is not well understood. Most potential mechanisms for sleep changes in psychiatric disorders deal specifically with insomnia and depression. Possible mechanisms include neurotransmitter imbalance (cholinergic-aminergic imbalance), circadian phase advance, and hypothalamic-pituitary-adrenal axis dysregulation (Benca, 2005a). Recent evidence implicating regions of the frontal lobe has emerged from imaging studies using positron emission tomography. As they progress from waking to non-REM (NREM) sleep, depressed subjects have smaller decreases in relative metabolism in regions of the frontal, parietal, and temporal cortex when compared to individuals who are healthy (Nofzinger et al., 2005). Normally, the transition from waking to NREM sleep is associated with decreases in these frontal lobe regions. What appears to occur with depression is that the decrease is less pronounced. Another finding of the study is that during both waking and NREM sleep, depressed patients show hypermetabolism in the brain's emotional pathways, including the amygdala, anterior cingulate cortex, and related structures. Because the amygdala also plays a role in sleep regulation (Jones, 2005), this finding suggests that sleep and mood disorders may be manifestations of dysregulation in overlapping neurocircuits. The authors hypothesize that increased metabolism in emotional pathways with depression may increase emotional arousal and thereby adversely affect sleep (Nofzinger et al., 2005).

Treatment

Comorbid psychiatric and sleep disorders are treated by a combination of medication and/or psychotherapy (Krahn, 2005; Benca, 2005a). A major problem is underdiagnosis and undertreatment of one or both of the comorbid disorders. One of the disorders may be missed or may be mistakenly dismissed as a condition that will recede once the other is treated. In the case of depression, for example, sleep abnormalities may continue once the depression episode has remitted (Fava, 2004). If untreated, residual insomnia is a risk factor for depression recurrence (Reynolds et al., 1997; Ohayon and Roth, 2003). Further, because sleep and psychiatric disorders, by themselves, are disabling, the treatment of the comorbidity may reduce needless disability. Insomnia, for example, worsens outcomes in depression, schizophrenia, and alcohol dependence. Treatment of both conditions can improve a patient's functioning and possibly improve adherence with therapy (Vincent and Hameed, 2003). Another concern is that medication for one disorder might exacerbate the other (e.g., prescription of sedating antidepressants for patients with hypersomnolence). The choice of medication for psychiatric disorder (or vice versa) should be influenced by the nature of the sleep complaint (e.g., more sedating antidepressant taken at night for insomnia; more alerting antidepressant for excessive daytime sleepiness).

Insomnia and Psychiatric Disorders

As mentioned above insomnia is associated with depression, acting as both a risk factor and a manifestation (Ford and Kamerow, 1989; Livingston et al., 1993; Breslau et al., 1996; Weissman et al., 1997; Chang et al., 1997; Ohayon and Roth, 2003; Cole and Dendukuri, 2003). Several studies done were longitudinal in design, including one that tracked more than 1,000 male physicians for 40 years (Chang et al., 1997). Another study, which followed 1,007 young adults at a health maintenance organization for 3.5 years, found that a history of insomnia at baseline not only predicted new onset depression, but also other psychiatric disorders (any anxiety disorder, alcohol abuse, drug abuse, and nicotine dependence) (Breslau et al., 1996) (Figure 3-6). The adjusted odds of developing a psychiatric disorder were highest for depression (OR = 3.95; 95% CI, 2.2–7.0). This figure is based on 16 percent of the sample who developed depression with a history of insomnia at baseline, as compared with 4.6 percent who developed depression without a history of insomnia. The study's general findings

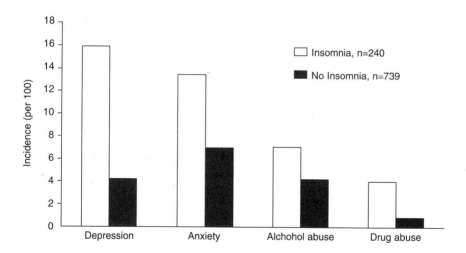

FIGURE 3-6 Incidence of psychiatric disorders during 3.5 years of follow-up of patients with a prior history of insomnia.
SOURCE: Breslau et al. (1996).

are supported by another large study of 10,000 adults by Weissman and colleagues (1997). That study found insomnia to have increased the risk of major depression by a similar magnitude (fivefold) and to have increased the risk of panic disorder (one of the anxiety disorders) even more strikingly, by 20-fold (OR = 20.3, 95% CI, 4.4–93.8). Insomnia is also a predictor of acute suicide among patients with mood disorders (Fawcett et al., 1990).

The striking association between insomnia and depression in so many studies suggests that insomnia is also an early marker for the onset of depression, and the two may be linked by a common pathophysiology. Although the pathophysiological relationship is not known, researchers are focusing on overlapping neural pathways for anxiety, arousal, and/or circadian disturbance (Benca, 2005b). One hypothesis is that common pathways are the amygdala and other limbic structures of the brain (Nofzinger et al., 2005). Another hypothesis is that chronic insomnia increases activity of the hypothalamic-pituitary-adrenal axis, which in turn contributes to depression (Perlis et al., 2005). The close association of insomnia and depression also raises the tantalizing possibility that treating insomnia may prevent some cases of depression (Riemann and Voderholzer, 2003), but limited data are available. The biological basis for the relationship between insomnia and new onset psychiatric disorders (other than depression) is also not known.

NARCOLEPSY AND HYPERSOMNIA

Manifestations and Prevalence

Narcolepsy and idiopathic hypersomnia are characterized by a clinically significant complaint of excessive daytime sleepiness that is neither explained by a circadian sleep disorder, sleep-disordered breathing, or sleep deprivation, nor is it caused by a medical condition disturbing sleep (AASM, 2005). The diagnosis of narcolepsy and hypersomnia is based principally on the Multiple Sleep Latency Test (MSLT), which objectively quantifies daytime sleepiness (Box 3-2) (Carskadon et al., 1986; Arand et al., 2005). Sleep logs or actigraphy (a movement detector coupled with software that uses movement patterns to provide estimate sleep and wake times) can also be used to exclude chronic sleep deprivation as a diagnosis prior to the MSLT. In many cases narcolepsy arises during the mid to late teenage years; however, frequently initial diagnosis is not correct, resulting in delays in diagnosis of 15 to 25 years after the onset of symptoms (Broughton et al., 1997). Onset of narcolepsy can also have a negative impact on school performance (see Chapter 4). Narcolepsy is associated with a number of symptoms (Anic-Labat et al., 1999; Overeem et al., 2002), including the following:

• Excessive daytime sleepiness, defined as a background of constant sleepiness with sleep attacks leading to unintended napping during the day. In most cases, naps are refreshing, but the rested feeling only lasts a short time. When severe, sleepiness can manifest as automatic behavior, a continuation of activities in a semiautomatic manner when sleepy, with no subsequent memory.

• Cataplexy, which are sudden and brief bilateral episodes of muscle weakness triggered by a strong emotional stimulus, such as laughing.

BOX 3-2
Clinical Laboratory Findings in Narcolepsy and Hypersomnia

The Multiple Sleep Latency Test (MSLT) objectively quantifies daytime sleepiness. It consists of five 20 minute daytime naps at 2-hour intervals. The amount of time it takes to fall asleep (sleep latency) and the occurrence of rapid eye movement (REM) sleep is recorded. Mean sleep latency of less than 8 minutes and two or more sleep onset rhythmic eye movement periods is diagnostic for narcolepsy. The MSLT must always be preceded by nocturnal sleep polysomnography to rule out other causes of short MSL or sleep onset rhythmic eye movement periods such as OSA, insufficient sleep, or delayed sleep phase syndrome. At least 6 hours of sleep must have occurred prior to the MSLT. Sleep logs or actigraphy for the preceding 2 weeks can be helpful to exclude chronic sleep deprivation. It must also be conducted after withdrawal of psychotropic medications (generally more than 2 weeks). Antidepressants, most notably, suppress REM sleep and/or may create REM rebound if stopped too recently prior to testing.

HLA-DQB1*0602 is the human leukocyte antigen DQB1 subtype associated with narcolepsy. Almost all cases with cataplexy are DQB1*0602 positive; approximately 40 percent of narcolepsy cases without cataplexy are HLA-DQB*0602 positive. The test is not highly predictive of narcolepsy, however, as 25 percent of the population is HLA-DQB1*0602 positive. Idiopathic and recurrent hypersomnia cases are not strongly associated with human leukocyte antigen.

Cerebrospinal fluid (CSF) hypocretin-1, also called orexin-A, is a neuropeptide involved in the cause of narcolepsy and cataplexy. It can be measured in the CSF, and this has been used to diagnose narcolepsy. Most cases with cataplexy (and HLA-DQB1*0602) have CSF hypocretin-1 levels below 30 percent of normal control value. This finding is very specific and sensitive for narcolepsy and cataplexy. Low CSF hypocretin is also diagnostic of narcolepsy without cataplexy, but is found in only a small portion of these cases (7 to 40 percent).

- Sleep paralysis, or muscle paralysis akin to REM sleep atonia while awake, when falling asleep, or waking up.
- Hypnagogic/hypnopompic hallucinations, which are dreamlike REM sleep experiences, often frightening, that occur when falling asleep or waking up.
- Insomnia, typically difficulty maintaining sleep.
- Autonomic behavior, or continue to function (talking, putting things away, etc.) during sleep episodes but awakens with no memory of performing such activities.
- REM behavior disorder, characterized by excessive motor activity during REM sleep (Anic-Labat et al., 1999; Overeem et al., 2002).

Narcolepsy can be diagnosed clinically, by using the MSLT, or by measuring cerebrospinal fluid (CSF) hypocretin-1 (Box 3-2).

Idiopathic hypersomnia is classically separated into two subtypes. The first, idiopathic hypersomnia with prolonged sleep time, is a rare disorder and is characterized by the following:

- Excessive daytime sleepiness occurs, as described above for narcolepsy, but in the typical form naps are unrefreshing.
- Excessive amounts of daily sleep, typically defined as more than 10 hours of sleep per day, as documented for long periods of time using daily logs and sleep studies.
- Sleep drunkenness (sometimes referred to as sleep inertia)—difficulty waking up and individual is foggy for long periods of time after wake onset.

The second subtype of idiopathic hypersomnia, idiopathic hypersomnia without long sleep time, is characterized by a complaint of excessive daytime sleepiness and a short mean sleep latency on the MSLT.

In most sleep disorders clinics with experience in this area, approximately one-third of hypersomnia cases are diagnosed with this condition (Aldrich, 1996). The prevalence is estimated to be around 0.01 percent. In contrast, the prevalence of idiopathic hypersomnia without prolonged sleep time may be more substantial, as most patients are likely not diagnosed (Arand et al., 2005).

Recurrent hypersomnia is periodic either in synchrony with menstruation (menstruation-linked periodic hypersomnia) or without any association and mostly in males with Klein-Levin syndrome (Billiard and Cadilhac, 1988; Arnulf et al., 2005a). Klein-Levin syndrome is characterized by recurrent episodes of dramatic hypersomnia lasting from 2 days to several weeks. These episodes are associated with behavioral and cognitive abnormalities, binge eating or hypersexuality, and alternate with long asymptomatic periods that last months or years (Arnulf et al., 2005a).

Narcolepsy and hypersomnia can affect children, adolescents, adults, and older persons. In most cases these disorders begin in adolescence. The prevalence of narcolepsy with definite cataplexy has been documented in adults by numerous population-based studies and occurs in 0.02 to 0.05 percent of the population of Western Europe and North America (Mignot, 1998). In contrast, very little is known about the prevalence of narcolepsy without cataplexy. Recent studies using the MSLT indicate that approximately 3.9 percent of the general population has MSLT score abnormalities consistent with narcolepsy without cataplexy (Singh et al., 2005).

Secondary cases of narcolepsy or hypersomnia are also common, but the overall prevalence is not known (Table 3-3). These can occur in the context of psychiatric disorders, for example depression; central nervous system tumors, most notably in the hypothalamus; neurodegenerative disorders, such as Parkinson's disease; inflammatory disorders, such as multiple sclerosis or paraneoplastic syndromes; traumatic disorders, such as head trauma; vascular disorders, such as those that are attributed to median thalamic stroke; and genetic disorders, including myotonic dystrophy or Prader-Willi syndrome (Billiard et al., 1994; Mignot et al., 2002a).

Etiology and Risk Factors

Similar to other sleep disorders, little is known about the pathophysiology and risk factors for narcolepsy and hypersomnia. Most of the knowledge in this area pertains to narcolepsy with cataplexy, which affects males and females equally. Symptoms usually arise during adolescence. Many contributing factors influence an individual's susceptibility, including both genetic and environmental factors (Mignot, 1998, 2001).

Virtually all individuals who suffer narcolepsy with cataplexy carry the haplotype HLA-DQB1*0602 and have severe neuronal loss in regions of the brain that are responsible for regulating the sleep-wake cycle. Approximately 70,000 hypothalamic neurons that are responsible for producing the neuropeptide hypocretin (orexin) are lost in individuals with narcolepsy with cataplexy (Thannickal et al., 2000; Peyron et al., 2000). Hypocretin is an excitatory neuropeptide that regulates the activity of other sleep regulatory networks. Consequently, in some cases low levels of hypocretin-1 in the CSF, may be used to diagnose narcolepsy (Kanbayashi et al., 2002; Krahn et al., 2002; Mignot et al., 2002a) (Table 3-3). The cause of hypocretin cell loss is unknown but it may be autoimmune due to the association with the HLA-DQB1*0602 (Juji et al., 1984; Mignot, 2001).

Less is known regarding the pathophysiology of narcolepsy without cataplexy. The etiology is likely heterogeneous. An unknown portion may be caused by partial or complete hypocretin deficiency (Kanbayashi et al., 2002; Krahn et al., 2002; Mignot et al., 2002a). However, it has been

TABLE 3-3 International Classification of Sleep Disorders: Definitions, Prevalence, and Pathophysiology of Narcolepsy and Hypersomnias

Condition	Diagnostic Criteria	North American Prevalence '	Pathophysiology and Etiology
Narcolepsy with cataplexy	Presence of definite cataplexy; usually abnormal MSLT results	0.02–0.18%	Hypocretin deficiency; 90% with low CSF HCRT-1 and positive for HLA-DQB1*0602
Narcolepsy without cataplexy	MSLT: mean sleep latency less than or equal to 8 minutes, 2 or greater SOREMPs; no or doubtful cataplexy	0.02%; many undiagnosed	Unknown, probably heterogeneous; 7–25% with low CSF HCRT-1, 40% HLA-DQB1*0602 positive
Secondary narcolepsy or hypersomnia	As above, but due to other known medical conditions (e.g., neurological)	Unknown	With or without hypocretin deficiency
Idiopathic hypersomnia with prolonged sleep	MSLT: short mean sleep latency, greater than two SOREMPs; long (10 hours or greater) unrefreshing nocturnal sleep	Rare, maybe 0.01–0.02%	Unknown, probable heterogeneous etiology
Idiopathic hypersomnia with normal sleep length	MSLT: short mean sleep latency, less than two SOREMPs; normal nightly sleep amounts (less than 10 hours)	Probably common, unknown prevalence	Unknown, probable heterogeneous etiology
Periodic hypersomnia (includes Kleine-Levin syndrome)	Recurrent (more than 1 time per year) sleepiness (lasting 2 to 28 days), normal function between occurrences	Rare, probably less than one per one million people	Unknown, probable heterogeneous etiology

NOTE: CSF, lumbar sac cerebrospinal fluid; HCRT, hypocretin; HLA, human leukocyte antigen; MSLT, Multiple Sleep Latency Test; SOREMP, sleep-onset REM period.
SOURCE: AASM (2005).

hypothesized that some individuals with partial cell loss may have normal CSF hypocretin-1 (Mignot et al., 2002a; Scammell, 2003). The pathophysiology of idiopathic hypersomnia is unknown. When the disorder is associated with prolonged sleep time, it typically starts during adolescence and is lifelong. It is essential to exclude secondary causes, such as head trauma or hypersomnia owing to depression (Roth, 1976; Billiard and Dauvilliers, 2001). Some cases with prolonged sleep times have been reported to be familial, suggesting a genetic origin. Even less is known about idiopathic hypersomnia with normal sleep time. This condition is more variable and symptomatically defined. The cause of Kleine-Levin syndrome is unknown (Arnulf et al., 2005b).

Treatment

Treatment for these conditions is symptomatically based. Even in the case of narcolepsy in which the disorder is caused by hypocretin deficiency, current treatment does not aim at improving the defective neurotransmission (Mignot et al., 1993; Nishino and Mignot, 1997; Wisor et al., 2001). Behavioral measures, such as napping, support groups, and work arrangements are helpful but rarely sufficient. In most cases, pharmacological treatment is needed (Nishino and Mignot, 1997; Lammers and Overeem, 2003). However, as with other pharmaceuticals designed to treat sleep problems, large-scale clinical trails have not examined the efficacy and safety of drugs to treat narcolepsy in children and adolescents.

In narcolepsy with cataplexy, pharmacological treatment for daytime sleepiness involves modafinil or amphetamine-like stimulants, which likely act through increasing dopamine transmission. Cataplexy and abnormal REM sleep symptoms, sleep paralysis and hallucinations, are typically treated with tricyclic antidepressants or serotonin and norepinephrine reuptake inhibitors. Adrenergic reuptake inhibition is believed to be the primary mode of action. Sodium oxybate, or gamma hydroxybutyric acid, is also used at night to consolidate disturbed nocturnal sleep. This treatment is also effective on cataplexy and other symptoms.

The treatment of narcolepsy without cataplexy and idiopathic hypersomnia uses similar compounds, most notably modafinil and amphetamine-like stimulants (Billiard and Dauvilliers, 2001). Treatments, with the possible exception of lithium, of periodic hypersomnia and Kleine-Levin syndrome type are typically ineffective (Arnulf et al., 2005a).

PARASOMNIAS

Manifestations and Prevalence

Parasomnias are unpleasant or undesirable behaviors or experiences that occur during entry into sleep, during sleep, or during arousals from sleep (AASM, 2005). They are categorized as primary parasomnias, which predominantly occur during the sleep state, and secondary parasomnias, which are complications associated with disorders of organ systems that occur during sleep. Primary parasomnias can further be classified depending on which sleep state they originate in, REM sleep, NREM, or others that can occur during either state (Table 3-4).

Parasomnias typically manifest themselves during transition periods from one state of sleep to another, during which time the brain activity is reorganizing (Mahowald and Schenck, 2005). Activities associated with parasomnias are characterized by being potentially violent or injurious, disruptive to other household members, resulting in excessive daytime sleepiness, or associated with medical, psychiatric, or neurological conditions (Mahowald and Ettinger, 1990).

Disorders of Arousal, NREM

Disorders of arousal are the most common type of parasomnia, occurring in as much as 4 percent of the adult population (Ohayon et al., 1999) and up to 17 percent of children (Klackenberg, 1982). Typically the arousals occur during the first 60 to 90 minutes of sleep and do not cause full awakenings, but rather partial arousal from deep NREM sleep. Disorders of arousal manifest in a variety of ways, from barely audible mumbling, disoriented sleepwalking, to frantic bouts of shrieking and flailing of limbs (Wills and Garcia, 2002).

Confusional Arousals

Individuals who experience confusional arousals exhibit confused mental and behavioral activity following arousals from sleep. They are often disoriented in time and space, display slow speech, and blunted answers to questions (AASM, 2005). Episodes of resistive and even violent behavior can last several minutes to hours. Confusional arousals are more than three to four times more prevalent in children compared to individuals 15 years or older (around 3 percent) (Ohayon et al., 2000). They can be precipitated by forced arousals, particularly early in an individual's sleep cycle.

TABLE 3-4 Selected Primary Sleep Parasomnias

Name	Description
Disorders of arousal associated with NREM sleep	
Confusional arousals	Individuals display mental confusion or confusional behavior during or following arousal, typically from SWS
Sleepwalking	Involves a series of behaviors initiated during arousals from SWS that culminate in walking around in an altered state of consciousness
Sleep terrors	Typically initiated by a loud scream associated with panic, followed by intense motor activity, which can result in injury
Disorders associated with REM sleep	
Nightmare disorder	Recurrent nightmares that are coherent dream sequences manifest as disturbing mental experiences that generally occur during REM sleep
REM sleep behavior disorder	A complex set of behaviors, including mild to harmful body movements associated with dreams and nightmares and loss of muscle atonia
Recurrent isolated sleep paralysis	Inability to speak or move, as in a temporary paralysis, at sleep onset or upon waking
Other parasomnias	
Enuresis	Involuntary release of urine
Nocturnal groaning (catathrenia)	Characterized by disruptive groaning that occurs during expiration, particularly during the second half of night
Sleep-related eating disorder	Marked by repeated episodes of involuntary eating and drinking during arousals from sleep
Sleep-related dissociative disorders	A dissociative episode that can occur in the period from wakefulness to sleep or from awakening from stages 1 or 2 or from REM sleep
Exploding head syndrome	Characterized by a sudden, loud noise or explosion in the head; this is an imagined, painless noise.
Sleep-related hallucinations	Hallucinatory images that occur at sleep onset or on awakening

NOTE: NREM, non-rapid eye movement; REM, rapid eye movement; SWS, slow-wave sleep.
SOURCES: Halasz et al. (1985), Terzano et al. (1988), Zucconi et al. (1995), Zadra et al. (1998), and AASM (2005).

Sleepwalking

Sleepwalking is characterized by a complex series of behaviors that culminate in walking around with an altered state of consciousness and impaired judgment (AASM, 2005). Individuals who are sleepwalking commonly perform routine and nonroutine behaviors at inappropriate times and have difficulty recalling episodic events. Like confusional arousals, the prevalence of sleepwalking is higher in children than adults (AASM, 2005).

There appears to be a genetic predisposition for sleepwalking. Children who have both parents affected by sleepwalking are 38 percent more likely to also be affected (Klackenberg, 1982; Hublin et al., 1997).

Sleep Terrors

Sleep terrors are characterized by arousal from SWS accompanied by a cry or piercing scream, in addition to autonomic nervous system and behavioral manifestations of intense fear (AASM, 2005). Individuals with sleep terrors are typically hard to arouse from sleep and, when they are awoken, are confused and disoriented. There does not appear to be a significant gender or age difference in prevalence or incidence of sleep terrors (AASM, 2005).

Disorders Associated with REM Sleep

Rapid Eye Movement Sleep Behavior Disorder

REM sleep behavior disorder is characterized by a complex set of behaviors that occur during REM sleep, including mild to harmful body movements associated with dreams and nightmares (AASM, 2005). Normally during REM sleep, muscles are temporarily paralyzed; however, in REM sleep behavior disorder this paralysis is absent, thus allowing individuals to "play out" their dreams. The overall prevalence in the general population is estimated to be less than half a percent, slightly higher in older persons (AASM, 2005), and affecting men more frequently than women.

REM sleep behavior disorder is frequently associated with neurological disorders and it has been suggested that it could be an early sign of neurodegeneration (Olson et al., 2000). At least 15 percent of individuals with Parkinson's disease (Comella et al., 1998; Gagnon et al., 2002) and 44 percent of individuals with multiple system atrophy (Plazzi et al., 1997; 1998) also suffer from REM sleep behavior disorder. There are a number of effective pharmacological treatments, including a long-acting benzodiazepine (Schenck and Mahowald, 1990), clonazepam (Schenck et al., 1993), and dopamine agonists (Bamford, 1993; Fantini et al., 2003).

Nightmare Disorder

Nightmare disorder is characterized by recurrent disturbances of dreaming that are disturbing mental experiences that seem real and sometimes cause the individual to wake up. If awoken, individuals commonly have difficulty returning to sleep. Nightmares often occur during the second half of a normal period of sleep. Dream content involves a distressing theme, typically imminent physical danger. During nightmares, individuals experience increased heart and respiration rates (Fisher et al., 1970; Nielsen and Zadra, 2000).

Nightmares commonly affect children and adolescents and decrease in frequency and intensity as an individual grows older (AASM, 2005). Drugs and alcohol can trigger nightmares. Prevalence rates are also higher in individuals suffering from acute stress disorder and posttraumatic stress disorder.

SLEEP AND NEUROLOGICAL DISORDERS

Individuals suffering from dementia commonly experience sleep abnormalities. Although there are a variety of conditions associated with dementia—Alzheimer's disease, Parkinson's disease, dementia with Lewy bodies, Huntington's disease, and Creutzfeldt-Jakob disease—there are some common patterns of sleep impairment associated with all dementias. Typically, sleep is more fragmented, leading to more awakenings and consequently less time asleep, and REM may be decreased (Petit et al., 2005). These sleep impairments usually worsen as the disease progresses.

Alzheimer's Disease

Manifestations and Prevalence

Alzheimer's disease is a neurodegenerative disorder characterized by memory loss and an intellectual decline that progresses with age and is caused by the degeneration of neurons in the brain. It is estimated that about 4 million individuals in the United States suffer from Alzheimer's disease. Approximately one-quarter of these individuals have sleep disturbances (Tractenberg et al., 2005; Moran et al., 2005). Alzheimer's disease causes an increase number of arousals and affects an individual's sleep architecture. As a result of an increase in duration and number of awakenings, individuals spend an increased percentage of time in stage 1 sleep and a reduced percentage in stage 2 and SWS (Prinz et al., 1982a,b; Reynolds et al., 1985; Montplaisir et al., 1995).

Etiology and Risk Factors

There is limited information regarding the etiology of sleep disorders associated with Alzheimer's disease and other conditions that cause dementia. Associations with sleep disturbance and other behavioral symptoms have been identified, including aggressiveness (Moran et al., 2005) and depression (Tractenberg et al., 2005). However, the pathophysiology of this association is not known. In addition to behavioral symptoms, OSA may also occur at a higher prevalence in individuals with Alzheimer's disease than in the general population (Bliwise, 2002).

Treatment

Treatment options for demented individuals who suffer sleep disorders are typically the same as those received by individuals who do not have dementia. The approach is to address the sleep disorder based on its symptoms while managing and treating the underlying medical or psychiatric disorder (Petit et al., 2005). However, treating an individual's sleep disorder is not effective in reducing dementia associated with Alzheimer's disease.

Parkinson's Disease

Manifestations and Prevalence

Sleep complaints and subsequent diminished quality of life are common in individuals who suffer from Parkinson's disease. Parkinson's disease is a neurological disorder that primarily affects the elderly—0.9 percent of people 65 to 69 years of age to upwards of 5 percent of people 80 to 84 years of age have Parkinson's disease (de Rijk et al., 1997). It is characterized by trouble initiating walking and other movements, muscle tremor, a slow gait, and reduced facial expressions. Sleep disturbances associated with Parkinson's disease include difficulty falling asleep, nocturnal akinesia, altered sleep architecture, abnormal motor activity, periodic limb movements, REM sleep behavior disorder (see above), and disturbed breathing. During the day, many Parkinson patients have excessive sleepiness.

Sleep disturbances typically increase with disease progression. Individuals suffer from increased sleep latency and frequent awakenings, spending as much as 30 to 40 percent of the night awake (Kales et al., 1971; Bergonzi et al., 1975). This causes reduced time spent in stages 3 and 4 and REM sleep and increased duration in stages 1 and 2 (Kales et al., 1971).

Etiology and Risk Factors

Sleep patterns are affected by abnormalities caused by neurodegeneration in regions of the brain that are involved in regulating the sleep-wake cycle. Dopaminergic neurons in the substantia nigra are dramatically reduced in number, as are noradrenerics neurons in the locus coeruleus (Jellinger, 1986) and cholinergic neurons in the pedunculopontine nucleus (Zweig et al., 1989). Braak and colleagues (2004) examined a large series of autopsy brains. They found that Lewy body degeneration begins in the lower brainstem and ascends to involve the substantia nigra only after several years, consistent with observations that REM alterations may precede the movement disorder by several years in many Parkinson's disease patients. REM sleep behavioral disorder is often seen in patients with Parkinson's disease and other parkinsonian syndromes, such as multiple systems atrophy and progressive supranuclear palsy. The ability to ameliorate the symptoms of REM sleep behavioral disorder with dopaminergic agonist drugs suggests that it may be an early sign of damage to the dopaminergic system (Trampus et al., 1991).

Treatment

Treating sleep disturbances associated with Parkinson's disease is complicated owing to the different actions associated with dopaminergic medications. Medications used to treat this disorder often include dopamine precursors (levodopa/carbidopa) and dopamine agonists (pramipexole and ropinirole). When used in low doses, these medications can promote sleep, but high doses may cause increased nocturnal wakefulness, decreased SWS, and decreased sleep continuity (Leeman et al., 1987; Monti et al., 1988; Cantor and Stern, 2002). In contrast, excessive daytime sleepiness, including sleep attacks, has also been described in association with dopamine agonists (Paus et al., 2003); therefore, many patients with Parkinson's disease require daytime stimulants such as modafinil or amphetamine to relieve excessive sleepiness.

Other classes of medication used to treat Parkinson's disease include monoamine oxidase-B inhibitors (selegiline), presynaptic relating agents (amatadine, anticholingeric agents), and catechol-O-methyltransferase (COMT) inhibitors (hyoscyaine, benztropine). All may potentially affect sleep (Chrisp et al., 1991), particularly with regard to decreasing REM sleep, but the sleep effects of these medications remain to be well described (Kaakkola, 2000).

Epilepsy

Manifestations and Prevalence

Epilepsy refers to a group of various disorders characterized by abnormal electrical activity in the brain that manifests itself in individuals as a loss of or impaired consciousness and abnormal movements and behaviors. Sleep, sleep deprivation, and seizure activity are tightly intertwined. After stroke and Alzheimer's disease, epilepsy is the third most common neurological disorder in the United States, with incidence between 1.5 to 3.1 percent (Shouse and Mahowald, 2005). It is estimated that sleep-related epilepsy may affect as many as 10 percent or more of epileptic individuals (AASM, 2005). Sixty percent of individuals who suffer partial complex localization related seizures—21.6 percent of the general epileptic population—exhibit convulsions only during sleep (Janz, 1962).

Disorders that cause seizures may affect an individual's sleep cycle, leading to sleep deprivation. Similarly, sleep and sleep deprivation increase the incidence of seizure activity. Sleep-related epilepsy normally presents with at least two of the following features: arousals, abrupt awakenings from sleep, generalized tonic-clonic movements of the limbs, focal limb movement, facial twitching, urinary incontinence, apnea, tongue biting, and postictal confusion and lethargy (AASM, 2005). These features cause sleep fragmentation and daytime fatigue.

There are a number of common epileptic syndromes that manifest solely or predominately during the night, including nocturnal frontal lobe epilepsy, benign epilepsy of childhood with centrotemporal spikes, early-onset or late-onset childhood occipital epilepsy, juvenile myoclonic epilepsy, and continuous spike waves during non-REM sleep. Nocturnal frontal lobe epilepsy is characterized by severe sleep disruption, injuries caused by involuntary movements, and occasional daytime seizures. Juvenile myoclonic epilepsy is characterized by synchronous involuntary muscle contractions that often occur during awakening. Continuous spike waves during non-REM sleep epilepsy are commonly associated with neurocognitive impairment and sometimes with impairment of muscle activity and control.

Etiology and Risk Factors

Risk factors for sleep-related epilepsy include stress, sleep deprivation, other sleep disorders, and irregular sleep-wake rhythms. The etiologies for nocturnal seizures are not clearly understood. Genetic factors are likely important; however, as of yet no pathogenic markers have been associated with sleep-related epilepsy. There are specific patterns of rhythmic activity among neurons within specific regions of the brain—the hypothalamus and brainstem—that regulate sleep and arousal. Association of specific neuronal activity between these different regions is important for regulating sleep, while bursts of disassociated neuronal activity may contribute to nocturnal seizures (Tassinari et al., 1972; Velasco and Velasco, 1982; Applegate et al., 1986; Shouse et al., 1996).

Treatment

Treatments for seizures caused by sleep-related epileptic syndromes are typically similar to those of other seizure disorders (Dreifuss and Porter, 1997). Individuals with epilepsy are susceptible to nocturnal sleep disturbance and daytime sleepiness associated with commonly used medications. However, daytime hypersomnolence is not always treatable with antiepileptic drugs (Palm et al., 1992). In particular, phenobarbital, a mainstay of treatment for many years, causes daytime sedation in a dose dependent manner (Brodie and Dichter, 1997). Daytime sedation is also observed with other antiepileptic agents including carbamazepine, alproate, phenytoin, and primidone. Some of the newer medication such as gabapentin, lamotrigine, bigabatrin, and zonisamide are often better tolerated (Salinsky et al., 1996). In addition to daytime sedation, these drugs also cause increased nocturnal sleep time. Vagal nerve stimulation, however, has been reported to improve daytime alertness (Rizzo et al., 2003), but it may also induce sleep apnea (Holmes et al., 2003).

Stroke

Manifestations and Prevalence

Stroke results in a sudden loss of consciousness, sensation, and voluntary movement caused by disruption of blood flow—and therefore oxygen supply—to the brain. Following a stroke an individual's sleep architecture is often altered, causing a decrease in the total sleep time, REM sleep, and SWS (Broughton and Baron, 1978). Insomnia is a common complication of stroke that may result from medication, inactivity, stress, depression, and brain damage.

The annual incidence of stroke is 2 to 18 per 1000 individuals, and sleep-wake disturbances are found in at least 20 percent of stroke patients (Bassetti, 2005). In addition, over 70 percent of individuals who have suffered a mild stroke and are under 75 years of age suffer fatigue (Carlsson et al., 2003).

Sleep-Disordered Breathing May Be a Risk Factor

Risk factors for stroke include heart disease, hypertension, alcohol abuse, transient ischemic attacks, and, as described above, possibly sleep-disordered breathing (Diaz and Sempere, 2004). Studies investigating the association between sleep-disordered breathing and stroke found that 60 to 70 percent of individuals who have suffered a stroke exhibit sleep-disordered breathing with an apnea-hypopnea index of 10 or greater (Dyken et al., 1996; Bassetti et al., 1996). Sleep-disordered breathing has also been found in a high frequency of individuals with transient ischemic attacks (McArdle et al., 2003), hypertension (Morrell et al., 1999), myocardial infarction, and heart failure (Good et al., 1996; Shamsuzzaman et al., 2003).

Treatment

There are no specific therapies that relieve sleep-related symptoms caused by a stroke. Rather, treatments depend on the specific symptoms and are similar to the treatments of sleep disorders that arise independent of a stroke. For example, CPAP is the treatment of choice for sleep disordered breathing, and insomnia and parasomnias are treated using similar temporary hypnotic drug therapies as typically used, zolpidem or benzodiazepines. However, treatments for hypersomnia are not always as effective following a stroke (Bassetti, 2005).

SUDDEN INFANT DEATH SYNDROME

Manifestations and Prevalence

Sudden infant death syndrome (SIDS), the sudden and unexpected death of infants less than a year old during sleep, has no known cause (American Academy of Pediatrics Task Force on Sudden Infant Death Syndrome, 2005; CDC, 2006). The syndrome is currently the third most common cause of infant death in the United States (CDC, 2006), responsible for approximately 3,000 infant deaths a year in this country (NICHD, 2006b). The majority of SIDS-related deaths occur in infants who are between 2 and 4 months old (NICHD, 2006a).

Etiology and Risk Factors

Although there are no known causes for SIDS, various hypotheses exist about the mechanisms underlying the syndrome. The leading theory is that developmental abnormalities in the infant's cardiorespiratory system increase the child's susceptibility to suffocation (Meny et al., 1994; Kinney et al., 1995; Verrier and Josephson, 2005). Infants who later die of SIDS have higher heart rates, narrower heart rate ranges, and problems with coordination of respiration, heart rate, and arterial blood pressure while sleeping (Kemp and Thach, 1991; Schechtman et al., 1995; Kinney et al., 1995; Verrier and Josephson, 2005). This lack of coordination in the cardiorespiratory system may be a result of defects in the region of the brain responsible for controlling breathing and arousal (Kinney et al., 1995; Panigraphy et al., 1997; AAP, 2000), possibly resulting in a baby being unable to wake up in response to troubled breathing.

Concordantly, risk factors attributed to SIDS typically relate to an infant's ability to breathe easily while sleeping. The chief risk factor for SIDS is a prone sleeping position, otherwise known as stomach sleeping (Dwyer et al., 1991; Ponsonby et al., 1993; Irgens et al., 1995). More recently, side sleeping is thought to be attended by an intermediate level of risk (American Academy of Pediatrics Task Force on Sudden Infant Death Syndrome, 2005; CDC, 2006). Other factors related to obstructed breathing space include bed sharing with adults or several family members, soft sleep surfaces and/or loose bedding and overheating while sleeping (Hauck and Kemp, 1998; AAP, 2000).

Vulnerability to SIDS seems to depend on both gender and ethnicity. Male infants are more likely to die of SIDS than female babies (NICHD, 2006a); African American infants have twice the likelihood as Caucasian infants of dying from SIDS (Hauck et al., 2003; Daley, 2004; NICHD, 2006a), while Native American infants are three times as likely to be victims of this syndrome (AAP, 2000). SIDS has also been reported to occur at increased frequency in family members with OSA (Tishler et al., 1996), suggesting that there may be common genetic risk factors for both conditions.

Finally, general measures of poor health form the final category of risk factors. Smoking, drinking, or drug use by the mother during gestation are linked to an increased chance of SIDS-related deaths in infants, as is infant exposure to smoke (Schoendorf and Kiely, 1992; AAP, 2000; Iyasu et al., 2002). Infants born with low body weight, prematurely, or to mothers under the age of 20 are also at higher risk of SIDS (Malloy and Hoffman, 1995; AAP, 2000).

Prevention

Preventive measures have reduced the incidence of SIDS in the United States by more than 50 percent. A number of national intervention programs currently exist through various organizations. Of these, the most prominent intervention program is NIH's "Back to Sleep" campaign (Chapter 5).

Additional preventive measures include no smoking, drinking, or drug use by the mother while pregnant; removal of loose bedding or other items that could suffocate an infant; and prevention of high temperatures in the baby's sleeping environment (NICHD, 2006a).

SLEEP AND MOVEMENT DISORDERS

Restless Legs Syndrome

Manifestations and Prevalence

RLS is a neurological condition characterized by an irresistible urge to move the legs (it also may affect the arms, trunk, or head and neck). It is also associated with paresthesias—uncomfortable feelings—which individuals describe as creepy-crawly, jittery, itchy, or burning feelings. The symptoms are partially or completely relieved by movement. The urge to move and unpleasant sensations worsen during periods of rest or inactivity, especially in the evening and at night, causing most individuals difficulty falling asleep (Michaud et al., 2000). The discomfort associated with RLS also causes individuals to wake frequently during the night (Montplaisir et al., 1997). Individuals with RLS often experience periodic limb movements; however, periodic limb movement disorder (see below) is not always associated RLS (Michaud et al., 2000).

The prevalence of RLS has been reported to be at minimum 5 percent (Lavigne and Montplaisir, 1994; Rothdach et al., 2000; NSF, 2005a; Montplaisir et al., 2005; Phillips et al., 2006), which makes it one of the most common movement disorders and sleep disorders. This condition may be found in in adolescents and teenagers (Kryger et al., 2002a) and is more common in older adults and females (Rothdach et al., 2000; Allen and Earley, 2001; Nichols et al., 2002), affecting over 20 percent of pregnant women. RLS symptoms associated with pregnancy are caused by transient low levels of ferritin and folate; therefore, they typically disappear within 4 weeks after delivery (Lee et al., 2001).

RLS may also be associated with attention-deficit hyperactivity disorder (ADHD). In a cross-sectional survey of 866 children, ADHD symptoms were almost twice as likely to occur with symptoms of RLS as would be expected by chance alone (Chervin et al., 2002).

Etiology and Risk Factors

The exact cause of RLS is not completely understood. It likely results from altered dopamine and iron metabolism, and there is evidence for a genetic contribution. More than 50 percent of idiopathic cases are associated with a positive family history of RLS (Ekbom, 1945; Walters et al., 1996; Montplaisir et al., 1997; Winkelmann et al., 2002; Allen et al., 2003), and these cases segregate in an autosomal dominant fashion with high penetrance (90 to 100 percent) (Winkelmann et al., 2002). Susceptibility gene loci have been identified on chromosomes 12q (Desautels et al., 2001), 14q (Bonati et al., 2003), and 9p (Chen et al., 2004); however, no genetic markers or abnormalities have been identified.

RLS commonly occurs in individuals with iron deficiency, including end-stage renal disease, iron-deficiency anemia, pregnancy, and gastric surgery. Iron deficiency, for example caused by repeated blood donation, may also be associated with RLS (Silber et al., 2003; Ulfberg and Nystrom, 2004; Kryger et al., 2003). It is hypothesized that low levels of iron impair transmission of dopamine signals, which contributes to RLS. Iron levels are reduced in the substantia nigra (Allen et al., 2001; Connor et al., 2003), which is a region of the brain responsible for controlling voluntary movement through neurons that rely on dopamine to communicate with each other. The iron deficiency is consistent with abnormal regulation of the transferrin receptor, which is responsible for transporting iron across cell membranes. Iron in turn is necessary for the synthesis of dopamine and the activity of the D_2 dopamine receptor (Turjanski et al., 1999). The association between dopamine, iron deficiency, and RLS is further supported by observations that dopamine antagonists usually make RLS symptoms worse (Winkelmann et al., 2001), while dopaminergic agonists are used to treat RLS (Walters et al., 1988; Wetter et al., 1999; Stiasny et al., 2001).

Idiopathic RLS is not associated with an increased mortality rate; however, in secondary cases of RLS, such as in individuals treated with long-term hemodialysis for end-stage renal disease, RLS is associated with a greater mortality risk (Winkelman et al., 1996). In a survey of 894 dialysis patients that rated symptoms of RLS, severe symptoms were associated with an increased hazard ratio (OR = 1.39; 95% CI, 1.08–1.79) (Unruh et al., 2004).

Treatment

There are both behavioral and pharmacological treatments for RLS; however, there have been no clinical trials reporting the efficacy of non-pharmacological strategies to reduce RLS symptoms. Mild to moderate symptoms can sometimes be treated by lifestyle changes, including maintaining a normal sleeping pattern, taking supplements to manage iron deficiencies, and minimizing consumption of alcohol, caffeine, and tobacco (NINDS, 2005).

RLS is primarily treated using one of four classes of prescription medications: dopaminergic agents, benzodiazepines, opioids, or anticonvulsants (central nervous system depressants). Dopaminergic agents are the primary treatment option for individuals with RLS (Hening et al., 2004). Medications include the dopamine precursor levodopa (L-dopa). Although associated with some adverse effects, administration of L-dopa significantly reduces symptoms of RLS and periodic limb movements that occur throughout the night (Brodeur et al., 1988). However, dopaminergic agents can also have a stimulating effect that may exacerbate insomnia. Benzodiazepines are effective in improving sleep continuity and are therefore frequently prescribed in combination with dopaminergic agents. Opioids may be prescribed in patients with severe symptoms to help to induce relaxation and minimize pain (Walters et al., 1993, 2001). However, opioids may also exacerbate sleep apnea; therefore, they should be used cautiously in patients who snore (Montplaisir et al., 2005). Anticonvulsants are commonly prescribed as an alternative to dopaminergic agents, owing to their ability to minimize leg pain (Montplaisir et al., 2005). It is believed that anticonvulsants, such as carbamazepine and gabapentin, are less potent than dopaminergic agents; however, there have been no comparative studies performed. Furthermore, there have been a limited number of studies that have examined the safety and efficacy of these treatments in children and adolescents.

Periodic Limb Movement Disorder

Periodic limb movement disorder is characterized by disruptions to sleep caused by periodic episodes of limb movements that occur during sleep, which cannot be explained by any other sleep disorder (AASM, 2005). Individuals with periodic limb movement disorder primarily complain of difficulty with sleep onset and sleep maintenance, insomnia, and/or hypersomnia. The periodic limb movements manifest themselves as rhythmic extensions of the big toe, dorsiflexions of the ankle, and occasional flexions of the knee and hip (Coleman, 1982). These are scored using the periodic limb movements index, which examines over the course of an hour the number of movements that are 0.5 to 5 seconds in duration, separated by an interval between 5 to 90 seconds, and in sequence of four or more an hour. An overnight index score of 5 or greater in children and 15 or greater in adults is considered pathogenic (AASM, 2005).

Periodic limb movements typically occur in the lower extremities and may result in autonomic arousal, cortical arousal, or an awakening. However, typically the individual is unaware of the movements. They are more frequent in the beginning of the night and cluster together. These events are associated with a fast heart rate, followed by a period of slow heart rate (Friedland et al., 1985). Periodic limb movements disorder is associated with above average rates of depression, memory impairment, attention deficits, oppositional behaviors, and fatigue (AASM, 2005). Similar to RLS, dopaminergic medications are helpful in alleviating the disorder's symptoms.

Periodic limb movements are believed to be very common, especially in older persons, occurring in 34 percent of individuals over the age of 60 (AASM, 2005). However, the disorder—periodic limb movements associated with sleep disruption—is not as common. Periodic limb movements are very common in RLS, occurring in 80 to 90 percent of individuals. It is also observed in individuals with narcolepsy, REM sleep behavior disorder (Folstein et al., 1975), OSA (Montplaisir et al., 1996), and hypersomnia (Whitehouse et al., 1982). Children with ADHD have an increased prevalence of periodic limb movements (Picchietti et al., 1998), and children with periodic limb movement disorders are more likely to have ADHD (Picchietti et al., 1999; Ozminkowski et al., 2004). Sleep-disordered breathing may be a modulator that increases the association between periodic limb movements and ADHD (Chervin and Archbold, 2001).

SLEEP AND MEDICAL DISORDERS

A number of different medical disorders and diseases, from a common cold to cancer, frequently alter an individual's sleep-wake cycle. These sleep problems often result from pain or infection associated with the primary condition. Although these are both known to cause problems with sleep-wake cycles, as will be shown below, very little is still known about the etiology.

Pain

Pain is described as an acute or chronic unpleasant sensory and emotional experience that varies from dull discomfort to unbearable agony that is associated with actual or potential tissue damage. It commonly causes sleep fragmentation and changes in an individual's sleep architecture. The symptoms depend on the type and severity of the pain. They include daytime fatigue and sleepiness, poor sleep quality, delay in sleep onset, and decreased cognitive and motor performance (Table 3-5) (Bonnet and Arand, 2003).

Chronic pain affects at least 10 percent of the general adult population (Harstall, 2003), of whom 50 percent complain of poor sleep (Atkinson et al., 1988; Dao et al., 1994; Morin et al., 1998; Roizenblatt et al., 2001; Riley et al., 2001; Dauvilliers and Touchon, 2001; McCracken and Iverson, 2002; Perlis et al., 2005), and 44 percent complain of insomnia (Moldofsky, 2001). There are a number of clinical pain conditions that individuals report affect their sleep quality—RLS, irritable bowel, gastric ulcer, cancer, musculoskeletal disorders, dental and orofacial pain, spinal cord damage, burns, and other trauma (Lavigne et al., 2005).

Although progress has been made, there are still many unanswered questions about how pain affects regions of the brain responsible for regulating the sleep-wake cycle. Neurons that carry pain information to the brain do communicate with regions of the brain that are responsible for arousal—raphe magnus "off" cells (Foo and Mason, 2003). However, it is not known if *hypocretin* and other genes that regulate the circadian rhythms are affected by acute or chronic pain. Further, it is not known whether the hypothalamus, which is involved in sleep homeostasis, is affected by chronic pain (Kshatri et al., 1998; Mignot et al., 2002b). Because little is known about the interaction between pain and the circuitry in the brain that is responsible for regulating the sleep-wake cycle, much of the management of sleep problems focuses on managing and alleviating the pain or sleep quality.

TABLE 3-5 Selected Sleep-Related Symptoms and Findings in the Presence of Pain

Bedtime symptoms
  • Delay in sleep onset
  • Anxiety, rumination
  • Intense fatigue and more intense pain

Sleep time findings
  • Lower sleep efficacy (less than 90%)
  • Longer percentage sleep time in stage 1, with less in stages 3 and 4
  • Numerous sleep stage shifts (stages 3 and 4 toward stages 2 or 1)
  • Fragmentation of sleep continuity (increase in number of microarousals, awakenings, sleep stage shifts, respiratory events, movement intrusions)
  • Alpha electroencephalographic intrusions in stages 3 and 4 with or without elevated phasic arousals (cyclic alternating pattern)
  • Absence of reduction in heart rate variability in sleep (cardiac sympathetic overactivation)
  • Nightmares, periodic leg movements, apnea, sweating, heart palpitations
  • Wake time in sleep with pain (e.g., neck, lower back, visceral, tooth)

Wake time symptoms
  • Unrefreshing sleep sensation, fatigue, headache, etc.
  • Sleepiness if driving
  • Anxiety and anger over fulfilling daytime requirements at home or work

SOURCE: Lavigne et al. (2005).

Infectious Disease

Infections caused by bacterial strains, viruses, and parasites may result in changes to sleep patterns. Although it is accepted that the activity of the immune system affects an individual's sleep-wake cycle, very little is known about how these two systems interact. This is complicated by the unique effects that specific infections have on sleep patterns and the absence of a large body of clinical research.

Bacterial Infections and Sleep

Bacterial infections typically cause an increase in the total time spent in SWS and a decreased duration of REM sleep (Toth, 1999; Toth and Opp, 2002). Alterations of sleep patterns can be affected by the type of bacterial infection (Opp and Toth, 2003). For example, gram-negative bacteria induce enhanced sleep more rapidly than do gram-positive bacteria. Differences in the process and progression of the disease also affect the sleep-wake cycle.

Viral Infections and Sleep

Viral infections also have effects on the sleep-wake cycle. Individuals inoculated with rhinovirus or influenza virus report less sleep during the incubation period, while during the symptomatic period they slept longer (Smith, 1992). However, compared to healthy individuals there were no reported difference in sleep quality and number of awakenings.

The human immunodeficiency virus (HIV) also has been shown to alter sleep patterns. Individuals spend increased time in SWS during the second half of night (Darko et al., 1995) and suffer from frequent arousals and decreased time in REM sleep (Norman et al., 1990). As the infection progresses to AIDS, individuals develop increased sleep fragmentation, significant reductions in SWS, and disruption to the entire sleep architecture (Norman et al., 1990; Darko et al., 1995).

Cancer

Many patients with cancer also suffer pain or depression, which contributes to difficulty sleeping. These require treatment as in other patients with pain or depression as causes of insomnia. Excessive sleepiness may be caused by injury to the ascending arousal system due to brain metastases or by leptomeningeal carcinomatosis. These signs often alert physicians to the need to treat the underlying spread of cancer to the central nervous system. Other patients with cancer may develop antitumor antibodies that attack the brain. In particular, anti-Ma-2 antibodies tend to cause hypothalamic lesions and may precipitate daytime sleepiness and even cataplexy (Rosenfeld et al., 2001). Treatment of the underlying cancer may reverse the symptoms in some cases.

Sleeping Sickness

Fungal and parasitic infections also can alter the sleep-wake cycle. For example, sleeping sickness, or African trypanosomiasis, commonly occurs in individuals who have been infected with the *Trypanosoma brucei* (*Tb*) parasite. It is characterized by episodes of nocturnal insomnia and daytime sleep, but not hypersomnia (Lundkvist et al., 2004).

Sleeping sickness is found primarily in sub-Saharan African countries, where *Tb* is transmitted to humans as a result of bites received from tsetse flies (Lundkvist et al., 2004). The prevalence of this disorder is not known; however, over 60 million people live in areas where the *Tb* parasite is endemic.

Sleeping sickness is associated with altered sleep architecture. EEG recordings of individuals with sleeping sickness from Gambia demonstrate periods of REM sleep that occur throughout the entire sleep-wake cycle, frequently without normal intermediate NREM periods (Buguet et al., 2001). Circadian fluctuations of hormones—cortisol, prolactin, and growth hormone—are also altered in individuals with sleeping sickness (Radomski et al., 1994). Therefore, it has been hypothesized that sleeping sickness may be a circadian rhythm disease that affects the neural pathways that interconnect the circadian-timing and sleep-regulating centers (Lundkvist et al., 2004).

Treatment Effects on Sleep

Numerous medical conditions are associated with a wide variety of sleep disorders including insomnia, hypersomnia, parasomnias, and sleep-related movement disorders. Although these disease-related sleep disorders have recently been receiving an increasing amount of attention, including addition to the latest International Classification of Sleep Disorders (AASM, 2005), the contribution that treatments for these medical conditions make to the development of sleep disturbances is less well appreciated. However, many medical therapies have iatrogenic effects on sleep-wake regulatory systems causing disturbed sleep, daytime sleepiness, and other related side effects.

Treatments for Cardiovascular Disease

Cardiovascular diseases, sometimes associated with sleep-related breathing disorders (Peters, 2005) (see above), are commonly treated with a wide range of medications including antihypertensives, hypolipidemics, and antiarrhythmics; each class of medication can adversely affect sleep and/or waking. For example, beta-antagonists, the mainstay of treatment for hypertension, are commonly associated with fatigue, insomnia, nightmares, and vivid dreams (McAinsh and Cruickshank, 1990). Sleep disturbances appear to be more severe with lipophilic drugs (e.g., propranolol) than with hydrophilic drugs (e.g., atenolol). However, even atenolol, one of the most hydrophilic beta-blockers, has been shown to increase total wake time (Van Den Heuvel et al., 1997). The mechanism underlying sleep disruption by beta-blocking agents may be their tendency to deplete melatonin, an important sleep-related hormone (Garrick et al., 1983; Dawson and Encel, 1993). Fatigue and somnolence have also been reported with other antihypertensive medications such as carvedilol, labetalol, clonidine, methyldopa, and reserpine (Paykel et al., 1982; Miyazaki et al., 2004). In contrast, angiotensin-converting enzyme inhibitors generally have very few effects on sleep (Reid, 1996). Hypolipidemic drugs, including atorvastatin and lovastatin, have also been associated with reports of insomnia, but placebo-controlled clinical trials of lovastatin, simvastatin, and pravastatin did not appear to increase sleep disturbance (Bradford et al., 1991; Keech et al., 1996). Amiodarone, a widely use antiarrhythmic agent (Hilleman et al., 1998), can cause nocturnal sleep disturbance, and digoxin has been associated with both insomnia and daytime fatigue (Weisberg et al., 2002).

Treatments for Cancer

Patients with cancer receive multiple types of treatments designed at controlling the disease process including chemotherapy, biotherapy, radiotherapy, and medications. All can have important adverse effects on regulating the sleep-wake cycle. For example, sleep problems have been reported in patients undergoing chemotherapy (Broeckel et al., 1998; Berger and Higginbotham, 2000; Lee et al., 2004). However, objective measures of sleep in the patients and analyses of clinical correlates are very limited. Thus, the mechanisms underlying these sleep problems are poorly understood. Menopausal symptoms arising from chemotherapy and hormonal therapy, especially those of a vasomotor type (e.g., hot flashes, sweating), may be a contributing factor (Rombaux et al., 2000; Mourits et al., 2001; Carpenter et al., 2002). Nocturnal sleep disturbances and daytime sleepiness have also been reported in patients undergoing radiotherapy (Beszterczey and Lipowski, 1977; Miaskowski and Lee, 1999).

Cytokines (biotherapy), a diverse group of peptide molecules that regulate cell functions, are sometimes used as adjunct therapy (Dunlop and Campbell, 2000). Interferon, interleukin-2, and tumor necrosis factor are associated with a variety of side effects including daytime sleepiness, disturbed sleep, and depression (Capuron et al., 2000). Although very effective in reducing cancer-related pain, opioids often cause sleep disturbance and are associated with decreased REM and SWS (Cronin et al., 2001).

Treatments for Renal Disease

RLS, periodic limb movement disorder, sleep apnea, and excessive daytime sleepiness affect up to 70 percent of patients with end-stage renal disease receiving treatment with hemodialysis (Parker et al., 2000; Parker, 2003). Hemodialysis may alter biological systems controlling processes that regulate the sleep-wake cycle via several potential mechanisms. The rapid fluid, electrolyte, and acid/base changes that occur are often associated with central nervous system symptoms such as headache, restlessness, changes in arousal, and fatigue during or immediately after treatment. Several studies have reported an increase in cytokine production secondary to blood interactions with bioincompatible aspects of hemodialysis (such as blood exposure to membranes, tubing, and cellular mechanical trauma) and backflow of endotoxins through the membrane (Panichi et al., 2000). Interleukin-1, tumor necrosis factor-α, and interleukin-6 are the major proinflammatory cytokines that may be involved (Pertosa et al., 2000). These substances have both somnogenic and pyrogenic properties and have been linked to a number of postdialytic symptoms (Konsman et al., 2002), including daytime sleepiness and sleep disturbances (Raison and Miller, 2001; Capuron et al., 2002). Dialysis-associated changes in melatonin levels and pattern of secretion and alterations in body temperature rhythm may also play a role in disrupting circadian systems (Vaziri et al., 1993, 1996; Parker et al., 2000; Parker, 2003).

Treatments for Rheumatologic and Immunologic Disorders

Numerous other classes of medications can alter sleep and waking. Corticosteroids are a class of medications that are used to treat a variety of medical conditions including rheumatologic and immunologic disorders, cancer, and asthma. Sleep disturbances, insomnia, daytime hyperactivity, and mild hypomania are common side effects (Wolkowitz et al., 1990); a significant decrease in REM sleep may also occur (Born et al., 1987). Theophylline, a respiratory stimulant and bronchodilator, is in the same class of medications as caffeine and can likewise disturb sleep—even in healthy subjects (Kaplan et al., 1993). Nonsteroidal anti-inflammatory agents may also affect sleep as they decrease the production of sleep-promoting prostaglandins, suppress normal surge of melatonin, and alter the daily rhythm of body temperature (Murphy et al., 1994, 1996). Pseudoephedrine and phenylpropanolamine, which have many of the same pharmacological properties of ephedrine, also cause sleep disruption—and many of these preparation are readily available over the counter (Lake et al., 1990; Bertrand et al., 1996).

Although the medications and treatments listed above are often necessary, it is essential for patients to be aware of potential side effects relating to the sleep-wake-related cycle. Unfortunately, patients often neglect to report such complaints as they think nothing can be done to alleviate the problems. However, numerous behavioral and pharmacological interventions are available to treat these iatrogenically induced problems with the sleep-wake cycle. In addition, administering treatment or medications at appropriate times of day in relationship to the sleep-wake schedule may potentially be beneficial and enhance clinical outcomes (Levi, 1994; Bliwise et al., 2001; Hermida and Smolensky, 2004). Research in this area is greatly needed.

BOX 3-3
Shift Work Disorder and Jet Lag

Shift Work Disorder

Shift work type circadian rhythm sleep disorder is characterized by complaints of insomnia or excessive sleepiness resulting from work hours that occur during the normal sleep period, including, night shifts, early morning shifts, and rotating shifts. Total sleep time is normally reduced by 1 to 4 hours and sleep quality is disturbed. During work shifts individuals can experience excessive sleepiness, reduced alertness, and reduced performance capacity. Individuals are also commonly more irritable, and the disorder may have negative social consequences. The condition is closely linked to work schedules; consequently, it abates in response to a conventional sleep schedule.

Jet Lag

Jet lag type is a temporary circadian rhythm sleep disorder that occurs when there is a transitory mismatch between the timing of the sleep-wake cycle caused by a change in time zone. Individuals with jet lag potentially experience disturbed sleep, decreased subjective alertness, general malaise, somatic symptoms such as gastrointestinal disturbance, and impaired daytime function. The severity and the duration of the symptoms are usually dependent on the number of time zones traveled and the direction of travel—eastern travel and travel through multiple time zones typically result in worse symptoms than western travel.

CIRCADIAN RHYTHM SLEEP DISORDERS

Circadian rhythm sleep disorders arise from chronic alterations, disruptions, or misalignment of the circadian clock in relation to environmental cues and the terrestrial light-dark cycle. The 2005 update of the International Classification of Sleep Disorders designated nine different circadian disorders, including delayed sleep phase type, advanced sleep phase type, nonentrained sleep-wake type, irregular sleep-wake type, shift work type, and jet lag type (Box 3-3) (AASM, 2005). These disorders may be comorbid with other neurological or psychiatric disorders, making the diagnosis and treatment difficult (Reid and Zee, 2005). Diagnosis with a circadian rhythm disorder requires meeting the following three criteria:

- Persistent or recurrent pattern of sleep disturbance due primarily to either an alteration of the circadian timekeeping system or a misalignment between endogenous circadian rhythm and exogenous factors that affect timing and duration of sleep.

• Circadian-related disruption leads to insomnia, excessive sleepiness, or both.

• The sleep disturbance is associated with impairment of social, occupational, or other functions (AASM, 2005).

The following sections will describe two of the nine more common types of circadian rhythm sleep disorders, delayed sleep phase type and advanced sleep phase type.

Delayed Sleep Phase Syndrome

Manifestations and Prevalence

The sleep pattern of individuals suffering from delayed sleep phase syndrome (or delayed sleep phase type) is characterized by sleep onset and wake times that are typically delayed 3 to 6 hours relative to conventional sleep-wake times (Figure 3-7). An individual's total sleep time is normal for his or her age (Weitzman et al., 1981), but individuals typically find it difficult to initiate sleep before 2:00 and 6:00 a.m., and prefer to wake up between 10:00 a.m. and 1:00 p.m. The impact of delayed sleep phase syndrome has not been fully investigated and is therefore limited. In a study that included 14 individuals it was reported that the syndrome may impair an individual's job performance and may be associated with marital problems and financial difficulty (Alvarez et al., 1992). A second study investigated the impact of delayed sleep phase syndrome in 22 adolescents and found an association with increased daytime irritability, poor school performance, and mental disturbances (Regestein and Monk, 1995; AASM, 2005).

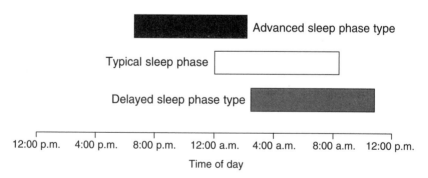

FIGURE 3-7 Representation of the temporal distribution of sleep.
SOURCE: Reid and Zee (2005).

The exact prevalence of delayed sleep phase syndrome in the general population is unknown. It is unclear what the prevalence of this disorder is; however, it may be more prevalent in adolescents and young adults (Weitzman et al., 1981; Pelayo et al., 1988; Regestein and Monk, 1995; AASM, 2005).

Etiology and Risk Factors

Night shift workers may be at higher risk for delayed sleep phase syndrome due to irregular circadian entrainment (Santhi et al., 2005). Similarly, individuals who live in extreme latitudes and are exposed to extended periods of light may also be at increased risk of suffering from delayed sleep phase syndrome (Lingjaerde et al., 1985; Pereira et al., 2005).

Biological, physiological, and genetic factors have been proposed to be responsible for causing delayed sleep phase syndrome. Behaviorally, late bedtimes and rise times delay an individual's exposure to light, which may prevent entraining of the circadian clock. Furthermore, exposure to dim light in the late evening and at night, may also affect the circadian phase (Zeitzer et al., 2000; Gronfier et al., 2004).

Biological alterations to the endogenous circadian system also contribute to delayed sleep phase syndrome. Although levels of melatonin typically increase in the evening hours, individuals with this syndrome have a hypersensitivity to nighttime bright light exposure in the suppression of melatonin (Czeisler et al., 1981). It has also been hypothesized that the disorder may result from a circadian phase that has a reduced sensitivity to photic entrainment, or the free-running period of the circadian cycle is prolonged (Czeisler et al., 1981). Consistent with these hypotheses, polymorphisms in circadian genes influence the entraining and free-running period of the circadian cycle and may be associated with delayed sleep phase syndrome (Takahashi et al., 2000; Iwase et al., 2002; Hohjoh et al., 2003; Archer et al., 2003; Pereira et al., 2005). A recent study has also identified a candidate gene, human *PER2*, that results in familial advanced sleep phase syndrome (Xu et al., 2005).

Treatment

Treatment for delayed sleep phase syndrome requires resynchronizing to a more appropriate phase to the 24-hour light-dark cycle. In addition to a structured sleep-wake schedule and good sleep hygiene practices, potential therapies include resetting the circadian pacemaker with bright light, melatonin, or a combination of both. However, studies that have investigated the efficacy of bright light have provided mixed results (Pelayo et al., 1988; Rosenthal et al., 1990; Akata et al., 1993; Weyerbrock et al., 1996), partially owing to limitations in their study design and the numbers of participants included in each study. Consequently, there are no standard criteria for its use. Similarly, there have been no large-scale controlled studies examining the efficacy of melatonin, and as of yet it has not been approved by the Food and Drug Administration for this indication (Reid and Zee, 2005).

Advanced Sleep Phase Syndrome

Manifestations and Prevalence

Advanced sleep phase syndrome (or advanced sleep phase type) is characterized by involuntary bedtimes and awake times that are more than 3 hours earlier than societal means (Figure 3-7) (Reid and Zee, 2005). As is the case with delayed sleep phase syndrome, the amount of sleep is not affected, unless evening activities result in later bedtimes. Therefore, the syndrome is primarily associated with impaired social and occupational activities.

The prevalence of advanced sleep phase syndrome is unknown; however, it has been estimated that as many as 1 percent of the middle-aged adults may suffer from it (Ando et al., 1995). One of the challenges in determining its prevalence is that affected individuals typically do not perceive it as a disorder and therefore do not seek medical treatment (Reid and Zee, 2005).

Etiology and Risk Factors

The causes of this syndrome are not known; however, as with delayed sleep phase type, biological and environmental factors likely contribute to the onset of advanced sleep phase type. Several familial cases of this syndrome have been reported (Jones et al., 1999; Ondze et al., 2001; Reid et al., 2001; Satoh et al., 2003), and these cases segregate in a dominant mode. Polymorphisms in circadian clock genes have been identified in a family with advanced sleep phase syndrome (Toh et al., 2001; Shiino et al., 2003). Changes in the activity of genes involved in circadian biology are consistent with observations that individuals with this syndrome have circadian rhythms that are less than 24 hours.

Treatment

Treatment options for individuals with advanced sleep phase syndrome are limited. Bright light therapy in the evening has been used successfully in a limited study to reduce awakenings (Campbell et al., 1993; Palmer et al., 2003). It is also hypothesized that administration of low levels of melatonin in the early morning may also be used (Lewy et al., 1996), though there are no published reports verifying this option.

REFERENCES

AAP (American Academy of Pediatrics). 2000. Changing concepts of sudden infant death syndrome: Implications for infant sleeping environment and sleep position. American Academy of Pediatrics. Task Force on Infant Sleep Position and Sudden Infant Death Syndrome. *Pediatrics* 105(3 Pt 1):650–656.

AASM (American Academy of Sleep Medicine). 2005. *The International Classification of Sleep Disorders.* Westchester, IL: American Academy of Sleep Medicine.

Akata T, Sekiguchi S, Takahashi M, Miyamoto M, Higuchi T, Machiyama Y. 1993. Successful combined treatment with vitamin B_{12} and bright artificial light of one case with delayed sleep phase syndrome. *Japanese Journal of Psychiatry and Neurology* 47(2):439–440.

Al-Delaimy WK, Manson JE, Willett WC, Stampfer MJ, Hu FB. 2002. Snoring as a risk factor for type II diabetes mellitus: A prospective study. *American Journal of Epidemiology* 155(5):387–393.

Aldrich MS. 1996. The clinical spectrum of narcolepsy and idiopathic hypersomnia. *Neurology* 46(2):393–401.

Ali NJ, Pitson DJ, Stradling JR. 1993. Snoring, sleep disturbance, and behaviour in 4–5 year olds. *Archives of Disease in Childhood* 68(3):360–366.

Allen RP, Earley CJ. 2001. Restless legs syndrome: A review of clinical and pathophysiologic features. *Journal of Clinical Neurophysiology* 18(2):128–147.

Allen RP, Barker PB, Wehrl F, Song HK, Earley CJ. 2001. MRI measurement of brain iron in patients with restless legs syndrome. *Neurology* 56(2):263–265.

Allen RP, Picchietti D, Hening WA, Trenkwalder C. 2003. Restless legs syndrome: Diagnostic criteria, special considerations, and epidemiology. A report from the restless legs syndrome diagnosis and epidemiology workshop at the National Institutes of Health. *Sleep Medicine* 4(2):101–119.

Alvarez B, Dahlitz MJ, Vignau J, Parkes JD. 1992. The delayed sleep phase syndrome: Clinical and investigative findings in 14 subjects. *Journal of Neurology, Neurosurgery, and Psychiatry* 55(8):665–670.

American Academy of Pediatrics Task Force on Sudden Infant Death Syndrome. 2005. The changing concept of sudden infant death syndrome: Diagnostic coding shifts, controversies regarding the sleeping environment, and new variables to consider in reducing risk. *Pediatrics* 116(5):1245–1255.

Amin RS, Carroll JL, Jeffries JL, Grone C, Bean JA, Chini B, Bokulic R, Daniels SR. 2004. Twenty-four-hour ambulatory blood pressure in children with sleep-disordered breathing. *American Journal of Respiratory and Critical Care Medicine* 169(8):950–956.

Amin RS, Kimball TR, Kalra M, Jeffries JL, Carroll JL, Bean JA, Witt SA, Glascock BJ, Daniels SR. 2005. Left ventricular function in children with sleep-disordered breathing. *American Journal of Cardiology* 95(6):801–804.

Ancoli-Israel S, Kripke DF, Klauber MR, Mason WJ, Fell R, Kaplan O. 1991. Sleep-disordered breathing in community-dwelling elderly. *Sleep* 14(6):486–495.

Ancoli-Israel S, Kripke DF, Klauber MR, Parker L, Stepnowsky C, Kullen A, Fell R. 1993. Natural history of sleep-disordered breathing in community dwelling elderly. *Sleep* 16(8 suppl):S25–S29.

Ancoli-Israel S, Klauber MR, Stepnowsky C, Estline E, Chinn A, Fell R. 1995. Sleep-disordered breathing in African-American elderly. *American Journal of Respiratory Critical Care Medicine* 152(6 Pt 1):1946–1949.

Ancoli-Israel S, Kripke DF, Klauber MR, Fell R, Stepnowsky C, Estline E, Khazeni N, Chinn A. 1996. Morbidity, mortality and sleep-disordered breathing in community dwelling elderly. *Sleep* 19(4):277–282.

Ando K, Kripke DF, Ancoli-Israel S. 1995. Estimated prevalence of delayed and advanced sleep phase syndromes. *Sleep Research* 24:509.

Andreas S, Schulz R, Werner GS, Kreuzer H. 1996. Prevalence of obstructive sleep apnoea in patients with coronary artery disease. *Coronary Artery Disease* 7(7):541–545.

Anic-Labat S, Guilleminault C, Kraemer HC, Meehan J, Arrigoni J, Mignot E. 1999. Validation of a cataplexy questionnaire in 983 sleep-disorders patients. *Sleep* 22(1): 77–87.

APA (American Psychiatric Association). 1994. *Diagnostic and Statistical Manual of Mental Disorders: DSM-IV*. 4th ed. Washington, DC: American Psychiatric Association.

Applegate CD, Burchfiel JL, Konkol RJ. 1986. Kindling antagonism: Effects of norepinephrine depletion on kindled seizure suppression after concurrent, alternate stimulation in rats. *Experiments in Neurology* 94(2):379–390.

Arand D, Bonnet M, Hurwitz T, Mitler M, Rosa R, Sangal RB. 2005. The clinical use of the MSLT and MWT. *Sleep* 28(1):123–144.

Archer SN, Robilliard DL, Skene DJ, Smits M, Williams A, Arendt J, von Schantz M. 2003. A length polymorphism in the circadian clock gene Per3 is linked to delayed sleep phase syndrome and extreme diurnal preference. *Sleep* 26(4):413–415.

Arnulf I, Mabrouk T, Mohamed K, Konofal E, Derenne JP, Couratier P. 2005a. Stages 1-2 non-rapid eye movement sleep behavior disorder associated with dementia: A new parasomnia? *Movement Disorders* 20(9):1223–1228.

Arnulf I, Zeitzer JM, File J, Farber N, Mignot E. 2005b. Kleine-Levin syndrome: A systematic review of 186 cases in the literature. *Brain* 128(Pt 12):2763–2776.

Atkinson JH, Slater MA, Grant I, Patterson TL, Garfin SR. 1988. Depressed mood in chronic low back pain: Relationship with stressful life events. *Pain* 35(1): 47–55.

Ayas NT, White DP, Manson JE, Stampfer MJ, Speizer FE, Malhotra A, Hu FB. 2003. A prospective study of sleep duration and coronary heart disease in women. *Archives of Internal Medicine* 163(2):205–209.

Babu AR, Herdegen J, Fogelfeld L, Shott S, Mazzone T. 2005. Type 2 diabetes, glycemic control, and continuous positive airway pressure in obstructive sleep apnea. *Archives of Internal Medicine* 165(4):447–452.

Baldwin DC Jr, Daugherty SR. 2004. Sleep deprivation and fatigue in residency training: Results of a national survey of first- and second-year residents. *Sleep* 27(2):217–223.

Bamford CR. 1993. Carbamazepine in REM sleep behavior disorder. *Sleep* 16(1):33–34.

Bassetti CL. 2005. Sleep and stroke. In: Kryger MH, Roth T, Dement WC, eds. *Principles and Practice of Sleep Medicine*. 4th ed. Philadelphia: Elsevier/Saunders. Pp. 811–830.

Bassetti C, Aldrich MS. 1999. Sleep apnea in acute cerebrovascular diseases: Final report on 128 patients. *Sleep* 22(2):217–223.

Bassetti C, Aldrich MS, Chervin RD, Quint D. 1996. Sleep apnea in patients with transient ischemic attack and stroke: A prospective study of 59 patients. *Neurology* 47(5):1167–1173.

Behlfelt K. 1990. Enlarged tonsils and the effect of tonsillectomy. Characteristics of the dentition and facial skeleton. Posture of the head, hyoid bone and tongue. Mode of breathing. *Swedish Dental Journal: Supplement* 72:1–35.

Benca RM. 2005a. Diagnosis and treatment of chronic insomnia: A review. *Psychiatry Services* 56(3):332–343.

Benca RM. 2005b. Mood disorder. In: Kryger MH, Roth T, Dement WC, eds. *Principles and Practice of Sleep Medicine*. 4th ed. Philadelphia: Elsevier/Saunders. Pp. 1311–1326.

Berger AM, Higginbotham P. 2000. Correlates of fatigue during and following adjuvant breast cancer chemotherapy: A pilot study. *Oncology Nursing Forum* 27(9):1443–1448.

Bergonzi P, Chiurulla C, Gambi D, Mennuni G, Pinto F. 1975. L-dopa plus dopa-decarboxylase inhibitor. Sleep organization in Parkinson's syndrome before and after treatment. *Acta Neurologica Belgica* 75(1):5–10.

Bertrand B, Jamart J, Marchal JL, Arendt C. 1996. Cetirizine and pseudoephedrine retard alone and in combination in the treatment of perennial allergic rhinitis: A double-blind multicentre study. *Rhinology* 34(2):91–96.

Beszterczey A, Lipowski ZJ. 1977. Insomnia in cancer patients. *Canadian Medical Association Journal* 116(4):355.

Billiard M, Cadilhac J. 1988. Recurrent hypersomnia [in French]. *Revue Neurologique* 144(4):249–258.

Billiard M, Dauvilliers Y. 2001. Idiopathic hypersomnia. *Sleep Medicine Reviews* 5(5):349–358.

Billiard M, Dolenc L, Aldaz C, Ondze B, Besset A. 1994. Hypersomnia associated with mood disorders: A new perspective. *Journal of Psychosomatic Research* 38(suppl 1):41–47.

Bixler EO, Vgontzas AN, Ten Have T, Tyson K, Kales A. 1998. Effects of age on sleep apnea in men: I. Prevalence and severity. *American Journal of Respiratory and Critical Care Medicine* 157(1):144–148.

Bixler EO, Vgontzas AN, Lin HM, Ten Have T, Leiby BE, Vela-Bueno A, Kales A. 2000. Association of hypertension and sleep-disordered breathing. *Archives of Internal Medicine* 160(15):2289–2295.

Bixler EO, Vgontzas AN, Lin HM, Ten Have T, Rein J, Vela-Bueno A, Kales A. 2001. Prevalence of sleep-disordered breathing in women: Effects of gender. *American Journal of Respiratory and Critical Care Medicine* 163(3 Pt 1):608–613.

Bliwise DL. 2002. Sleep apnea, APOE4 and Alzheimer's disease: 20 years and counting? *Journal of Psychosomatic Research* 53(1):539–546.

Bliwise DL, Bliwise NG, Partinen M, Pursley AM, Dement WC. 1988. Sleep apnea and mortality in an aged cohort. *American Journal of Public Health* 78(5):544–547.

Bliwise DL, Kutner NG, Zhang R, Parker KP. 2001. Survival by time of day of hemodialysis in an elderly cohort. *Journal of the American Medical Association* 286(21):2690–2694.

Bonati MT, Ferini-Strambi L, Aridon P, Oldani A, Zucconi M, Casari G. 2003. Autosomal dominant restless legs syndrome maps on chromosome 14q. *Brain* 126(6):1485–1492.

Bonnet MH, Arand DL. 2003. Clinical effects of sleep fragmentation versus sleep deprivation. *Sleep Medicine Reviews* 7(4):297–310.

Born J, Zwick A, Roth G, Fehm-Wolfsdorf G, Fehm HL. 1987. Differential effects of hydrocortisone, fluocortolone, and aldosterone on nocturnal sleep in humans. *Acta Endocrinologica (Copenhagen)* 116(1):129–137.

Braak H, Ghebremedhin E, Rub U, Bratzke H, Del Tredici K. 2004. Stages in the development of Parkinson's disease-related pathology. *Cell and Tissue Research* 318(1):121–134.

Bradford RH, Shear CL, Chremos AN, Dujovne C, Downton M, Franklin FA, Gould AL, Hesney M, Higgins J, Hurley DP, et al. 1991. Expanded clinical evaluation of lovastatin (EXCEL) study results. I. Efficacy in modifying plasma lipoproteins and adverse event profile in 8245 patients with moderate hypercholesterolemia. *Archives of Internal Medicine* 151(1):43–49.

Bradley TD, Logan AG, Kimoff RJ, Series F, Morrison D, Ferguson K, Belenkie I, Pfeifer M, Fleetham J, Hanly P, Smilovitch M, Tomlinson G, Floras JS. 2005. Continuous positive airway pressure for central sleep apnea and heart failure. *New England Journal of Medicine* 353(19):2025–2033.

Breslau N, Roth T, Rosenthal L, Andreski P. 1996. Sleep disturbance and psychiatric disorders: A longitudinal epidemiological study of young adults. *Biological Psychiatry* 39(6): 411–418.

Brodeur C, Montplaisir J, Godbout R, Marinier R. 1988. Treatment of restless legs syndrome and periodic movements during sleep with L-dopa: A double-blind, controlled study. *Neurology* 38(12):1845–1848.

Brodie MJ, Dichter MA. 1997. Established antiepileptic drugs. *Seizure* 6(3):159–174.

Broeckel JA, Jacobsen PB, Horton J, Balducci L, Lyman GH. 1998. Characteristics and correlates of fatigue after adjuvant chemotherapy for breast cancer. *Journal of Clinical Oncology* 16(5):1689–1696.

Brooks B, Cistulli PA, Borkman M, Ross G, McGhee S, Grunstein RR, Sullivan CE, Yue DK. 1994. Obstructive sleep apnea in obese noninsulin-dependent diabetic patients: Effect of continuous positive airway pressure treatment on insulin responsiveness. *Journal of Clinical Endocrinology and Metabolism* 79(6):1681–1685.

Broughton R, Baron R. 1978. Sleep patterns in the intensive care unit and on the ward after acute myocardial infarction. *Electroencephalography and Clinical Neurophysiology* 45(3):348–360.

Broughton RJ, Fleming JA, George CF, Hill JD, Kryger MH, Moldofsky H, Montplaisir JY, Morehouse RL, Moscovitch A, Murphy WF. 1997. Randomized, double-blind, placebo-controlled crossover trial of modafinil in the treatment of excessive daytime sleepiness in narcolepsy. *Neurology* 49(2):444–451.

Buguet A, Bourdon L, Bouteille B, Cespuglio R, Vincendeau P, Radomski MW, Dumas M. 2001. The duality of sleeping sickness: Focusing on sleep. *Sleep Medicine Reviews* 5(2):139–153.

Buxbaum SG, Elston RC, Tishler PV, Redline S. 2002. Genetics of the apnea hypopnea index in Caucasians and African Americans: I. Segregation analysis. *Genetic Epidemiology* 22(3):243–253.

Campbell SS, Dawson D, Anderson MW. 1993. Alleviation of sleep maintenance insomnia with timed exposure to bright light. *Journal of American Geriatric Society* 41(8):829–836.

Cantor CR, Stern MB. 2002. Dopamine agonists and sleep in Parkinson's disease. *Neurology* 58(4 Suppl 1):S71–S78.

Caples SM, Gami AS, Somers VK. 2005. Obstructive sleep apnea. *Annals of Internal Medicine* 142(3):187–197.

Capuron L, Ravaud A, Dantzer R. 2000. Early depressive symptoms in cancer patients receiving interleukin 2 and/or interferon alfa-2b therapy. *Journal of Clinical Oncology* 18(10): 2143–2151.

Capuron L, Gumnick JF, Musselman DL, Lawson DH, Reemsnyder A, Nemeroff CB, Miller AH. 2002. Neurobehavioral effects of interferon-alpha in cancer patients: Phenomenology and paroxetine responsiveness of symptom dimensions. *Neuropsychopharmacology* 26(5):643–652.

Carlsson GE, Moller A, Blomstrand C. 2003. Consequences of mild stroke in persons < 75 years—a 1-year follow-up. *Cerebrovascular Disease* 16(4):383–388.

Carpenter JS, Johnson D, Wagner L, Andrykowski M. 2002. Hot flashes and related outcomes in breast cancer survivors and matched comparison women. *Oncological Nursing Forum* 29(3): E16–E25.

Carskadon MA. 1990. Patterns of sleep and sleepiness in adolescents. *Pediatrician* 17(1):5–12.

Carskadon MA, Dement WC, Mitler MM, Roth T, Westbrook PR, Keenan S. 1986. Guidelines for the multiple sleep latency test (MSLT): A standard measure of sleepiness. *Sleep* 9(4):519–524.

Carskadon MA, Acebo C, Jenni OG. 2004. Regulation of adolescent sleep: Implications for behavior. *Annals of the New York Academy of Sciences* 1021:276–291.

CDC (Centers for Disease Control and Prevention). 2005. Percentage of adults who reported an average of ≤ 6 hours of sleep per 24-hour period, by sex and age group—United States, 1985 and 2004. *Morbidity and Mortality Weekly Report* 54(37):933.

CDC. 2006. *Sudden Infant Death Syndrome (SIDS)*. [Online]. Available: http://www.cdc.gov/SIDS/index.htm [accessed January 17, 2006].

Chang PP, Ford DE, Mead LA, Cooper-Patrick L, Klag MJ. 1997. Insomnia in young men and subsequent depression. The Johns Hopkins precursors study. *American Journal of Epidemiology* 146(2):105–114.

Chen S, Ondo WG, Rao S, Li L, Chen Q, Wang Q. 2004. Genomewide linkage scan identifies a novel susceptibility locus for restless legs syndrome on chromosome 9p. *American Journal of Human Genetics* 74(5):876–885.

Chervin RD, Archbold KH. 2001. Hyperactivity and polysomnographic findings in children evaluated for sleep-disordered breathing. *Sleep* 24(3):313–320.

Chervin RD, Hedger AK, Dillon JE, Pituch KJ, Panahi P, Dahl RE, Guilleminault C. 2002. Associations between symptoms of inattention, hyperactivity, restless legs, and periodic leg movements. *Sleep: Journal of Sleep Research and Sleep Medicine* 25(2):213–218.

Chin K, Nakamura T, Takahashi K, Sumi K, Ogawa Y, Masuzaki H, Muro S, Hattori N, Matsumoto H, Niimi A, Chiba T, Nakao K, Mishima M, Ohi M, Nakamura T. 2003. Effects of obstructive sleep apnea syndrome on serum aminotransferase levels in obese patients. *American Journal of Medicine* 114(5):370–376.

Chrisp P, Mammen GJ, Sorkin EM. 1991. Selegiline. A review of its pharmacology, symptomatic benefits and protective potential in Parkinson's disease. *Drugs and Aging* 1(3):228–248.

Cole MG, Dendukuri N. 2003. Risk factors for depression among elderly community subjects: A systematic review and meta-analysis. *American Journal of Psychiatry* 160(6):1147–1156.

Coleman RM. 1982. Periodic movements in sleep (nocturnal myoclonus) and restless legs syndrome. In: Guilleminault C, ed. *Sleep and Waking Disorders: Indications and Techniques*. Menlo Park, CA: Addison-Wesley. Pp. 265–295.

Comella CL, Nardine TM, Diederich NJ, Stebbins GT. 1998. Sleep-related violence, injury, and REM sleep behavior disorder in Parkinson's disease. *Neurology* 51(2):526–529.

Connor JR, Boyer PJ, Menzies SL, Dellinger B, Allen RP, Ondo WG, Earley CJ. 2003. Neuropathological examination suggests impaired brain iron acquisition in restless legs syndrome. *Neurology* 61(3):304–309.

Cronin AJ, Keifer JC, Davies MF, King TS, Bixler EO. 2001. Postoperative sleep disturbance: Influences of opioids and pain in humans. *Sleep* 24(1):39–44.

Czeisler CA, Richardson GS, Zimmerman JC, Moore-Ede MC, Weitzman ED. 1981. Entrainment of human circadian rhythms by light-dark cycles: A reassessment. *Photochemistry and Photobiology* 34(2): 239–247.

D'Alessandro R, Magelli C, Gamberini G, Bacchelli S, Cristina E, Magnani B, Lugaresi E. 1990. Snoring every night as a risk factor for myocardial infarction: A case-control study. *British Medical Journal* 300(6739):1557–1558.

Daley KC. 2004. Update on sudden infant death syndrome. *Current Opinion in Pediatrics* 16(2):227–232.

Dao TT, Lavigne GJ, Charbonneau A, Feine JS, Lund JP. 1994. The efficacy of oral splints in the treatment of myofascial pain of the jaw muscles: A controlled clinical trial. *Pain* 56(1):85–94.

Darko DF, Mitler MM, Henriksen SJ. 1995. Lentiviral infection, immune response peptides and sleep. *Advances in Neuroimmunology* 5(1): 57–77.

Dauvilliers Y, Touchon J. 2001. Sleep in fibromyalgia: Review of clinical and polysomnographic data [in French]. *Neurophysiologie Clinique* 31(1):18–33.

116   SLEEP DISORDERS AND SLEEP DEPRIVATION

Dauvilliers Y, Morin C, Cervena K, Carlander B, Touchon J, Besset A, Billiard M. 2005. Family studies in insomnia. *Journal of Psychosomatic Research* 58(3):271–278.

Dawson D, Encel N. 1993. Melatonin and sleep in humans. *Journal of Pineal Research* 15(1): 1–12.

de Rijk MC, Tzourio C, Breteler MM, Dartigues JF, Amaducci L, Lopez-Pousa S, Manubens-Bertran JM, Alperovitch A, Rocca WA. 1997. Prevalence of parkinsonism and Parkinson's disease in Europe: The EUROPARKINSON Collaborative Study. European Community Concerted Action on the Epidemiology of Parkinson's disease. *Journal of Neurology, Neurosurgery, and Psychiatry* 62(1):10–15.

Desautels A, Turecki G, Montplaisir J, Sequeira A, Verner A, Rouleau GA. 2001. Identification of a major susceptibility locus for restless legs syndrome on chromosome 12q. *American Journal of Human Genetics* 69(6):1266–1270.

Diaz J, Sempere AP. 2004. Cerebral ischemia: New risk factors. *Cerebrovascular Disease* 17(suppl 1):43–50.

Dinges DF, Pack F, Williams K, Gillen KA, Powell JW, Ott GE, Aptowicz C, Pack AI. 1997. Cumulative sleepiness, mood disturbance, and psychomotor vigilance performance decrements during a week of sleep restricted to 4–5 hours per night. *Sleep* 20(4):267–277.

Dinges D, Ball E, Fredrickson P, Kiley J, Kryger MH, Richardson GS, Rogus S, Sheldon S, Wooten V, Zepf B. 1999. Recognizing problem sleepiness in your patients. *American Family Physician* 59(4):937–944.

Dinges D, Rogers N, Baynard. 2005. Chronic sleep deprivation. In: Kryger MH, Roth T, Dement WC, eds. *Principles and Practice of Sleep Medicine*. 4th ed. Philadelphia: Elsevier/Saunders. Pp. 67–76.

Doherty LS, Kiely JL, Swan V, McNicholas WT. 2005. Long-term effects of nasal continuous positive airway pressure therapy on cardiovascular outcomes in sleep apnea syndrome. *Chest* 127(6):2076–2084.

Drake CL, Roehrs T, Richardson G, Walsh JK, Roth T. 2004. Shift work sleep disorder: Prevalence and consequences beyond that of symptomatic day workers. *Sleep* 27(8):1453–1462.

Dreifuss FE, Porter RJ. 1997. Choice of antiepileptic drugs. In: Engel J, Pedley TA, eds. *Epilepsy: A Comprehensive Textbook*. Philadelphia: Lippincott-Raven. Pp. 1233–1236.

Dunlop RJ, Campbell CW. 2000. Cytokines and advanced cancer. *Journal of Pain and Symptom Management* 20(3):214–232.

Duran J, Esnaola S, Rubio R, Iztueta A. 2001. Obstructive sleep apnea-hypopnea and related clinical features in a population-based sample of subjects aged 30 to 70 yr. *American Journal of Respiratory and Critical Care Medicine* 163(3):685–689.

Dwyer T, Ponsonby AL, Newman NM, Gibbons LE. 1991. Prospective cohort study of prone sleeping position and sudden infant death syndrome. *Lancet* 337(8752):1244–1247.

Dyken ME, Somers VK, Yamada T, Ren ZY, Zimmerman MB. 1996. Investigating the relationship between stroke and obstructive sleep apnea. *Stroke* 27(3):401–407.

Eaker ED, Pinsky J, Castelli WP. 1992. Myocardial infarction and coronary death among women: Psychosocial predictors from a 20-year follow-up of women in the Framingham Study. *American Journal of Epidemiology* 135(8):854–864.

Edinger JD, Means MK. 2005. Overview of insomnia: Definitions, epidemiology, differential diagnosis, and assessment. In: Kryger MH, Roth T, Dement WC, eds. *Principles and Practice of Sleep Medicine*. 4th ed. Philadelphia: Elsevier/Saunders. Pp. 702–713.

Ekbom KA. 1945. Restless legs. *Acta Medica Scandinavia Supplement* 158:1–123.

Fantini ML, Gagnon JF, Filipini D, Montplaisir J. 2003. The effects of pramipexole in REM sleep behavior disorder. *Neurology* 61(10):1418–1420.

Faulx MD, Larkin EK, Hoit BD, Aylor JE, Wright AT, Redline S. 2004. Sex influences endothelial function in sleep-disordered breathing. *Sleep* 27(6):1113–1120.

Fava M. 2004. Daytime sleepiness and insomnia as correlates of depression. *Journal of Clinical Psychiatry* 65(suppl 16):27–32.

Fawcett J, Scheftner WA, Fogg L, Clark DC, Young MA, Hedeker D, Gibbons R. 1990. Time-related predictors of suicide in major affective disorder. *American Journal of Psychiatry* 147(9):1189–1194.

Ferguson KA, Lowe AA. 2005. Oral appliances for sleep-disordered breathing. In: Kryger MH, Roth T, Dement WC, eds. *Principles and Practice of Sleep Medicine*. 4th ed. Philadelphia: Elsevier/Saunders. Pp. 1098–1108.

Ferguson KA, Ono T, Lowe AA, Ryan CF, Fleetham JA. 1995. The relationship between obesity and craniofacial structure in obstructive sleep apnea. *Chest* 108(2):375–381.

Fisher C, Byrne J, Edwards A, Kahn E. 1970. A psychophysiological study of nightmares. *Journal of American Psychoanalysis Association* 18(4):747–782.

Foley DJ, Monjan AA, Brown SL, Simonsick EM, Wallace RB, Blazer DG. 1995. Sleep complaints among elderly persons: An epidemiologic study of three communities. *Sleep* 18(6):425–432.

Foley DJ, Masaki K, White L, Larkin EK, Monjan A, Redline S. 2003. Sleep-disordered breathing and cognitive impairment in elderly Japanese-American men. *Sleep* 26(5):596–599.

Folstein MF, Folstein SE, McHugh PR. 1975. "Mini-mental state". A practical method for grading the cognitive state of patients for the clinician. *Journal of Psychiatric Research* 12(3):189–198.

Foo H, Mason P. 2003. Brainstem modulation of pain during sleep and waking. *Sleep Medicine Reviews* 7(2):145–154.

Ford DE, Kamerow DB. 1989. Epidemiologic study of sleep disturbances and psychiatric disorders. An opportunity for prevention? *Journal of the American Medical Association* 262(11):1479–1484.

Fredriksen K, Rhodes J, Reddy R, Way N. 2004. Sleepless in Chicago: Tracking the effects of adolescent sleep loss during the middle school years. *Child Development* 75(1):84–95.

Friedland RP, Brun A, Budinger TF. 1985. Pathological and positron emission tomographic correlations in Alzheimer's disease. *Lancet* 1(8422):228.

Gagnon JF, Bedard MA, Fantini ML, Petit D, Panisset M, Rompre S, Carrier J, Montplaisir J. 2002. REM sleep behavior disorder and REM sleep without atonia in Parkinson's disease. *Neurology* 59(4):585–589.

Gami AS, Howard DE, Olson EJ, Somers VK. 2005. Day-night pattern of sudden death in obstructive sleep apnea. *New England Journal of Medicine* 352(12):1206–1214.

Garrick NA, Tamarkin L, Taylor PL, Markey SP, Murphy DL. 1983. Light and propranolol suppress the nocturnal elevation of serotonin in the cerebrospinal fluid of rhesus monkeys. *Science* 221(4609):474–476.

Giles DE, Kupfer DJ, Rush AJ, Roffwarg HP. 1998. Controlled comparison of electrophysiological sleep in families of probands with unipolar depression. *American Journal of Psychiatry* 155(2):192–199.

Gislason T, Benediktsdottir B. 1995. Snoring, apneic episodes, and nocturnal hypoxemia among children 6 months to 6 years old. An epidemiologic study of lower limit of prevalence. *Chest* 107(4):963–966.

Good DC, Henkle JQ, Gelber D, Welsh J, Verhulst S. 1996. Sleep-disordered breathing and poor functional outcome after stroke. *Stroke* 27(2):252–259.

Gottlieb DJ, Punjabi NM, Newman AB, Resnick HE, Redline S, Baldwin CM, Nieto FJ. 2005. Association of sleep time with diabetes mellitus and impaired glucose tolerance. *Archives of Internal Medicine* 165(8):863–867.

Gronfier C, Wright KP Jr, Kronauer RE, Jewett ME, Czeisler CA. 2004. Efficacy of a single sequence of intermittent bright light pulses for delaying circadian phase in humans. *American Journal of Physiology—Endocrinology and Metabolism* 287(1):174–181.

Grunstein R. 2005a. Continuous positive airway pressure treatment for obstructive sleep apnea-hypopnea syndrome. In: Kryger MH, Roth T, Dement WC, eds. *Principles and Practice of Sleep Medicine.* 4th ed. Philadelphia: Elsevier/Saunders. Pp. 1066–1080.

Grunstein R. 2005b. Endocrine disorders. In: Kryger MH, Roth T, Dement WC, eds. *Principles and Practice of Sleep Medicine.* 4th ed. Philadelphia: Elsevier/Saunders. Pp. 1237–1245.

Grunstein R, Wilcox I, Yang TS, Gould Y, Hedner J. 1993. Snoring and sleep apnoea in men: Association with central obesity and hypertension. *International Journal of Obesity-Related Metabolic Disorders* 17(9):533–540.

Guilleminault C, Connolly SJ, Winkle RA. 1983. Cardiac arrhythmia and conduction disturbances during sleep in 400 patients with sleep apnea syndrome. *American Journal of Cardiology* 52(5):490–494.

Guilleminault C, Partinen M, Hollman K, Powell N, Stoohs R. 1995. Familial aggregates in obstructive sleep apnea syndrome. *Chest* 107(6):1545–1551.

Gupta NK, Mueller WH, Chan W, Meininger JC. 2002. Is obesity associated with poor sleep quality in adolescents? *American Journal of Human Biology* 14(6):762–768.

Hajak G, Muller WE, Wittchen HU, Pittrow D, Kirch W. 2003. Abuse and dependence potential for the non-benzodiazepine hypnotics Zolpidem and Zopiclone: A review of case reports and epidemiological data. *Addiction* 98(10):1371–1378.

Halasz P, Ujszaszi J, Gadoros J. 1985. Are microarousals preceded by electroencephalographic slow wave synchronization precursors of confusional awakenings? *Sleep* 8(3):231–238.

Haponik EF. 1992. Sleep disturbances of older persons: Physicians' attitudes. *Sleep* 15(2):168–172.

Harma M, Tenkanen L, Sjoblom T, Alikoski T, Heinsalmi P. 1998. Combined effects of shift work and life-style on the prevalence of insomnia, sleep deprivation and daytime sleepiness. *Scandinavian Journal of Work, Environment and Health* 24(4):300–307.

Harsch IA, Schahin SP, Radespiel-Troger M, Weintz O, Jahreiss H, Fuchs FS, Wiest GH, Hahn EG, Lohmann T, Konturek PC, Ficker JH. 2004. Continuous positive airway pressure treatment rapidly improves insulin sensitivity in patients with obstructive sleep apnea syndrome. *American Journal of Respiratory and Critical Care Medicine* 169(2):156–162.

Harstall C, Ospina M. 2003. How prevalent is chronic pain? *Pain: Clinical Updates* 11(2):1–4.

Harvey AG. 2000. Sleep hygiene and sleep-onset insomnia. *Journal of Nervous and Mental Disease* 188(1):53–55.

Hasler G, Buysse DJ, Klaghofer R, Gamma A, Ajdacic V, Eich D, Rossler W, Angst J. 2004. The association between short sleep duration and obesity in young adults: A 13-year prospective study. *Sleep* 27(4):661–666.

Hasler G, Buysse DJ, Gamma A, Ajdacic V, Eich D, Rossler W, Angst J. 2005. Excessive daytime sleepiness in young adults: A 20-year prospective community study. *Journal of Clinical Psychiatry* 66(4):521–529.

Hauck FR, Kemp JS. 1998. Bedsharing promotes breastfeeding and AAP Task Force on Infant Positioning and SIDS. *Pediatrics* 102(3 Pt 1):662–664.

Hauck FR, Herman SM, Donovan M, Iyasu S, Merrick MC, Donoghue E, Kirschner RH, Willinger M. 2003. Sleep environment and the risk of sudden infant death syndrome in an urban population: The Chicago Infant Mortality Study. *Pediatrics* 111(5 Part 2):1207–1214.

Hauri PJ. 1997. Can we mix behavioral therapy with hypnotics when treating insomniacs? *Sleep* 20(12):1111–1118.

He J, Kryger MH, Zorick FJ, Conway W, Roth T. 1988. Mortality and apnea index in obstructive sleep apnea. Experience in 385 male patients. *Chest* 94(1):9–14.

Hening WA, Allen RP, Earley CJ, Picchietti DL, Silber MH, Restless Legs Syndrome Task Force of the Standards of Practice Committee of the American Academy of Sleep Medicine. 2004. An update on the dopaminergic treatment of restless legs syndrome and periodic limb movement disorder. *Sleep* 27(3):560–583.

Hermida RC, Smolensky MH. 2004. Chronotherapy of hypertension. *Current Opinion in Nephrology and Hypertension* 13(5):501–505.

Hilleman D, Miller MA, Parker R, Doering P, Pieper JA. 1998. Optimal management of amiodarone therapy: Efficacy and side effects. *Pharmacotherapy* 18(6 Pt 2):138S–145S.

Hohagen F, Rink K, Kappler C, Schramm E, Riemann D, Weyerer S, Berger M. 1993. Prevalence and treatment of insomnia in general practice. A longitudinal study. *European Archives of Psychiatry and Clinical Neuroscience* 242(6):329–336.

Hohjoh H, Takasu M, Shishikura K, Takahashi Y, Honda Y, Tokunaga K. 2003. Significant association of the arylalkylamine N-acetyltransferase (AA-NAT) gene with delayed sleep phase syndrome. *Neurogenetics* 4(3):151–153.

Holmes MD, Chang M, Kapur V. 2003. Sleep apnea and excessive daytime somnolence induced by vagal nerve stimulation. *Neurology* 61(8):1126–1129.

Hu FB, Willett WC, Manson JE, Colditz GA, Rimm EB , Speizer FE, Hennekens CH, Stampfer MJ. 2000. Snoring and risk of cardiovascular disease in women. *Journal of the American College of Cardiologist* 35(2):308–313.

Hublin C, Kaprio J, Partinen M, Heikkila K, Koskenvuo M. 1997. Prevalence and genetics of sleepwalking: A population-based twin study. *Neurology* 48(1):177–181.

Hung J, Whitford EG, Parsons RW, Hillman DR. 1990. Association of sleep apnoea with myocardial infarction in men. *Lancet* 336(8710):261–264.

Ip MS, Lam B, Ng MM, Lam WK, Tsang KW, Lam KS. 2002. Obstructive sleep apnea is independently associated with insulin resistance. *American Journal of Respiratory and Critical Care Medicine* 165(5):670–676.

Irgens LM, Markestad T, Baste V, Schreuder P, Skjaerven R, Oyen N. 1995. Sleeping position and sudden infant death syndrome in Norway 1967-91. *Archives of Disease in Childhood* 72(6):478–482.

Iwase T, Kajimura N, Uchiyama M, Ebisawa T, Yoshimura K. 2002. Mutation screening of the human CLOCK gene in circadian rhythm sleep disorders. *Psychiatry Research* 109(2):121–128.

Iyasu S, Randall LL, Welty TK, Hsia J, Kinney HC, Mandell F, McClain M, Randall B, Habbe D, Wilson H, Willinger M. 2002. Risk factors for sudden infant death syndrome among northern plains Indians. *Journal of the American Medical Association* 288(21):2717–2723.

Janz D. 1962. The grand mal epilepsies and the sleeping-waking cycle. *Epilepsia* 3:69–109.

Javaheri S, Parker TJ, Liming JD, Corbett WS, Nishiyama H, Wexler L, Roselle GA. 1998. Sleep apnea in 81 ambulatory male patients with stable heart failure: Types and their prevalences, consequences, and presentations. *Circulation* 97(21):2154–2159.

Jeans WD, Fernando DC, Maw AR, Leighton BC. 1981. A longitudinal study of the growth of the nasopharynx and its contents in normal children. *British Journal of Radiology* 54(638):117–121.

Jellinger K. 1986. Pathology of Parkinsonism. Fahn S, Marsden C, Goldstein M, Calne D, eds. *Recent Developments in Parkinson's Disease.* New York: Raven Press. Pp. 33–66.

Jennum P, Hein HO, Suadicani P, Gyntelberg F. 1995. Risk of ischemic heart disease in self-reported snorers. A prospective study of 2,937 men aged 54 to 74 years: The Copenhagen male study. *Chest* 108(1):138–142.

Johnson JG, Cohen P, Kasen S, First MB, Brook JS. 2004. Association between television viewing and sleep problems during adolescence and early adulthood. *Archives of Pediatrics and Adolescent Medicine* 158(6):562–568.

Jones BE. 2005. Basic mechanisms of sleep-wake states. In: Kryger MH, Roth T, Dement WC, eds. *Principles and Practice of Sleep Medicine*. 4th ed. Philadelphia: Elsevier/Saunders. Pp. 136–153.

Jones CR, Campbell SS, Zone SE, Cooper F, DeSano A, Murphy PJ, Jones B, Czajkowski L, Ptacek LJ. 1999. Familial advanced sleep-phase syndrome: A short-period circadian rhythm variant in humans. *Nature Medicine* 5(9):1062–1065.

Juji T, Satake M, Honda Y, Doi Y. 1984. HLA antigens in Japanese patients with narcolepsy. All the patients were DR2 positive. *Tissue Antigens* 24(5):316–319.

Kaakkola S. 2000. Clinical pharmacology, therapeutic use and potential of COMT inhibitors in Parkinson's disease. *Drugs* 59(6):1233–1250.

Kales A, Ansel RD, Markham CH, Scharf MB, Tan TL. 1971. Sleep in patients with Parkinson's disease and normal subjects prior to and following levodopa administration. *Clinical Pharmacology and Therapeutics* 12(2):397–406.

Kalra M, Inge T, Garcia V, Daniels S, Lawson L, Curti R, Cohen A, Amin R. 2005. Obstructive sleep apnea in extremely overweight adolescents undergoing bariatric surgery. *Obesity Research* 13(7):1175–1179.

Kanbayashi T, Inoue Y, Chiba S, Aizawa R, Saito Y, Tsukamoto H, Fujii Y, Nishino S, Shimizu T. 2002. CSF hypocretin-1 (orexin-A) concentrations in narcolepsy with and without cataplexy and idiopathic hypersomnia. *Journal of Sleep Research* 11(1):91–93.

Kaplan J, Fredrickson PA, Renaux SA, O'Brien PC. 1993. Theophylline effect on sleep in normal subjects. *Chest* 103(1):193–195.

Kapsimalis F, Kryger MH. 2002. Gender and obstructive sleep apnea syndrome, part 1: Clinical features. *Sleep* 25(4):412–419.

Kapur VK, Redline S, Nieto F, Young TB, Newman AB, Henderson JA. 2002. The relationship between chronically disrupted sleep and healthcare use. *Sleep* 25(3):289–296.

Katz DA, McHorney CA. 1998. Clinical correlates of insomnia in patients with chronic illness. *Archives of Internal Medicine* 158(10):1099–1107.

Katz I, Stradling J, Slutsky AS, Zamel N, Hoffstein V. 1990. Do patients with obstructive sleep apnea have thick necks? *American Review of Respiratory Disease* 141(5 Pt 1):1228–1231.

Keech AC, Armitage JM, Wallendszus KR, Lawson A, Hauer AJ, Parish SE, Collins R. 1996. Absence of effects of prolonged simvastatin therapy on nocturnal sleep in a large randomized placebo-controlled study. Oxford Cholesterol Study Group. *British Journal of Clinical Pharmacology* 42(4):483–490.

Kemp JS, Thach BT. 1991. Sudden death in infants sleeping on polystyrene-filled cushions. *New England Journal of Medicine* 324(26):1858–1864.

Kinney HC, Filiano JJ, Sleeper LA, Mandell F, Valdes-Dapena M, White WF. 1995. Decreased muscarinic receptor binding in the arcuate nucleus in sudden infant death syndrome. *Science* 269(5229):1446–1450.

Klackenberg G. 1982. Somnambulism in childhood—prevalence, course and behavioral correlations. A prospective longitudinal study (6–16 years). *Acta Paediatrica Scandinavia* 71(3):495–499.

Kleitman N. 1987. *Sleep and Wakefulness*. Chicago: University of Chicago Press.

Klerman EB, Dijk DJ. 2005. Interindividual variation in sleep duration and its association with sleep debt in young adults. *Sleep* 28(10):1253–1259.

Konsman JP, Parnet P, Dantzer R. 2002. Cytokine-induced sickness behaviour: Mechanisms and implications. *Trends in Neuroscience* 25(3):154–159.

Krahn LE. 2005. Psychiatric disorders associated with disturbed sleep. *Seminars in Neurology* 25(1):90–96.

Krahn LE, Pankratz VS, Oliver L, Boeve BF, Silber MH. 2002. Hypocretin (orexin) levels in cerebrospinal fluid of patients with narcolepsy: Relationship to cataplexy and HLA DQB1*0602 status. *Sleep* 25(7):733–736.

Kripke DF, Ancoli-Israel S, Klauber MR, Wingard DL, Mason WJ, Mullaney DJ. 1997. Prevalence of sleep-disordered breathing in ages 40-64 years: A population-based survey. *Sleep* 20(1):65–76.

Kripke DF, Garfinkel L, Wingard DL, Klauber MR, Marler MR. 2002. Mortality associated with sleep duration and insomnia. *Archives in General Psychiatry* 59(2):131–136.

Kryger MH, Otake K, Foerster J. 2002. Low body stores of iron and restless legs syndrome: A correctable cause of insomnia in adolescents and teenagers. *Sleep Medicine* 3(2):127–132.

Kryger MH, Shepertycky M, Foerster J, Manfreda J. 2003. Sleep disorders in repeat blood donors. *Sleep* 26(5):625–626.

Kshatri AM, Baghdoyan HA, Lydic R. 1998. Cholinomimetics, but not morphine, increase antinociceptive behavior from pontine reticular regions regulating rapid-eye-movement sleep. *Sleep* 21(7):677–685.

Lake CR, Rosenberg DB, Gallant S, Zaloga G, Chernow B. 1990. Phenylpropanolamine increases plasma caffeine levels. *Clinical Pharmacology and Therapeutics* 47(6):675–685.

Lammers GJ, Overeem S. 2003. Pharmacological management of narcolepsy. *Expert Opinions in Pharmacotherapy* 4(10):1739–1746.

Larkin EK, Rosen CL, Kirchner HL, Storfer-Isser A, Emancipator JL, Johnson NL, Zambito AM, Tracy RP, Jenny NS, Redline S. 2005. Variation of C-reactive protein levels in adolescents: Association with sleep-disordered breathing and sleep duration. *Circulation* 111(15):1978–1984.

Lavie P, Lavie L, Herer P. 2005. All-cause mortality in males with sleep apnoea syndrome: Declining mortality rates with age. *European Respiratory Journal* 25(3):514–520.

Lavigne GJ, Montplaisir JY. 1994. Restless legs syndrome and sleep bruxism: Prevalence and association among Canadians. *Sleep* 17(8):739–743.

Lavigne GL, McMillan D, Zucconi M. 2005. Pain and sleep. In: Kryger MH, Roth T, Dement WC, eds. *Principles and Practice of Sleep Medicine*. 4th ed. Philadelphia: Elsevier Saunders. Pp. 1246–1255.

Lee KA, Zaffke ME, Baratte-Beebe K. 2001. Restless legs syndrome and sleep disturbance during pregnancy: The role of folate and iron. *Journal of Women's Health and Gender-based Medicine* 10(4):335–341.

Lee KA, Landis C, Chasens ER, Dowling G, Merritt S, Parker KP, Redeker N, Richards KC, Rogers AE, Shaver JF, Umlauf MG, Weaver TE. 2004. Sleep and chronobiology: Recommendations for nursing education. *Nursing Outlook* 52(3):126–133.

Leeman AL, O'Neill CJ, Nicholson PW, Deshmukh AA, Denham MJ, Royston JP, Dobbs RJ, Dobbs SM. 1987. Parkinson's disease in the elderly: Response to and optimal spacing of night time dosing with levodopa. *British Journal of Clinical Pharmacology* 24(5):637–643.

Levi F. 1994. Chronotherapy of cancer: Biological basis and clinical application [in French]. *Pathologie-Biologie (Paris)* 42(4):338–341.

Lewy AJ, Ahmed S, Sack RL. 1996. Phase shifting the human circadian clock using melatonin. *Behavioural Brain Research* 73(1–2):131–134.

Li KK, Kushida C, Powell NB, Riley RW, Guilleminault C. 2000. Obstructive sleep apnea syndrome: A comparison between Far-East Asian and white men. *Laryngoscope* 110(10 Pt 1):1689–1693.

Lindberg E, Janson C, Svardsudd K, Gislason T, Hetta J, Boman G. 1998. Increased mortality among sleepy snorers: A prospective population-based study. *Thorax* 53(8):631–637.

Lingjaerde O, Bratlid T, Hansen T. 1985. Insomnia during the "dark period" in northern Norway. An explorative, controlled trial with light treatment. *Acta Psychiatrica Scandinavia* 71(5):506–512.

Liu X. 2004. Sleep and adolescent suicidal behavior. *Sleep* 27(7):1351–1358.

Liu X, Uchiyama M, Kim K, Okawa M, Shibui K, Kudo Y, Doi Y, Minowa M, Ogihara R. 2000. Sleep loss and daytime sleepiness in the general adult population of Japan. *Psychiatry Research* 93(1):1–11.

Liu Y, Tanaka H, Fukuoka Heart Study Group. 2002. Overtime work, insufficient sleep, and risk of non-fatal acute myocardial infarction in Japanese men. *Occupational and Environmental Medicine* 59(7):447–451.

Livingston G, Blizard B, Mann A. 1993. Does sleep disturbance predict depression in elderly people? A study in inner London. *British Journal of General Practice* 43(376): 445–448.

Locard E, Mamelle N, Billette A, Miginiac M, Munoz F, Rey S. 1992. Risk factors of obesity in a five-year-old population: Parental versus environmental factors. *International Journal of Obesity and Related Metabolic Disorders* 16(10):721–729.

Lundkvist GB, Kristensson K, Bentivoglio M. 2004. Why trypanosomes cause sleeping sickness. *Physiology (Bethesda)* 19(4):198–206.

Mahowald MW, Ettinger MG. 1990. Things that go bump in the night: The parasomnias revisited. *Journal of Clinical Neurophysiology* 7(1):119–143.

Mahowald MW, Schenck CH. 2005. Insights from studying human sleep disorders. *Nature* 437(7063):1279–1285.

Malloy MH, Hoffman HJ. 1995. Prematurity, sudden infant death syndrome, and age of death. *Pediatrics* 96(3 Pt 1):464–471.

Marcus CL, Greene MG, Carroll JL. 1998. Blood pressure in children with obstructive sleep apnea. *American Journal of Respiratory and Critical Care Medicine* 157(4 Pt 1):1098–1103.

Marcus CL, Chapman D, Ward SD, McColley SA, Herrerias CT, Stillwell PC, Howenstine M, Light MJ, McColley SA, Schaeffer DA, Wagener JS, Laskosz LN. 2002. Clinical practice guideline: Diagnosis and management of childhood obstructive sleep apnea syndrome. *Pediatrics* 109(4):704–712.

Marin JM, Carrizo SJ, Vicente E, Agusti AG. 2005. Long-term cardiovascular outcomes in men with obstructive sleep apnoea-hypopnoea with or without treatment with continuous positive airway pressure: An observational study. *Lancet* 365(9464):1046–1053.

Martin BC, Warram JH, Krolewski AS, Bergman RN, Soeldner JS, Kahn CR. 1992. Role of glucose and insulin resistance in development of type 2 diabetes mellitus: Results of a 25-year follow-up study. *Lancet* 340(8825):925–929.

McAinsh J, Cruickshank JM. 1990. Beta-blockers and central nervous system side effects. *Pharmacology and Therapeutics* 46(2):163–197.

McArdle N, Riha RL, Vennelle M, Coleman EL, Dennis MS, Warlow CP, Douglas NJ. 2003. Sleep-disordered breathing as a risk factor for cerebrovascular disease: A case-control study in patients with transient ischemic attacks. *Stroke* 34(12):2916–2921.

McClusky HY, Milby JB, Switzer PK, Williams V, Wooten V. 1991. Efficacy of behavioral versus triazolam treatment in persistent sleep-onset insomnia. *American Journal of Psychiatry* 148(1):121–126.

McCracken LM, Iverson GL. 2002. Disrupted sleep patterns and daily functioning in patients with chronic pain. *Pain Research and Management: The Journal of the Canadian Pain Society* 7(2):75–79.

Meier-Ewert HK, Ridker PM, Rifai N, Regan MM, Price NJ, Dinges DF, Mullington JM. 2004. Effect of sleep loss on C-reactive protein, an inflammatory marker of cardiovascular risk. *Journal of the American College of Cardiologists* 43(4):678–683.

Mellinger GD, Balter MB, Uhlenhuth EH. 1985. Insomnia and its treatment: Prevalence and correlates. *Archives of General Psychiatry* 42(3):225–232.

Meny RG, Carroll JL, Carbone MT, Kelly DH. 1994. Cardiorespiratory recordings from infants dying suddenly and unexpectedly at home. *Pediatrics* 93(1):44–49.

Miaskowski C, Lee KA. 1999. Pain, fatigue, and sleep disturbances in oncology outpatients receiving radiation therapy for bone metastasis: A pilot study. *Journal of Pain and Symptom Management* 17(5):320–332.

Michaud M, Chabli A, Lavigne G, Montplaisir J. 2000. Arm restlessness in patients with restless legs syndrome. *Movement Disorders* 15(2):289–293.

Mignot E. 1998. Genetic and familial aspects of narcolepsy. *Neurology* 50(2 suppl 1):S16–S22.

Mignot E. 2001. A hundred years of narcolepsy research. *Archives of Italian Biology* 139(3): 207–220.

Mignot E, Renaud A, Nishino S, Arrigoni J, Guilleminault C, Dement WC. 1993. Canine cataplexy is preferentially controlled by adrenergic mechanisms: Evidence using monoamine selective uptake inhibitors and release enhancers. *Psychopharmacology (Berlin)* 113(1):76–82.

Mignot E, Lammers GJ, Ripley B, Okun M, Nevsimalova S, Overeem S, Vankova J, Black J, Harsh J, Bassetti C, Schrader H, Nishino S. 2002a. The role of cerebrospinal fluid hypocretin measurement in the diagnosis of narcolepsy and other hypersomnias. *Archives of Neurology* 59(10):1553–1562.

Mignot E, Taheri S, Nishino S. 2002b. Sleeping with the hypothalamus: Emerging therapeutic targets for sleep disorders. *Nature Neuroscience* 5(suppl):1071–1075.

Mitler MM, O'Malley MB. 2005. Wake-promoting medications: Efficacy and adverse effects. In: Kryger MH, Roth T, Dement WC, eds. *Principles and Practice of Sleep Medicine*. 4th ed. Philadelphia: Elsevier/Saunders. Pp. 484–498.

Miyazaki S, Uchida S, Mukai J, Nishihara K. 2004. Clonidine effects on all-night human sleep: Opposite action of low- and medium-dose clonidine on human NREM-REM sleep proportion. *Psychiatry and Clinical Neuroscience* 58(2):138–144.

Moldofsky H. 2001. Sleep and pain. *Sleep Medicine Reviews* 5(5):385–396.

Mondini S, Guilleminault C. 1985. Abnormal breathing patterns during sleep in diabetes. *Annals of Neurology* 17(4):391–395.

Monk TH. 2005. Shift work: Basic principles. In: Kryger MH, Roth T, Dement WC, eds. *Principles and Practice of Sleep Medicine*. 4th ed. Philadelphia: Elsevier/Saunders. Pp. 673–679.

Monti JM, Hawkins M, Jantos H, D'Angelo L, Fernandez M. 1988. Biphasic effects of dopamine D-2 receptor agonists on sleep and wakefulness in the rat. *Psychopharmacology (Berlin)* 95(3):395–400.

Montplaisir J, Petit D, Lorrain D, Gauthier S, Nielsen T. 1995. Sleep in Alzheimer's disease: Further considerations on the role of brainstem and forebrain cholinergic populations in sleep-wake mechanisms. *Sleep* 18(3):145–148.

Montplaisir J, Petit D, McNamara D, Gauthier S. 1996. Comparisons between SPECT and quantitative EEG measures of cortical impairment in mild to moderate Alzheimer's disease. *European Neurology* 36(4):197–200.

Montplaisir J, Boucher S, Poirier G, Lavigne G, Lapierre O, Lesperance P. 1997. Clinical, polysomnographic, and genetic characteristics of restless legs syndrome: A study of 133 patients diagnosed with new standard criteria. *Movement Disorders* 12(1):61–65.

Montplaisir J, Allen RP, Walters AD, Lerini-Strambi L. 2005. Restless legs syndrome and periodic limb movements during sleep. In: Kryger MH, Roth T, Dement WC, eds. *Principles and Practice of Sleep Medicine*. 4th ed. Philadelphia: Elsevier/Saunders. Pp. 839–852.

Mooe T, Rabben T, Wiklund U, Franklin KA, Eriksson P. 1996a. Sleep-disordered breathing in men with coronary artery disease. *Chest* 109(3):659–663.

Mooe T, Rabben T, Wiklund U, Franklin KA, Eriksson P. 1996b. Sleep-disordered breathing in women: Occurrence and association with coronary artery disease. *American Journal of Medicine* 101(3):251–256.

Moran M, Lynch CA, Walsh C, Coen R, Coakley D, Lawlor BA. 2005. Sleep disturbance in mild to moderate Alzheimer's disease. *Sleep Medicine* 6(4):347–352.

Morin CM. 2005. Psychological and behavioral treatments for primary insomnia. In: Kryger MH, Roth T, Dement WC, eds. *Principles and Practice of Sleep Medicine.* 4th ed. Philadelphia: Elsevier/Saunders. Pp. 726–737.

Morin CM, Gibson D, Wade J. 1998. Self-reported sleep and mood disturbance in chronic pain patients. *Clinical Journal of Pain* 14(4):311–314.

Morin CM, Mimeault V, Gagne A. 1999. Nonpharmacological treatment of late-life insomnia. *Journal of Psychosomatic Research* 46(2):103–116.

Morrell MJ, Heywood P, Moosavi SH, Guz A, Stevens J. 1999. Unilateral focal lesions in the rostrolateral medulla influence chemosensitivity and breathing measured during wakefulness, sleep, and exercise. *Journal of Neurology, Neurosurgery, and Psychiatry* 67(5):637–645.

Morrison DN, Mcgee R, Stanton WR. 1992. Sleep problems in adolescence. *Journal of the American Academy of Child and Adolescent Psychiatry* 31(1):94–99.

Morton S, Rosen C, Larkin E, Tishler P, Aylor J, Redline S. 2001. Predictors of sleep-disordered breathing in children with a history of tonsillectomy and/or adenoidectomy. *Sleep* 24(7):823–829.

Moser NJ, Phillips BA, Berry DT, Harbison L. 1994. What is hypopnea, anyway? *Chest* 105(2):426–428.

Mourits MJ, De Vries EG, Willemse PH, Ten Hoor KA, Hollema H, Van der Zee AG. 2001. Tamoxifen treatment and gynecologic side effects: A review. *Obstetrics and Gynecology* 97(5 Pt 2):855–866.

Murdey ID, Cameron N, Biddle SJ, Marshall SJ, Gorely T. 2005. Short-term changes in sedentary behaviour during adolescence: Project STIL (Sedentary Teenagers and Inactive Lifestyles). *Annals of Human Biology* 32(3):283–296.

Murphy PJ, Badia P, Myers BL, Boecker MR, Wright KP Jr. 1994. Nonsteroidal anti-inflammatory drugs affect normal sleep patterns in humans. *Physiology and Behavior* 55(6):1063–1066.

Murphy PJ, Myers BL, Badia P. 1996. Nonsteroidal anti-inflammatory drugs alter body temperature and suppress melatonin in humans. *Physiology and Behavior* 59(1):133–139.

Namen AM, Wymer A, Case D, Haponik EF. 1999. Performance of sleep histories in an ambulatory medicine clinic: Impact of simple chart reminders. *Chest* 116(6):1558–1563.

Namen AM, Landry SH, Case LD, McCall WV, Dunagan DP, Haponik EF. 2001. Sleep histories are seldom documented on a general medical service. *Southern Medical Journal* 94(9):874–879.

Narkiewicz K, Somers VK. 2003. Sympathetic nerve activity in obstructive sleep apnoea. *Acta Physiologica Scandinavica* 177(3):385–390.

Narkiewicz K, Kato M, Phillips BG, Pesek CA, Davison DE, Somers VK. 1999. Nocturnal continuous positive airway pressure decreases daytime sympathetic traffic in obstructive sleep apnea. *Circulation* 100(23):2332–2335.

Netzer NC, Hoegel JJ, Loube D, Netzer CM, Hay B, Alvarez-Sala R, Strohl KP, Sleep in Primary Care International Study Group. 2003. Prevalence of symptoms and risk of sleep apnea in primary care. *Chest* 124(4):1406–1414.

Newman AB, Spiekerman CF, Enright P, Lefkowitz D, Manolio T, Reynolds CF, Robbins J. 2000. Daytime sleepiness predicts mortality and cardiovascular disease in older adults. The Cardiovascular Health Study Research Group. *Journal of the American Geriatric Society* 48(2):115–123.

NHLBI (National Heart, Lung, and Blood Institute). 2003. *National Sleep Disorders Research Plan, 2003.* Bethesda, MD: National Institutes of Health.

NICHD (National Institute of Child Health and Human Development). 2006a. *Safe Sleep for Your Baby: Ten Ways to Reduce the Risk of Sudden Infant Death Syndrome (SIDS)*. [Online]. Available: http://www.nichd.nih.gov/sids/reduce_infant_risk.htm [accessed January 17, 2006].

NICHD. 2006b. *SIDS Facts*. [Online]. Available: www.nichd.nih.gov/sids/PART_II.pdf [accessed March 13, 2006].

Nichols DA, Allen RP, Grauke JH, Brown JB, Rice ML, Hyde PR, Dement WC, Kushida CA. 2002. Restless legs syndrome symptoms in primary care: A prevalence study. *Archives of Internal Medicine* 163(18):2323–2329.

Nielsen TA, Zadra A. 2000. Dreaming disorders. In: Kryger MH, Roth T, Dement WC, eds. *Principles and Practice of Sleep Medicine*. 3rd ed. Philadelphia: Elsevier Saunders. Pp. 753–772.

Nieto FJ, Young TB, Lind BK, Shahar E, Samet JM, Redline S, D'Agostino RB, Newman AB, Lebowitz MD, Pickering TG. 2000. Association of sleep-disordered breathing, sleep apnea, and hypertension in a large community-based study. Sleep Heart Health Study. *Journal of the American Medical Association* 283(14):1829–1836.

Nieto FJ, Herrington DM, Redline S, Benjamin EJ, Robbins JA. 2004. Sleep apnea and markers of vascular endothelial function in a large community sample of older adults. *American Journal of Respiratory and Critical Care Medicine* 169(3):354–360.

NIH (National Institutes of Health). 2005. *NIH State-of-the-Science Conference Statement on Manifestations and Management of Chronic Insomnia in Adults* [Online]. Available: http://consensus.nih.gov/2005/2005InsomniaSOS026html.htm [accessed March 6, 2006].

NINDS (National Institute of Neurological Disorders and Stroke). 2005. *Restless Legs Syndrome Fact Sheet*. [Online]. Available: http://www.ninds.nih.gov/disorders/restless_legs/detail_restless_legs.htm [accessed June 13, 2005].

Nishino S, Mignot E. 1997. Pharmacological aspects of human and canine narcolepsy. *Progress in Neurobiology* 52(1):27–78.

Nofzinger EA, Buysse DJ, Germain A, Carter CS, Luna B, Price JC, Meltzer CC, Miewald JM, Reynolds CF, and Kupfer DJ. 2004a. Increased activation of anterior paralimbic and executive cortex from waking to REM sleep in depression. *Archives of General Psychiatry* 61(7):695–702.

Nofzinger EA, Buysse DJ, Germain A, Price JC, Miewald JM, and Kupfer DJ. 2004b. Functional neuroimaging evidence for hyperarousal in insomnia. *American Journal of Psychiatry* 161(11):2126–2128.

Nofzinger EA, Buysse DJ, Germain A, Price JC, Meltzer CC, Miewald JM, Kupfer DJ. 2005. Alterations in regional cerebral glucose metabolism across waking and non-rapid eye movement sleep in depression. *Archives of General Psychiatry* 62(4):387–396.

Norman SE, Chediak AD, Kiel M, Cohn MA. 1990. Sleep disturbances in HIV-infected homosexual men. *AIDS* 4(8):775–781.

Nowell PD, Buysse DJ, Reynolds CF III, Hauri PJ, Roth T, Stepanski EJ, Thorpy MJ, Bixler E, Kales A, Manfredi RL, Vgontzas AN, Stapf DM, Houck PR, Kupfer DJ. 1997. Clinical factors contributing to the differential diagnosis of primary insomnia and insomnia related to mental disorders. *American Journal of Psychiatry* 154(10):1412–1416.

NSF (National Sleep Foundation). 2000a. *2000 Omnibus Sleep in America Poll*. [Online]. Available: www.sleepfoundation.org/publications/2001poll.html [accessed May 25, 2005].

NSF. 2005b. *2005 Sleep in America Poll*. [Online]. Available: http://www.sleepfoundation.org/_content/hottopics/2005_summary_of_findings.pdf [accessed June 7, 2005].

NSF. 2005c. *Shift work: Coping*. [Online]. Available: http://www.sleepfoundation.org/sleeptionary/index.php?id=20&subsection=coping [accessed June 7, 2005].

Ohayon MM. 2002. Epidemiology of insomnia: What we know and what we still need to learn. *Sleep Medicine Reviews* 6(2):97–111.

Ohayon MM, Roth T. 2003. Place of chronic insomnia in the course of depressive and anxiety disorders. *Journal of Psychiatric Research* 37(1):9–15.

Ohayon MM, Caulet M, Guilleminault C. 1997. How a general population perceives its sleep and how this relates to the complaint of insomnia. *Sleep* 20(9):715–723.

Ohayon MM, Guilleminault C, Priest RG. 1999. Night terrors, sleepwalking, and confusional arousals in the general population: Their frequency and relationship to other sleep and mental disorders. *Journal of Clinical Psychiatry* 60(4):268–277.

Ohayon MM, Priest RG, Zulley J, Smirne S. 2000. The place of confusional arousals in sleep and mental disorders: Findings in a general population sample of 13,057 subjects. *Journal of Nervous Mental Disease* 188(6):340–348.

Olson EJ, Boeve BF, Silber MH. 2000. Rapid eye movement sleep behaviour disorder: Demographic, clinical and laboratory findings in 93 cases. *Brain* 123 (Pt 2):331–339.

Ondze B, Espa F, Ming LC, Chakkar B, Besset A, Billiard M. 2001. Advanced sleep phase syndrome [in French]. *Reviews of Neurology* 157(11 Pt 2):S130–S134.

Opp MR, Toth LA. 2003. Neural-immune interactions in the regulation of sleep. *Frontiers of Bioscience* 8:d768–d779.

Overeem S, Scammell TE, Lammers GJ. 2002. Hypocretin/orexin and sleep: Implications for the pathophysiology and diagnosis of narcolepsy. *Current Opinion in Neurology* 15(6): 739–745.

Ozminkowski R, Wang S, Trautman H, Orsini L. 2004. Estimating the cost burden of insomnia for health plans. *Journal of Managed Care Pharmacy* 10(5):467.

Palm L, Anderson H, Elmqvist D, Blennow G. 1992. Daytime sleep tendency before and after discontinuation of antiepileptic drugs in preadolescent children with epilepsy. *Epilepsia* 33(4):687–691.

Palmer CR, Kripke DF, Savage HC Jr, Cindrich LA, Loving RT, Elliott JA. 2003. Efficacy of enhanced evening light for advanced sleep phase syndrome. *Behavioral Sleep Medicine* 1(4):213–226.

Palmer LJ, Buxbaum SG, Larkin E, Patel SR, Elston RC, Tishler PV, Redline S. 2003. A whole-genome scan for obstructive sleep apnea and obesity. *American Journal of Human Genetics* 72(2):340–350.

Palmer LJ, Buxbaum SG, Larkin EK, Patel SR, Elston RC, Tishler PV, Redline S. 2004. Whole genome scan for obstructive sleep apnea and obesity in African-American families. *American Journal of Respiratory and Critical Care Medicine* 169(12):1314–1321.

Panichi V, Migliori M, De Pietro S, Taccola D, Andreini B, Metelli MR, Giovannini L, Palla R. 2000. The link of biocompatibility to cytokine production. *Kidney International Supplement* 76(suppl):S96–S103.

Panigraphy A, Filiano JJ, Sleep LA, Mandell F, Valdes-Dapena M, Krous HF, Rava LA, White WF, Kinney HC. 1997. Decreased kainate receptor binding in the arcuate nucleus of the sudden infant death syndrome. *Journal of Neuropathology and Experimental Neurology* 56(11):1253–1261.

Parker KP. 2003. Sleep disturbances in dialysis patients. *Sleep Medicine Reviews* 7(2): 131–143.

Parker KP, Bliwise DL, Rye DB. 2000. Hemodialysis disrupts basic sleep regulatory mechanisms: Building hypotheses. *Nursing Research* 49(6):327–332.

Parra O, Arboix A, Bechich S, Garcia-Eroles L, Montserrat JM, Lopez JA, Ballester E, Guerra JM, Sopena JJ. 2000. Time course of sleep-related breathing disorders in first-ever stroke or transient ischemic attack. *American Journal of Respiratory and Critical Care Medicine* 161(2):375–380.

Partinen M, Hublin C. 2005. Epidemiology of sleep disorders. In: Kryger MH, Roth T, Dement WC, eds. *Principles and Practice of Sleep Medicine*. 4th ed. Philadelphia: Elsevier/Saunders. Pp. 626–647.

Patel SR, White DP, Malhotra A, Stanchina ML, Ayas NT. 2003. Continuous positive airway pressure therapy for treating sleepiness in a diverse population with obstructive sleep apnea: Results of a meta-analysis. *Archives of Internal Medicine* 163(5): 565–571.

Patel SR, Ayas NT, Malhotra MR, White DP, Schernhammer ES, Speizer FE, Stampfer MJ, Hu FB. 2004. A prospective study of sleep duration and mortality risk in women. *Sleep* 27(3):440–444.

Paus S, Brecht HM, Koster J, Seeger G, Klockgether T, Wullner U. 2003. Sleep attacks, daytime sleepiness, and dopamine agonists in Parkinson's disease. *Movement Disorders* 18(6):659–667.

Paykel ES, Fleminger R, Watson JP. 1982. Psychiatric side effects of antihypertensive drugs other than reserpine. *Journal of Clinical Psychopharmacology* 2(1):14–39.

Pelayo R, Thorpy MJ, Govinsky P. 1988. Prevalence of delayed sleep phase syndrome among adolescents. *Sleep Research* 17:392.

Peppard PE, Young T, Palta M, Skatrud J. 2000. Prospective study of the association between sleep-disordered breathing and hypertension. *New England Journal of Medicine* 342(19): 1378–1384.

Pereira DS, Tufik S, Louzada FM, Benedito-Silva AA, Lopez AR, Lemos NA, Korczak AL, D'Almeida V, Pedrazzoli M. 2005. Association of the length polymorphism in the human Per3 gene with the delayed sleep-phase syndrome: Does latitude have an influence upon it? *Sleep* 28(1):29–32.

Perlis ML, Smith MT, Pigeon WR. 2005. Etiology and pathophysiology of insomnia. In: Kryger MH, Roth T, Dement WC, eds. *Principles and Practice of Sleep Medicine*. 4th ed. Philadelphia: Elsevier/Saunders. Pp. 714–725.

Pertosa G, Grandaliano G, Gesualdo L, Schena FP. 2000. Clinical relevance of cytokine production in hemodialysis. *Kidney International Supplement* 76:S104–S111.

Peters RW. 2005. Obstructive sleep apnea and cardiovascular disease. *Chest* 127(1):1–3.

Petit D, Montplaisir J, Boeve B. 2005. Alzheimer's disease and other dementias. In: Kryger MH, Roth T, Dement WC, eds. *Principles and Practice of Sleep Medicine*. 4th ed. Philadelphia: Elsevier/Saunders. Pp. 853–862.

Peyron C, Faraco J, Rogers W, Ripley B, Overeem S. 2000. A mutation in a case of early onset narcolepsy and a generalized absence of hypocretin peptides in human narcoleptic brains. *Nature Medicine* 6(9):991–997.

Phillips BG, Hisel TM, Kato M, Pesek CA, Dyken ME, Narkiewicz K, Somers VK. 1999. Recent weight gain in patients with newly diagnosed obstructive sleep apnea. *Journal of Hypertension* 17(9):1297–1300.

Phillips BG, Kato M, Narkiewicz K, Choe I, Somers VK. 2000. Increases in leptin levels, sympathetic drive, and weight gain in obstructive sleep apnea. *American Journal of Physiology—Heart and Circulatory Physiology* 279(1): H234–H237.

Phillips B, Hening W, Britz P, Mannino D. 2006. Prevalence and correlates of restless legs syndrome: 2 Results from the 2005 National Sleep Foundation poll. *Chest* 129(1): 76–80.

Picchietti DL, England SJ, Walters AS, Willis K, Verrico T. 1998. Periodic limb movement disorder and restless legs syndrome in children with attention-deficit hyperactivity disorder. *Journal of Child Neurology* 13(12): 588–594.

128   SLEEP DISORDERS AND SLEEP DEPRIVATION

Picchietti DL, Underwood DJ, Farris WA, Walters AS, Shah MM, Dahl RE, Trubnick LJ, Bertocci MA, Wagner M, Hening WA. 1999. Further studies on periodic limb movement disorder and restless legs syndrome in children with attention-deficit hyperactivity disorder. *Movement Disorders* 14(6):1000–1007.
Pilcher JJ, Huffcutt AI. 1996. Effects of sleep deprivation on performance: A meta-analysis. *Sleep* 19(4):318–326.
Pillar G, Lavie P. 1995. Assessment of the role of inheritance in sleep apnea syndrome. *American Journal of Respiratory and Critical Care Medicine* 151(3 Pt 1): 688–691.
Plazzi G, Corsini R, Provini F, Pierangeli G, Martinelli P, Montagna P, Lugaresi E, Cortelli P. 1997. REM sleep behavior disorders in multiple system atrophy. *Neurology* 48(4):1094–1097.
Plazzi G, Cortelli P, Montagna P, De Monte A, Corsini R, Contin M, Provini F, Pierangeli G, Lugaresi E. 1998. REM sleep behaviour disorder differentiates pure autonomic failure from multiple system atrophy with autonomic failure. *Journal of Neurology, Neurosurgery and Psychiatry* 64(5):683–685.
Ponsonby AL, Dwyer T, Gibbons LE, Cochrane JA, Wang YG. 1993. Factors potentiating the risk of sudden infant death syndrome associated with the prone position. *New England Journal of Medicine* 329(6):377–382.
Powell NB, Riley RW, Guilleminault C. 2005. Surgical management of sleep-disordered breathing. In: Kryger MH, Roth T, Dement WC, eds. *Principles and Practice of Sleep Medicine.* 4th ed. Philadelphia: Elsevier/Saunders. Pp. 1081–1097.
Prinz PN, Peskind ER, Vitaliano PP, Raskind MA, Eisdorfer C, Zemcuznikov N, Gerber CJ. 1982a. Changes in the sleep and waking EEGs of nondemented and demented elderly subjects. *Journal of the American Geriatrics Society* 30(2):86–93.
Prinz PN, Vitaliano PP, Vitiello MV, Bokan J, Raskind M, Peskind E, Gerber C. 1982b. Sleep, EEG and mental function changes in senile dementia of the Alzheimer's type. *Neurobiology of Aging* 3(4):361–370.
Punjabi NM, Beamer BA. 2005. Sleep apnea and metabolic dysfunction. In: Kryger MH, Roth T, Dement WC, eds. *Principles and Practice of Sleep Medicine.* 4th ed. Philadelphia: Elsevier/Saunders. Pp. 1034–1042.
Punjabi NM, Sorkin JD, Katzel LI, Goldberg AP, Schwartz AR, Smith PL. 2002. Sleep-disordered breathing and insulin resistance in middle-aged and overweight men. *American Journal of Respiratory and Critical Care Medicine* 165(5):677–682.
Punjabi NM, Shahar E, Redline S, Gottlieb DJ, Givelber R, Resnick HE, Sleep Heart Health Study Investigators. 2004. Sleep-disordered breathing, glucose intolerance, and insulin resistance: The Sleep Heart Health Study. *American Journal of Epidemiology* 160(6):521–530.
Qureshi AI, Giles WH, Croft JB, Bliwise DL. 1997. Habitual sleep patterns and risk for stroke and coronary heart disease: A 10-year follow-up from NHANES I. *Neurology* 48(4):904–911.
Radomski MW, Buguet A, Bogui P, Doua F, Lonsdorfer A, Tapie P, Dumas M. 1994. Disruptions in the secretion of cortisol, prolactin, and certain cytokines in human African trypanosomiasis patients. *Bulletin de la Societe de Pathologie Exotique (Paris)* 87(5): 376–379.
Raison CL, Miller AH. 2001. The neuroimmunology of stress and depression. *Seminars in Clinical Neuropsychiatry* 6(4):277–294.
Rao U, Dahl RE, Ryan ND, Birmaher B, Williamson DE, Giles DE, Rao R, Kaufman J, Nelson B. 1996. The relationship between longitudinal clinical course and sleep and cortisol changes in adolescent depression. *Biological Psychiatry* 40(6):474–484.

Redline S, Tishler PV, Tosteson TD, Williamson J, Kump K, Browner I, Ferrette V, Krejci P. 1995. The familial aggregation of obstructive sleep apnea. *American Journal of Respiratory and Critical Care Medicine* 151(3 Pt 1):682–687.

Redline S, Tishler PV, Hans MG, Tosteson TD, Strohl KP, Spry K. 1997. Racial differences in sleep-disordered breathing in African-Americans and Caucasians. *American Journal of Respiratory and Critical Care Medicine* 155(1):186–192.

Redline S, Tishler PV, Schluchter M, Aylor J, Clark K, Graham G. 1999. Risk factors for sleep-disordered breathing in children: Associations with obesity, race, and respiratory problems. *American Journal of Respiratory and Critical Care Medicine* 159(5):1527–1532.

Redline S, Kapur VK, Sanders MH, Quan SF, Gottlieb DJ, Rapoport DM, Bonekat WH, Smith PL, Kiley JP, Iber C. 2000. Effects of varying approaches for identifying respiratory disturbances on sleep apnea assessment. *American Journal of Respiratory and Critical Care Medicine* 161(2 Pt 1):369–374.

Regestein QR, Monk TH. 1995. Delayed sleep phase syndrome: A review of its clinical aspects. *American Journal of Psychiatry* 152(4):602–608.

Reid JL. 1996. New therapeutic agents for hypertension. *British Journal of Clinical Pharmacology* 42(1):37–41.

Reid KJ, Zee PC. 2005. Circadian disorders of the sleep-wake cycle. In: Kryger MH, Roth T, Dement WC, eds. *Principles and Practice of Sleep Medicine*. 4th ed. Philadelphia: Elsevier/Saunders. Pp. 691–701.

Reid KJ, Chang AM, Dubocovich ML, Turek FW, Takahashi JS, Zee PC. 2001. Familial advanced sleep phase syndrome. *Archives of Neurology* 58(7):1089–1094.

Reynolds CF III, Kupfer DJ, Taska LS, Hoch CC, Spiker DG, Sewitch DE, Zimmer B, Marin RS, Nelson JP, Martin D, Morycz R. 1985. EEG sleep in elderly depressed, demented, and healthy subjects. *Biological Psychiatry* 20(4):431–442.

Reynolds CF III, Frank E, Houck PR, Mazumdar S, Dew MA, Cornes C, Buysse DJ, Begley A, Kupfer DJ. 1997. Which elderly patients with remitted depression remain well with continued interpersonal psychotherapy after discontinuation of antidepressant medication? *American Journal of Psychiatry* 154(7):958–962.

Riemann D, Voderholzer U. 2003. Primary insomnia: A risk factor to develop depression? *Journal of Affective Disorders* 76(1-3):255–259.

Riley JL III, Benson MB, Gremillion HA, Myers CD, Robinson ME, Smith CL Jr, Waxenberg LB. 2001. Sleep disturbance in orofacial pain patients: Pain-related or emotional distress? *Cranio* 19(2):106–113.

Rizzo P, Beelke M, De Carli F, Canovaro P, Nobili L, Robert A, Tanganelli P, Regesta G, Ferrillo F. 2003. Chronic vagus nerve stimulation improves alertness and reduces rapid eye movement sleep in patients affected by refractory epilepsy. *Sleep* 26(5):607–611.

Robinson GV, Pepperell JC, Segal HC, Davies RJ, Stradling JR. 2004a. Circulating cardiovascular risk factors in obstructive sleep apnoea: Data from randomised controlled trials. *Thorax* 59(9):777–782.

Robinson GV, Stradling JR, Davies RJ. 2004b. Sleep 6: Obstructive sleep apnoea/hypopnoea syndrome and hypertension. *Thorax* 59(12):1089–1094.

Roizenblatt S, Moldofsky H, Benedito-Silva AA, Tufik S. 2001. Alpha sleep characteristics in fibromyalgia. *Arthritis and Rheumatism* 44(1):222–230.

Rombaux P, Hamoir M, Plouin-Gaudon I, Liistro G, Aubert G, Rodenstein D. 2000. Obstructive sleep apnea syndrome after reconstructive laryngectomy for glottic carcinoma. *European Archives of Otorhinolaryngology* 257(9):502–506.

Rosen CL, D'Andrea L, Haddad GG. 1992. Adult criteria for obstructive sleep apnea do not identify children with serious obstruction. *American Review of Respiratory Diseases* 146(5 Pt 1):1231–1234.

Rosen CL, Larkin EK, Kirchner HL, Emancipator JL, Bivins SF, Surovec SA, Martin RJ, Redline S. 2003. Prevalence and risk factors for sleep-disordered breathing in 8- to 11-year-old children: Association with race and prematurity. *Journal of Pediatrics* 142(4): 383–389.

Rosenfeld MR, Eichen JG, Wade DF, Posner JB, Dalmau J. 2001. Molecular and clinical diversity in paraneoplastic immunity to Ma proteins. *Annals of Neurology* 50(3):339–348.

Rosenthal NE, Joseph-Vanderpool JR, Levendosky AA, Johnston SH, Allen R, Kelly KA, Souetre E, Schultz PM, Starz KE. 1990. Phase-shifting effects of bright morning light as treatment for delayed sleep phase syndrome. *Sleep* 13(4):354–361.

Roth B. 1976. Narcolepsy and hypersomnia: Review and classification of 642 personally observed cases. *Schweizer Archiv fur Neurologie, Neurochirurgie und Psychiatrie* 119(1): 31–41.

Roth T, Ancoli-Israel S. 1999. Daytime consequences and correlates of insomnia in the United States: Results of the 1991 National Sleep Foundation Survey. II. *Sleep* 22(suppl 2):S354–S358.

Rothdach AJ, Trenkwalder C, Haberstock J, Keil U, Berger K. 2000. Prevalence and risk factors of RLS in an elderly population: The MEMO study. Memory and morbidity in Augsburg elderly. *Neurology* 54(5):1064–1068.

Ryan ND, Puig-Antich J, Ambrosini P, Rabinovich H, Robinson D, Nelson B, Iyengar S, Twomey J. 1987. The clinical picture of major depression in children and adolescents. *Archives of General Psychiatry* 44(10):854–861.

Salinsky MC, Oken BS, Binder LM. 1996. Assessment of drowsiness in epilepsy patients receiving chronic antiepileptic drug therapy. *Epilepsia* 37(2):181–187.

Santhi N, Duffy JF, Horowitz TS, Czeisler CA. 2005. Scheduling of sleep/darkness affects the circadian phase of night shift workers. *Neuroscience Letters* 384(3):316–320.

Satoh K, Mishima K, Inoue Y, Ebisawa T, Shimizu T. 2003. Two pedigrees of familial advanced sleep phase syndrome in Japan. *Sleep* 26(4):416–417.

Scammell TE. 2003. The neurobiology, diagnosis, and treatment of narcolepsy. *Annals of Neurology* 53(2):154–166.

Schechtman VL, Harper RK, Harper RM. 1995. Aberrant temporal patterning of slow-wave sleep in siblings of SIDS victims. *Electroencephalography and Clinical Neurophysiology* 94(2):95–102.

Schenck C, Mahowald M. 1990. A polysomnographic neurologic, psychiatric and clinical outcome report on 70 consecutive cases with REM sleep behavior disorder (RBD): sustained clonazepam efficacy in 89.5% of 57 treated patients. *Cleveland Clinic Journal of Medicine* 57(10):10–24.

Schenck CH, Hurwitz TD, Mahowald MW. 1993. Symposium: Normal and abnormal REM sleep regulation: REM sleep behaviour disorder: An update on a series of 96 patients and a review of the world literature. *Journal of Sleep Research* 2(4):224–231.

Schmidt-Nowara WW, Coultas DB, Wiggins C, Skipper BE, Samet JM. 1990. Snoring in a Hispanic-American population. Risk factors and association with hypertension and other morbidity. *Archives of Internal Medicine* 150(3):597–601.

Schoendorf KC, Kiely JL. 1992. Relationship of sudden infant death syndrome to maternal smoking during and after pregnancy. *Pediatrics* 90(6):905–908.

Schwartz SW, Cornoni-Huntley J, Cole SR, Hays JC, Blazer DG, Schocken DD. 1998. Are sleep complaints an independent risk factor for myocardial infarction? *Annals of Epidemiology* 8(6):384–392.

Sekine M, Yamagami T, Handa K, Saito T, Nanri S, Kawaminami K, Tokui N, Yoshida K, Kagamimori S. 2002. A dose-response relationship between short sleeping hours and childhood obesity: Results of the Toyama birth cohort study. *Child: Care, Health and Development* 28(2):163–170.

Shahar E, Whitney CW, Redline S, Lee ET, Newman AB, Javier Nieto F, O'Connor GT, Boland LL, Schwartz JE, Samet JM. 2001. Sleep-disordered breathing and cardiovascular disease: Cross-sectional results of the Sleep Heart Health Study. *American Journal of Respiratory and Critical Care Medicine* 163(1):19–25.

Shahar E, Redline S, Young T, Boland LL, Baldwin CM, Nieto FJ, O'Connor GT, Rapoport DM, Robbins JA. 2003. Hormone replacement therapy and sleep-disordered breathing. *American Journal of Respiratory and Critical Care Medicine* 167(9):1186–1192.

Shamsuzzaman AS, Gersh BJ, Somers VK. 2003. Obstructive sleep apnea: Implications for cardiac and vascular disease. *Journal of the American Medical Association* 290(14):1906–1914.

Shepertycky MR, Banno K, Kryger MH. 2005. Differences between men and women in the clinical presentation of patients diagnosed with obstructive sleep apnea syndrome. *Sleep* 28(3):309–314.

Shiino Y, Nakajima S, Ozeki Y, Isono T, Yamada N. 2003. Mutation screening of the human period 2 gene in bipolar disorder. *Neuroscience Letters* 338(1):82–84.

Shouse MN, Mahowald M. 2005. Epilepsy, sleep, and sleep disorders. In: Kryger MH, Roth T, Dement WC, eds. *Principles and Practice of Sleep Medicine.* 4th ed. Philadelphia: Elsevier/Saunders. Pp. 863–878.

Shouse MN, da Silva AM, Sammaritano M. 1996. Circadian rhythm, sleep, and epilepsy. *Journal of Clinical Neurophysiology* 13(1):32–50.

Silber MH, Richardson JW. 2003. Multiple blood donations associated with iron deficiency in patients with restless legs syndrome. *Mayo Clinic Proceedings* 78(1):52–54.

Simon GE, VonKorff M. 1997. Prevalence, burden, and treatment of insomnia in primary care. *American Journal of Psychiatry* 154(10):1417–1423.

Sin DD, Fitzgerald F, Parker JD, Newton G, Floras JS, Bradley TD. 1999. Risk factors for central and obstructive sleep apnea in 450 men and women with congestive heart failure. *American Journal of Respiratory and Critical Care Medicine* 160(4):1101–1106.

Singh M, Drake C, Roehrs T, Koshorek G, Roth T. 2005. The prevalence of SOREMPs in the general population. *Sleep* 28(abstract suppl):A221.

Smith A. 1992. Sleep, colds, and performance. In: Broughton RJ, Ogilvie R, eds. *Sleep Arousal and Performance.* Boston: Birkhouser.

Smith MT, Perlis ML, Park A, Smith MS, Pennington J, Giles DE, Buysse DJ. 2002. Comparative meta-analysis of pharmacotherapy and behavior therapy for persistent insomnia. *American Journal of Psychiatry* 159(1):5–11.

Somers VK, Mark AL, Abboud FM 1988. Sympathetic activation by hypoxia and hypercapnia—implications for sleep apnea. *Clinical and Experimental Hypertension: Part A, Theory and Practice* 10(suppl 1):413–422.

Somers VK, Dyken ME, Mark AL, Abboud FM. 1992. Parasympathetic hyperresponsiveness and bradyarrhythmias during apnoea in hypertension. *Clinical Autonomic Research* 2(3):171–176.

Somers VK, Dyken ME, Clary MP, Abboud FM. 1995. Sympathetic neural mechanisms in obstructive sleep apnea. *Journal of Clinical Investigation* 96(4):1897–1904.

Spiegel K, Leproult R, Van Cauter E. 1999. Impact of sleep debt on metabolic and endocrine function. *Lancet* 354(9188):1435–1439.

Spiegel K, Tasali E, Penev P, Van Cauter E. 2004. Brief communication: Sleep curtailment in healthy young men is associated with decreased leptin levels, elevated ghrelin levels, and increased hunger and appetite. *Annals of Internal Medicine* 141(11):846–850.

Stiasny K, Wetter TC, Winkelmann J, Brandenburg U, Penzel T, Rubin M, Hundemer HP, Oertel WH, Trenkwalder C. 2001. Long-term effects of pergolide in the treatment of restless legs syndrome. *Neurology* 56(10):1399–1402.

Strine TW, Chapman DP. 2005. Associations of frequent sleep insufficiency with health-related quality of life and health behaviors. *Sleep Medicine* 6(1):23–27.

Strohl KP, Redline S. 1996. Recognition of obstructive sleep apnea. *American Journal of Respiratory and Critical Care Medicine* 154(2 Pt 1):279–289.

Strollo PJ, Atwood CW Jr, Sanders MH. 2005. Medical therapy for obstructive sleep apnea-hypopnea syndrome. In: Kryger MH, Roth T, Dement WC, eds. *Principles and Practice of Sleep Medicine*. 4th ed. Philadelphia: Elsevier/Saunders. Pp. 1053–1065.

Sulit LG, Storfer-Isser A, Rosen CL, Kirchner HL, Redline S. 2005. Associations of obesity, sleep-disordered breathing, and wheezing in children. *American Journal of Respiratory and Critical Care Medicine* 171(6):659–664.

Szymczak JT, Jasinska M, Pawlak E, Zwierzykowska M. 1993. Annual and weekly changes in the sleep-wake rhythm of school children. *Sleep* 16(5):433–435.

Taasan VC, Block AJ, Boysen PG, Wynne JW. 1981. Alcohol increases sleep apnea and oxygen desaturation in asymptomatic men. *American Journal of Medicine* 71(2):240–245.

Taheri S, Lin L, Austin D, Young T, Mignot E. 2004. Short sleep duration is associated with reduced leptin, elevated ghrelin, and increased body mass index. *Public Library of Science Medicine* 1(3):210–217.

Takahashi Y, Hohjoh H, Matsuura K. 2000. Predisposing factors in delayed sleep phase syndrome. *Psychiatry and Clinical Neuroscience* 54(3):356–358.

Tamakoshi A, Ohno Y, JACC Study Group. 2004. Self-reported sleep duration as a predictor of all-cause mortality: Results from the JACC study, Japan. *Sleep* 27(1):51–54.

Tassinari CA, Mancia D, Bernardina BD, Gastaut H. 1972. *Pavor nocturnus* of non-epileptic nature in epileptic children. *Electroencephalography and Clinical Neurophysiology* 33(6):603–607.

Terzano MG, Parrino L, Spaggiari MC. 1988. The cyclic alternating pattern sequences in the dynamic organization of sleep. *Electroencephalography and Clinical Neurophysiology* 69(5):437–447.

Thannickal TC, Moore RY, Nienhuis R, Ramanathan L, Gulyani S, Aldrich M, Cornford M, Siegel JM. 2000. Reduced number of hypocretin neurons in human narcolepsy. *Neuron* 27(3):469–474.

Thorpy MJ. 2005. Classification of sleep disorders. In: Kryger MH, Roth T, Dement WC, eds. *Principles and Practice of Sleep Medicine*. 4th ed. Philadelphia: Elsevier/Saunders. Pp. 615–625.

Tishler PV, Redline S, Ferrette V, Hans MG, Altose MD. 1996. The association of sudden unexpected infant death with obstructive sleep apnea. *American Journal of Respiratory and Critical Care Medicine* 153(6 Pt 1):1857–1863.

Tochikubo O, Ikeda A, Miyajima E, Ishii M. 1996. Effects of insufficient sleep on blood pressure monitored by a new multibiomedical recorder. *Hypertension* 27(6):1318–1324.

Toh KL, Jones CR, He Y, Eide EJ, Hinz WA, Virshup DM, Ptacek LJ, Fu YH. 2001. An hPer2 phosphorylation site mutation in familial advanced sleep phase syndrome. *Science* 291(5506):1040–1043.

Toth LA. 1999. Microbial modulation of sleep. In: Lydic R, Baghdoyan HA, eds. *Handbook of Behavioral State Control: Cellular and Molecular Mechanisms*. Boca Raton, FL: CRC Press.

Toth LA, Opp MR. 2002. Infection and sleep. In: Lee CT, Sateia M, Carskadon M. *Sleep Medicine*. Philadelphia, PA: Hanley and Belfus.

Tractenberg RE, Singer CM, Kaye JA. 2005. Symptoms of sleep disturbance in persons with Alzheimer's disease and normal elderly. *Journal of Sleep Research* 14(2):177–185.

Trampus M, Ferri N, Monopoli A, Ongini E. 1991. The dopamine D1 receptor is involved in the regulation of REM sleep in the rat. *European Journal of Pharmacology* 194(2–3):189–194.

Tune GS. 1968. Sleep and wakefulness in normal human adults. *British Medical Journal* 2(600):269–271.

Turek FW, Joshu C, Kohsaka A, Lin E, Ivanova G, McDearmon E, Laposky A, Losee-Olson S, Easton A, Jensen DR, Eckel RH, Takahashi JS, Bass J. 2005. Obesity and metabolic syndrome in circadian Clock mutant mice. *Science* 308(5724):1043–1045.

Turjanski N, Lees AJ, Brooks DJ. 1999. Striatal dopaminergic function in restless legs syndrome: 18F-dopa and 11C-raclopride PET studies. *Neurology* 52(5):932–937.

Ulfberg J, Nystrom B. 2004. Restless legs syndrome in blood donors. *Sleep Medicine* 5(2):115–118.

United States Census Bureau. 1990. *Time Leaving Home to Go to Work for the United States: 1990 Census.* [Online] Available: http://www.census.gov/population/socdemo/journey/usdeptim.txt [accessed March 7, 2006].

Unruh ML, Levey AS, D'Ambrosio C, Fink NE, Powe NR, Meyer KB. 2004. Restless legs symptoms among incident dialysis patients: Association with lower quality of life and shorter survival. *American Journal of Kidney Diseases* 43(5):900–909.

Van Den Heuvel CJ, Reid KJ, Dawson D. 1997. Effect of atenolol on nocturnal sleep and temperature in young men: Reversal by pharmacological doses of melatonin. *Physiology and Behavior* 61(6):795–802.

Vaziri ND, Oveisi F, Wierszbiezki M, Shaw V, Sporty LD. 1993. Serum melatonin and 6-sulfatoxymelatonin in end-stage renal disease: Effect of hemodialysis. *Artificial Organs* 17(9):764–769.

Vaziri ND, Oveisi F, Reyes GA, Zhou XJ. 1996. Dysregulation of melatonin metabolism in chronic renal insufficiency: Role of erythropoietin-deficiency anemia. *Kidney International* 50(2):653–656.

Veasey S, Rosen R, Barzansky B, Rosen I, Owens J. 2002. Sleep loss and fatigue in residency training: A reappraisal. *Journal of the American Medical Association* 288(9):1116–1124.

Velasco M, Velasco F. 1982. Brain stem regulation of cortical and motor excitability: Effects on experimental and focal motor seizures. In: Sterman MB, Shouse MN, Passouant P, eds. *Sleep and Epilepsy.* New York: Academic Press. Pp. 53–61.

Verrier RL, Josephson ME. 2005. Cardiac arrhythmogenesis during sleep: Mechanisms, diagnosis, and therapy. In: Kryger MH, Roth T, Dement WC, eds. *Principles and Practice of Sleep Medicine.* 4th ed. Philadelphia: Elsevier/Saunders. Pp. 1171–1191.

Vgontzas AN, Kales A. 1999. Sleep and its disorders. *Annual Review of Medicine* 50(1):387–400.

Vgontzas AN, Tan TL, Bixler EO, Martin LF, Shubert D, Kales A. 1994. Sleep apnea and sleep disruption in obese patients. *Archives of Internal Medicine* 154(15):1705–1711.

Vgontzas AN, Bixler EO, Lin HM, Prolo P, Mastorakos G, Vela-Bueno A, Kales A, Chrousos GP. 2001. Chronic insomnia is associated with nyctohemeral activation of the hypothalamic-pituitary-adrenal axis: Clinical implications. *Journal of Clinical Endocrinology and Metabolism* 86(8): 3787–3794.

Vincent NK, Hameed H. 2003. Relation between adherence and outcome in the group treatment of insomnia. *Behavioral Sleep Medicine* 1(3):125–139.

Vioque J, Torres A, Quiles J. 2000. Time spent watching television, sleep duration and obesity in adults living in Valencia, Spain. *International Journal of Obesity and Related Metabolic Disorders* 24(12):1683–1688.

von Kries R, Toschke AM, Wurmser H, Sauerwald T, Koletzko B. 2002. Reduced risk for overweight and obesity in 5- and 6-y-old children by duration of sleep—a cross-sectional study. *International Journal of Obesity and Related Metabolic Disorders: Journal of the International Association for the Study of Obesity* 26(5):710–716.

Walsh JK, Dement WC, Dinges DF. 2005. Sleep medicine, public policy, and public health. In: Kryger MH, Roth T, Dement WC, eds. *Principles and Practice of Sleep Medicine*. 4th ed. Philadelphia: Elsevier/Saunders. Pp. 648–656.

Walters AS, Hening WA, Kavey N, Chokroverty S, Gidro-Frank S. 1988. A double-blind randomized crossover trial of bromocriptine and placebo in restless legs syndrome. *Annals of Neurology* 24(3):455–458.

Walters AS, Wagner ML, Hening WA, Grasing K, Mills R, Chokroverty S, Kavey N. 1993. Successful treatment of the idiopathic restless legs syndrome in a randomized double-blind trial of oxycodone versus placebo. *Sleep* 16(4):327–332.

Walters AS, Hickey K, Maltzman J, Verrico T, Joseph D, Hening W, Wilson V, Chokroverty S. 1996. A questionnaire study of 138 patients with restless legs syndrome: The "night-walkers" survey. *Neurology* 46(1):92–95.

Walters AS, Winkelmann J, Trenkwalder C, Fry JM, Kataria V, Wagner M, Sharma R, Hening W, Li L. 2001. Long-term follow-up on restless legs syndrome patients treated with opioids. *Movement Disorders* 16(6):1105–1109.

Weisberg RB, Bruce SE, Machan JT, Kessler RC, Culpepper L, Keller MB. 2002. Non-psychiatric illness among primary care patients with trauma histories and posttraumatic stress disorder. *Psychiatric Services* 53(7): 848–854.

Weissman MM, Greenwald S, Nino-Murcia G, Dement WC. 1997. The morbidity of insomnia uncomplicated by psychiatric disorders. *General Hospital Psychiatry* 19(4):245–250.

Weitzman ED, Czeisler CA, Coleman RM, Spielman AJ, Zimmerman JC, Dement W, Richardson G, Pollak CP. 1981. Delayed sleep phase syndrome. A chronobiological disorder with sleep-onset insomnia. *Archives of General Psychiatry* 38(7):737–746.

Wesensten NJ, Belenky G, Kautz MA, Thorne DR, Reichardt RM, Balkin TJ. 2002. Maintaining alertness and performance during sleep deprivation: Modafinil versus caffeine. *Psychopharmacology (Berlin)* 159(3):238–247.

Wetter TC, Stiasny K, Winkelmann J, Buhlinger A, Brandenburg U, Penzel T, Medori R, Rubin M, Oertel WH, Trenkwalder C. 1999. A randomized controlled study of pergolide in patients with restless legs syndrome. *Neurology* 52(5):944–950.

Weyerbrock A, Timmer J, Hohagen F, Berger M, Bauer J. 1996. Effects of light and chrono-therapy on human circadian rhythms in delayed sleep phase syndrome: Cytokines, cortisol, growth hormone, and the sleep-wake cycle. *Biological Psychiatry* 40(8):794–797.

White DP. 2005. Central sleep apnea. In: Kryger MH, Roth T, Dement WC, eds. *Principles and Practice of Sleep Medicine*. 4th ed. Philadelphia: Elsevier/Saunders. Pp. 969–982.

Whitehouse PJ, Price DL, Struble RG, Clark AW, Coyle JT, Delon MR. 1982. Alzheimer's disease and senile dementia: Loss of neurons in the basal forebrain. *Science* 215(4537):-1237–1239.

Wills L, Garcia J. 2002. Parasomnias: Epidemiology and management. *CNS Drugs* 16(12):803–810.

Winkelman JW, Chertow GM, Lazarus JM. 1996. Restless legs syndrome in end–stage renal disease. *American Journal of Kidney Disease* 28(3):372–378.

Winkelmann J, Schadrack J, Wetter TC, Zieglgansberger W, Trenkwalder C. 2001. Opioid and dopamine antagonist drug challenges in untreated restless legs syndrome patients. *Sleep Medicine* 2(1):57–61.

Winkelmann J, Muller-Myhsok B, Wittchen HU, Hock B, Prager M, Pfister H, Strohle A, Eisensehr I, Dichgans M, Gasser T, Trenkwalder C. 2002. Complex segregation analysis of restless legs syndrome provides evidence for an autosomal dominant mode of inheritance in early age at onset families. *Annals of Neurology* 52(3):297–302.

Wisor JP, Nishino S, Sora I, Uhl GH, Mignot E, Edgar DM. 2001. Dopaminergic role in stimulant-induced wakefulness. *Journal of Neuroscience* 21(5):1787–1794.

Wolfson AR, Carskadon MA. 1998. Sleep schedules and daytime functioning in adolescents. *Child Development* 69(4):875–887.

Wolkowitz OM, Rubinow D, Doran AR, Breier A, Berrettini WH, Kling MA, Pickar D. 1990. Prednisone effects on neurochemistry and behavior. Preliminary findings. *Archives of General Psychiatry* 47(10):963–968.

Xu Y, Padiath QS, Shapiro RE, Jones CR, Wu SC, Saigoh N, Saigoh K, Ptacek LJ, Fu YH. 2005. Functional consequences of a CKIdelta mutation causing familial advanced sleep phase syndrome. *Nature* 434(7033):640–644.

Yaggi HK, Concato J, Kernan WN, Lichtman JH, Brass LM, Mohsenin V. 2005. Obstructive sleep apnea as a risk factor for stroke and death. *New England Journal of Medicine* 353(19):2034–2041.

Young T, Javaheri S. 2005. Systemic and pulmonary hypertension in obstructive sleep apnea. In: Kryger MH, Roth T, Dement WC, eds. *Principles and Practice of Sleep Medicine.* 4th ed. Philadelphia: Elsevier/Saunders. Pp. 1192–1202.

Young T, Palta M, Dempsey J, Skatrud J, Weber S, Badr S. 1993. The occurrence of sleep-disordered breathing among middle-aged adults. *New England Journal of Medicine* 328(17):1230–1235.

Young T, Blustein J, Finn L, Palta M. 1997a. Sleep-disordered breathing and motor vehicle accidents in a population-based sample of employed adults. *Sleep* 20(8):608–613.

Young T, Evans L, Finn L, Palta M. 1997b. Estimation of the clinically diagnosed proportion of sleep apnea syndrome in middle-aged men and women. *Sleep* 20(9):705–706.

Young T, Peppard PE, Gottlieb DJ. 2002a. Epidemiology of obstructive sleep apnea: A population health perspective. *American Journal of Respiratory and Critical Care Medicine* 165(9):1217–1239.

Young T, Shahar E, Nieto FJ, Redline S, Newman AB, Gottlieb DJ, Walsleben JA, Finn L, Enright P, Samet JM, Sleep Heart Health Study Research Group. 2002b. Predictors of sleep-disordered breathing in community-dwelling adults: The Sleep Heart Health Study. *Archives of Internal Medicine* 162(8):893–900.

Young T, Rabago D, Zgierska A, Austin D, Laurel F. 2003. Objective and subjective sleep quality in premenopausal, perimenopausal, and postmenopausal women in the Wisconsin Sleep Cohort Study. *Sleep* 26(6):667–672.

Zadra AL, Nielsen TA, Donderi DC. 1998. Prevalence of auditory, olfactory, and gustatory experiences in home dreams. *Perceptual and Motor Skills* 87(3 Pt 1):819–826.

Zeitzer JM, Dijk DJ, Kronauer R, Brown E, Czeisler C. 2000. Sensitivity of the human circadian pacemaker to nocturnal light: Melatonin phase resetting and suppression. *Journal of Physiology* 526 (Pt 3):695–702.

Zucconi M, Oldani A, Ferini-Strambi L, Smirne S. 1995. Arousal fluctuations in non-rapid eye movement parasomnias: The role of cyclic alternating pattern as a measure of sleep instability. *Journal of Clinical Neurophysiology* 12(2):147–154.

Zweig RM, Jankel WR, Hedreen JC, Mayeux R, Price DL. 1989. The pedunculopontine nucleus in Parkinson's disease. *Annals of Neurology* 26(1):41–44.

4

Functional and Economic Impact of Sleep Loss and Sleep-Related Disorders

CHAPTER SUMMARY   *Sleep loss and sleep disorders affect an individual's performance, safety, and quality of life. Almost 20 percent of all serious car crash injuries in the general population are associated with driver sleepiness, independent of alcohol effects. Further, sleep loss and sleep disorders have a significant economic impact. The high estimated costs to society of leaving the most prevalent sleep disorders untreated are far more than the costs that would be incurred by delivering adequate treatment. Hundreds of billions of dollars a year are spent on direct medical costs associated with doctor visits, hospital services, prescriptions, and over-the-counter drugs. Compared to healthy individuals, individuals suffering from sleep loss, sleep disorders, or both are less productive, have an increased health care utilization, and an increased likelihood of accidents.*

The public health consequences of sleep loss, night work, and sleep disorders are far from benign. Some of the most devastating human and environmental health disasters have been partially attributed to sleep loss and night shift work-related performance failures, including the tragedy at the Bhopal, India, chemical plant; the nuclear reactor meltdowns at Three Mile Island and Chernobyl; as well as the grounding of the *Star Princess* cruise ship and the Exxon *Valdez* oil tanker (NCSDS, 1994; NTSB, 1997; Moss and Sills, 1981; United States Senate Committee on Energy and National Resources, 1986; USNRC, 1987; Dinges et al., 1989). Each of these incidents not only cost millions of dollars to clean up, but also had a significant impact on the environment and the health of local communities.

Less visible consequences of sleep conditions take a toll on nearly every key indicator of public health: mortality, morbidity, performance, accidents and injuries, functioning and quality of life, family well-being, and health care utilization. This chapter begins with an overview of the consequences of sleep loss and sleep disorders on an individual's performance, safety, and quality of life. Drawing on the available body of evidence, the chapter then describes the economic impact of sleep loss and sleep disorders.

PERFORMANCE AND COGNITION DEFICITS

Nearly all types of sleep problems are associated with performance deficits in occupational, educational, and other settings. The deficits include attention, vigilance, and other measures of cognition, including memory and complex decision making. This section addresses sleep loss and then turns to sleep-disordered breathing and other sleep disorders.

Sleep Loss Affects Cognitive Performance

Sleep loss had been largely dismissed as the cause of poor cognitive performance by early, yet poorly designed, research. The prevailing view until the 1990s was that people adapted to chronic sleep loss without adverse cognitive effects (Dinges et al., 2005). More recent research has revealed sleep loss-induced neurobehavioral effects, which often go unrecognized by the affected individuals. The neurobehavioral impact extends from simple measures of cognition (i.e., attention and reaction time) to far more complex errors in judgment and decision making, such as medical errors, discussed below and in Box 4-1. Performance effects of sleep loss include the following:

- Involuntary microsleeps occur.
- Attention to intensive performance is unstable, with increased errors of omission and commission.

BOX 4-1
Reducing Interns' Work Hours in Intensive Care Units Lowers Medical Errors

The longstanding debate over medical residents' lengthy work hours pits patient safety advocates against those who view the practice as necessary for continuity of care, preparation for medical practice, and cost containment (Steinbrook, 2002). After years of debate, and the threat of federal regulations, the Accreditation Council for Graduate Medical Education changed its requirements in 2003 to restrict residents' work hours to about 80 hours per week (ACGME, 2003). The policy permits no more than a maximum shift duration of 24 hours and overnight call no more than every third night.

Does this revised policy protect patients? The Harvard Work Hours, Health and Safety Study compared a schedule of about 80 hours per week (termed the *traditional schedule*) with a reduced schedule that eliminated shifts of 24 hours or more and kept work hours under 63 per week. The trial was conducted in intensive care units because they typically have the longest hours and the highest rates of errors.

The intervention schedule not only enhanced interns' sleep duration and lowered their rate of attentional failures, but also reduced the rate of serious medical errors, according to two articles published in 2004 in the *New England Journal of Medicine*. In the first article, the investigators used a within-subjects design (n = 20 interns) and validated sleep duration by polysomnography and attentional failures by slow-rolling eye movements recorded during continuous electro-oculography. Under the intervention schedule, the article reported that residents slept nearly 6 more hours per week, and they experienced half the rate of attentional failures during on-call nights than under the traditional schedule (Lockley et al., 2004).

The second article on medical errors reported results after randomizing interns to either the traditional or reduced schedule (Landrigan et al., 2004). Two physicians who directly observed the interns without awareness of their schedules identified serious medical errors, defined as causing or having the potential to cause harm to a patient. Errors were recorded by type (medication, diagnosis, and procedure) and in terms of number, or rate per 1,000 patient days. The study covered a total of 2,203 patient-days involving 634 admissions. Under the traditional schedule, interns made nearly 21 percent more medication errors and at least five times more diagnostic errors. Overall, the unitwide rate of serious medical errors was 22 percent higher in the traditional versus the intervention schedule ($P < .001$) as shown in the table below. The investigators concluded that reducing interns' hours can lower the occurrence of serious medical errors in the intensive care unit.

continued

BOX 4-1 continued

Incidence of Serious Medical Errors (rate/1,000 patient days)

Variable	Traditional Schedule	Intervention Schedule	P Value
Serious medical errors made by interns			
Serious medical errors	176 (136.0)	91 (100.1)	< 0.001
Preventable adverse events	27 (20.9)	15 (16.5)	0.21
Intercepted serious errors	91 (70.3)	50 (55.0)	0.02
Nonintercepted serious errors	58 (44.8)	26 (28.6)	< 0.001
Types of serious medical errors made by interns			
Medication	129 (99.7)	75 (82.5)	0.03
Procedural	11 (8.5)	6 (6.6)	0.34
Diagnostic	24 (18.6)	3 (3.3)	< 0.001
Other	12 (9.3)	7 (7.7)	0.47
All serious medical errors, unitwide			
Serious medical errors	250 (193.2)	144 (158.4)	< 0.001
Preventable adverse events	50 (38.6)	35 (38.5)	0.91
Intercepted serious errors	123 (95.1)	63 (69.3)	< 0.001
Nonintercepted serious errors	77 (59.5)	46 (50.6)	0.14
Types of serious medical errors made by interns			
Medication	175 (135.2)	105 (115.5)	0.03
Procedural	18 (13.9)	11 (12.1)	0.48
Diagnostic	28 (21.6)	10 (11.0)	< 0.001
Other	29 (22.4)	18 (19.8)	0.45

SOURCE: Landrigan et al. (2004).

- Cognitive slowing occurs in subject-paced tasks, while time pressure increases cognitive errors.
- Response time slows.
- Performance declines in short-term recall of working memory.
- Performance requiring divergent thinking deteriorates.
- Learning (acquisition) of cognitive tasks is reduced.
- An increase in response suppression errors in tasks requiring normal primarily prefrontal cortex function.

• The likelihood of response preservation on ineffective solutions is increased.

• Compensatory efforts to remain behaviorally effective are increased.

• Although tasks may be done well, performance deteriorates as tasks duration increases (Durmer and Dinges, 2005).

Attention and reaction time are altered by experimental sleep loss, which leads to cumulative, dose-dependent deterioration of attention and reaction time (Figure 4-1). Deterioration is measured in part using the psy-

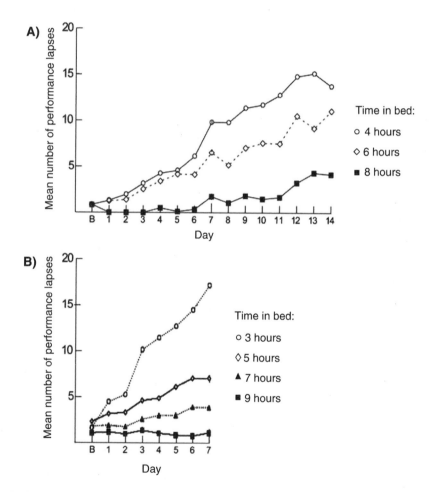

FIGURE 4-1 Repeated nights of sleep loss have cumulative cognitive impairment.
NOTE: B, baseline day.
SOURCES: (A) Van Dongen et al. (2003); (B) Belenky et al. (2003).

chomotor vigilance task (PVT), a test that requires continuous attention to detect randomly occurring stimuli and that is impervious to aptitude and learning effects. In one study 48 healthy subjects were randomized to 4, 6, or 8 hours time in bed for 14 days (Van Dongen et al., 2003). Investigators found a dose-dependent effect, which increased over time (Figure 4-1A). Performance deficits in individuals who slept 6 hours or less per night were similar to those observed in individuals after two nights of *total* sleep deprivation. Most striking was that study subjects remained largely unaware of their performance deficits, as measured by subjective sleepiness ratings. A second study (Belenky et al., 2003) showed a similar dose-dependent, cumulative effect over 7 days of sleep loss in 66 healthy volunteers (Figure 4-1B). Subjects were followed for 3 days after the period of sleep restriction, during which time they recovered, but not enough to return to their baseline levels. Imaging studies have demonstrated a physiological basis for cognitive impairments with sleep loss that has been linked with metabolic declines in the frontal lobe of the brain (Thomas et al., 2000). Although there is not a large body of evidence, associations are also likely between sleep loss and increased risk taking (Roehrs et al., 2004).

Sleep Loss in Adolescents and Academic Performance

Sleep loss in adolescence is common and grows progressively worse over the course of adolescence, according to studies from numerous countries (Wolfson and Carskadon, 2003; Howell et al., 2004). Average sleep duration diminishes by 40 to 50 minutes from ages 13 to 19. Despite the physiological need for about 9 hours of sleep, sleep duration, across this age span, averages around 7 hours and about a quarter of high school and college students are sleep deprived (Wolfson and Carskadon, 1998). Research indicates that patterns of shortened sleep occur in the preadolescent period and may be most marked in African American boys, compared to white children or African American girls (Spilsbury et al., 2004). The decline in adolescent sleep duration is attributed to psychological and social changes, including growing desire for autonomy, increased academic demands, and growing social and recreational opportunities, all of which take place in spite of no change in rise time for school (Figure 4-2) (Wolfson and Carskadon, 1998). Furthermore, the need to earn income adds to the burden. Students who worked 20 or more hours weekly, compared with those who worked less than 20 hours, were found to go to bed later, sleep fewer hours, oversleep, and fall asleep more in class (Millman et al., 2005).

Sleep loss affects alertness, attention, and other cognitive functions in adolescents (Randazzo et al., 1998), but demonstrating a causal relationship between sleep loss and academic performance has been difficult. Most studies attempting to link the two are cross-sectional in design, based on

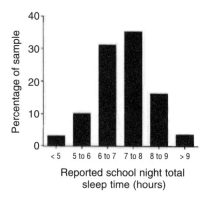

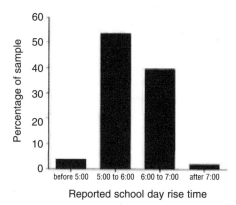

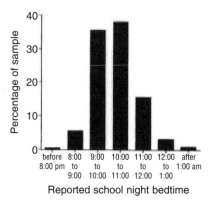

FIGURE 4-2 Sample distribution of sleep patterns.
SOURCE: Wolfson and Carskadon (1998).

self-reporting of grades and sleep times, and lack a control for potential confounders (Wolfson and Carskadon, 2003). An association between short sleep duration and lower academic performance has been demonstrated (Wolfson and Carskadon, 1998; Drake et al., 2003; Shin et al., 2003), but the question of causality has not been resolved by longitudinal studies. A 3-year study of 2,200 middle school students did not find that sleep loss resulted in lower academic performance. It only found a cross-sectional association at the beginning of the study. However, by the end of the study, as sleep time worsened, grades did not proportionately decrease (Fredriksen et al., 2004). A study of the Minneapolis School District, which delayed start times for its high schools by almost 1.5 hours (from 7:15 a.m. to 8:40 a.m.), found significant improvements in sleep time, attendance, and fewer symptoms of depressed mood (Wahlstrom et al., 2001). Further, there was a trend toward better grades, but not of statistical significance. The study compared grades over the 3 years prior to the change with grades 3 years afterwards.

Much of the difficulty in studying sleep loss and its relation to academic performance stems from multiple, often unmeasured, environmental factors that affect sleep (such as school demands, student employment after school, family influences, TV viewing, and Internet access). These are set against the rapid developmental and physiological changes occurring in adolescence. Another difficulty is the challenge of objectively assessing school performance (Wolfson and Carskadon, 2003).

Additional robust intervention studies are needed to determine the effect of having later school start times on student performance. However, a confounder to later school start times is the potential onset of sleep phase delay during middle school (seventh and eighth grade). Moving middle school start time early to compensate for later high school start time may be problematic for the middle school children. There have been no studies that have examined effects of early start time on elementary-aged children (Wolfson and Carskadon, 2003). An alternative to changing the school starting times might be to implement bright light therapy in early morning classes for high school students as a means to change the circadian timing system of these students and thereby enable earlier sleep schedules (Wolfson and Carskadon, 2003).

Sleep Loss and Medical Errors

The Institute of Medicine's report *To Err Is Human* estimated that as many as 98,000 deaths—due to medical errors—occur annually in United States hospitals (IOM, 2000). Long work hours and extended shifts among hospital workers are now known to contribute to the problem. Since the report's release, several new studies, discussed below, have found strong relationships between sleep loss, shift duration, and medical errors among medical residents.

Medical residents work longer hours than virtually all other occupational groups (Steinbrook, 2002). During the first year, medical residents frequently work a 24-hour shift every third night (i.e., 96-hours per week). Two studies found that sleep-deprived surgical residents commit up to twice the number of errors in a simulated laparoscopic surgery (Grantcharov et al., 2001; Eastridge et al., 2003). In a survey of 5,600 medical residents, conducted by the Accreditation Council for Graduate Medical Education, total work time was inversely correlated with reported sleep time. Residents who worked more than 80 hours per week were 50 percent more likely than those working less than 80 hours to report making a significant medical error that led to an adverse patient outcome (Baldwin and Daugherty, 2004). The strongest evidence tying medical errors to sleep-related fatigue from extended work hours comes from an intervention trial designed to limit residents' work hours (Box 4-1). Earlier attempts to demonstrate patient safety benefits by reducing resident hours were beset by methodological problems (Fletcher et al., 2004).

Residents are not the only health professionals to report medical errors in association with short sleep. Nurses who completed logbooks recording their schedule length, sleep, and errors, reported 3.3 times more medical errors during 12.5 hour shifts than 8.5 hour shifts (Rogers et al., 2004). Nearly 40 percent of the nurses reported having 12-hour shifts; and although their sleep duration was not directly studied, the findings suggest that fatigue is a major factor.

Obstructive Sleep Apnea Is Associated with Development, Cognition, and Behavior in Children

Children with obstructive sleep apnea (OSA) often have problems in development, cognition, behavior, and academic performance, according to detailed reviews of the evidence (Schechter, 2002; Bass et al., 2004). The risk of neurobehavioral abnormalities in children with severe OSA is about three times greater than in children without OSA (Schechter, 2002). The contribution of overnight reduction of oxygen levels in the blood (hypoxemia) in comparison to sleep disruption is unclear. One study shows an association with the lowest level of oxygen during sleep and scores in arithmetic (Urschitz et al., 2005), but other studies show cognitive or behavioral deficits in children who snore without severe sleep apnea (Kennedy et al., 2004; Rosen et al., 2004; Gottlieb et al., 2004; O'Hara et al., 2005). Outcome measures used in numerous studies include intelligence quotient, learning and vocabulary, attention, symptoms of attention deficit hyperactivity disorder (ADHD), and academic performance. For example, two historical cohort studies found decrements in intelligence quotient, impaired learning, and vocabulary in children with polysomnography-confirmed cases (Rhodes et al., 1995; Blunden et al., 2000). A study of younger children with sleep apnea also did not find a relationship with academic performance, after adjusting for the effects of socioeconomic status (Chervin et al., 2003). O'Brien and colleagues (2004) found that 35 children with sleep-disordered breathing, compared with matched controls, showed significant deficits in neurocognition, including overall cognitive ability, as well as attention and executive function, but the study did not find behavioral differences. A previous study by the same researchers found higher symptoms of ADHD, according to parents' reports, in children with OSA (O'Brien et al., 2003). Several other studies have found greater symptoms of ADHD in children with OSA than controls (Weissbluth and Liu, 1983; Stradling et al., 1990; Chervin et al., 1997).

The neurobehavioral effects of OSA may be partially reversible with tonsillectomy and adenoidectomy, a surgical procedure that opens the airway. Treatment is related to partial improvement in school performance, cognition, or behavior (Ali et al., 1996; Friedman et al., 2003). A limitation to this work is that it is often difficult to control for the many confounders that influence cognitive function, with a recent study showing that after robustly adjusting for neighborhood socioeconomic status (Emancipator et al., 2006), effects were much attenuated, although they persisted in a subgroup of children who had been born prematurely. No randomized controlled study has been conducted to address the potential reversibility of cognitive deficits with sleep-disordered breathing; such data would more definitively address this situation. Gozal (1998) studied 54 children with sleep-disordered breathing and low school performance. Half of them underwent surgical tonsillectomy and adenoidectomy to treat OSA. Children undergoing the interventions improved their academic performance, compared to untreated children. One problem with the study design; however, was that surgical treatment was not randomly assigned (parents elected whether or not their children could receive surgery). Given the high proportion of children with sleep-disordered breathing, especially in vulnerable groups such as children in minority populations and those born prematurely, there is a large need to address the role of sleep-disordered breathing and its reversibility in these important outcomes.

Sleep-Disordered Breathing and Cognitive Impairment in Adults

Several cross-sectional studies indicate that sleep-disordered breathing in adults is associated with impaired cognitive function (Greenberg et al., 1987; Bedard et al., 1991; Naegele et al., 1995; Redline et al., 1997; Kim et al., 1997). Cognitive deficits, in turn, partially contribute to poorer work performance (Ulfberg et al., 1996), accidents and injuries, and deterioration of the quality of life (see later sections).

A meta-analysis of the case-control studies found that the magnitude of the cognitive disturbance was greatest in individuals with severe OSA. Cognitive domains most affected were attention and executive function (the capacity to plan and organize complex tasks) with only milder effects on memory (Engleman et al., 2000). The meta-analysis also found some cognitive benefit associated with continuous positive airway pressure (CPAP) treatment. In a series of randomized, placebo-controlled crossover trials, people with mild OSA exhibited a trend toward better performance. The failure to detect a robust effect may have been due to the fact that the patients had mild disease, were nonadherent to therapy, or that they had a possibly irreversible component to the cognitive impairment. The cognitive deficits with sleep-disordered breathing are thought to be related to both sleep fragmentation and hypoxemia (Weaver and George, 2005). However, one study showed no clear threshold level between level of hypoxia and performance deficits (Adams et al., 2001). Animal models of chronic episodic hypoxia have led to the hypothesis that cognitive deficits in humans result from injury of nerve cells in the prefrontal cortex (Beebe and Gozal, 2002), the area of the brain responsible for problem solving, emotion, and complex thought.

MOTOR VEHICLE CRASHES AND OTHER INJURIES

Motor Vehicle Crashes

Sleepiness is a significant, and possibly growing, contributor to serious motor vehicle injuries. Almost 20 percent of all serious car crash injuries in the general population are associated with driver sleepiness, independent of alcohol effects (Connor et al., 2002). Driver sleepiness is most frequently a manifestation of sleep loss, as discussed below, but other sleep disorders, which have lower prevalence, contribute to the problem, including sleep-disordered breathing, restless legs syndrome, and narcolepsy.

The 20 percent figure, cited above, is the population-attributable risk, which is a key public health measure indicating what percentage of car crash injuries, including fatal injuries of passengers, could be avoided by eliminating driver sleepiness. The finding was based on a population-based case-control study in a region of New Zealand in which 571 car drivers and a matched control sample were asked detailed questions about measures of acute sleepiness while driving (Connor et al., 2002). The study adjusted for potential confounding factors, including alcohol. Crashes examined in this study involved a hospitalization or death. The greatest risk factor for the crashes was sleep loss and time of day (driving between 2:00 a.m. to 5:00 a.m.), but sleep apnea symptoms were not risk factors.

Indications are that the public health burden of sleepiness-related injuries is likely increasing, given recent trends in drowsy driving. The National Sleep Foundation found that self-reported drowsy driving has increased significantly over the past years, from 51 percent of respondents in 2001 to 60 percent in 2005 (NSF, 2005). Similarly striking was that more than 10 percent of the entire sample reported nodding off or falling asleep while driving at least 1 to 2 days per month.

The impact of driver sleepiness is similar in magnitude to that of alcohol consumption. A study of all crashes between 1990 to 1992 reported to North Carolina's uniform reporting system found that fall-asleep crashes (ones in which a law officer determines the driver to be asleep or fatigued) and alcohol-related crashes were similar in terms of serious injuries (13.5 and 17.8 percent of crashes from all causes, respectively) and fatalities (1.4 and 2.1 percent of all fatalities, respectively) (Pack et al., 1995). In actual driving performance on a closed course, sleep-deprived adults performed as poorly as did alcohol-challenged adults (Powell et al., 2001). After a night of total sleep deprivation, impairments in lane-keeping ability were similar to those found with blood alcohol content of 0.07 percent (Fairclough and Graham, 1999).

Fall-asleep crashes have distinct patterns by type, age, and time of day. According to the North Carolina study, fall-asleep crashes are largely off-the-road and at higher speeds (in excess of 50 mph) (Pack et al., 1995). Adolescents and young adults between the ages of 16 and 29 are the most likely to be involved in crashes caused by the driver falling asleep (Horne and Reyner, 1995; Pack et al., 1995). They account for about 50 percent of all crashes (Horne and Reyner, 1995; Pack et al., 1995). Fall-asleep crashes occur at two periods of day that coincide with circadian variation in sleepiness, in the early morning (2:00 a.m. to 8:00 a.m.) (Pack et al., 1995; Connor et al., 2002) and during the midafternoon (Horne and Reyner, 1995; Pack et al., 1995; Carskadon, 2004). The most common reasons behind fall-asleep crashes are working multiple jobs, night shift work, and sleep duration of less than 5 hours (Connor et al., 2002; Stutts et al., 2003).

Sleep apnea accounts for a small, but measurable percentage of motor vehicle crashes, primarily in drivers above the age of 25 (Sassani et al., 2004). Individuals with sleep apnea are at twice the risk of having a traffic accident as unaffected individuals (Teran-Santos et al., 1999)—the higher the apnea-hypopnea index, the higher the risk (Young et al., 1997a). Sleepy drivers tend to display reduced vigilance, slow reaction times, and loss of steering control. Steering impairment in OSA, sleep deprivation, and alcohol intoxication was compared in a controlled clinical trial. Untreated OSA and sleep deprivation were similar in producing progressive steering deterioration throughout the drive, whereas alcohol-impaired individuals steered equally throughout the drive (Hack et al., 2001). Occupational groups at high risk of sleep-related crashes are night shift workers (Horne and Reyner, 1995; Ohayon et al., 2002; Drake et al., 2004), medical residents and house staff (Marcus and Loughlin, 1996; Barger et al., 2005), and commercial truck drivers (Walsh et al., 2005).

Commercial truck drivers have attracted the most study because of the prevalence, severity, and public health impact of crashes involving commercial trucks. There are an estimated 110,000 injuries and 5,000 fatalities each year in motor vehicle accidents involving commercial trucks (CNTS, 1996). The National Transportation Safety Board (NTSB) determined that fatigue (including sleepiness) was the probable cause of 57 percent of crashes leading to a truck driver's death (NTSB, 1990a,b). Although this figure is not universally accepted, the definition of *fatigue* by the NTSB is equivalent to the term *sleepiness* or *sleep-related fatigue* used by sleep experts (i.e., fatigue that results in human performance failure) (Walsh et al., 2005). For each truck driver fatality, another three to four people are killed (NHTSA, 1994).

A congressionally mandated study of 80 long-haul truck drivers in the United States and Canada found that drivers had short sleep duration, averaging 5.2 hours in bed and 4.8 hours of sleep per day (Federal Motor Carrier Safety Administration, 1996). Sleep duration was verified electrophysiologically over the 5-day study. Further, commercial drivers have a high prevalence of sleep apnea (Stoohs et al., 1995). Recent studies have found that sleep apnea affects 8 to 15 percent of commercial drivers in the United States and Australia (Gurubhagavatula et al., 2004; Howard et al., 2004).

Work-Related Injuries

Sleep-related fatigue is an independent risk factor in work-related injuries and fatalities, according to two large and well-designed studies (Akerstedt et al., 2002; Swaen et al., 2003). Swaen and coworkers prospectively studied a cohort of more than 7,000 workers in numerous industries in the Netherlands over a 1-year period before studying the occurrence of occupational accidents. During the year they collected information about sleep patterns and other potential risk factors for work-related injuries. The 108 employees who reported being injured during the next year could be assessed for risk factors without recall bias affecting the results. The study found a dose-response relationship between two sleep-related fatigue measures and injuries. For example, highly fatigued workers were 70 percent more likely to be involved in accidents than were workers reporting low fatigue levels, after adjustment for other risk factors. Workers with chronic insomnia were also far more likely than those who were good sleepers to report industrial accidents or injuries (Leger et al., 2002). Finally, disturbed sleep plays a role in occupational fatalities. In a large 20-year prospective study in Sweden of nearly 50,000 individuals, those reporting disturbed sleep were nearly twice as likely to die in a work-related accident (OR = 1.89, 95% CI 1.22–2.94) (Akerstedt et al., 2002). Similarly, workers who report snoring and excessive daytime sleepiness, indications of sleep apnea, are twice as likely to be involved in workplace accidents, as verified by registry data and after adjusting for all potential confounders (Lindberg et al., 2001).

Falls in Older People

Falls are a common and costly problem in older people (65 years and older), whether in the community or in long-term care facilities. Each year, more than 30 percent of older people fall (Hausdorff et al., 2001). Falls are the leading cause of death for this particular age group (Murphy, 2000). Although most falls are not directly fatal, they are a leading cause of injuries and trauma-related hospital admissions (Alexander et al., 1992).

Insomnia increases the risk of falling (Brassington et al., 2000). One of the major questions raised by this finding is what is responsible for the increased risk of falls—the underlying insomnia or the use of medication to treat it? Until recently, most of the studies addressing this question were not large enough to yield an answer. In 2005, a large, prospective study of 34,000 nursing home residents across the state of Michigan ruled out use of hypnotic medications as a risk factor for falls (Avidan et al., 2005). In fact, the study found that treated insomnia, and untreated insomnia, but not hypnotic medications, were predictors of falls. Although the results of this study did not find that insomnia increased the risk of hip fractures, other studies have found an association (Fitzpatrick et al., 2001). Preliminary data from the Study of Osteoporosis in Women also indicate an increased risk of falls associated with decreased sleep efficiency and sleep time (as measured objectively using actigraphy) in a large group of older women, with effects persisting after adjustment of health status and mood and other confounders (Stone et al., 2004).

Interventions

There have been a few studies that have examined the effect of interventions on improving the outcomes associated with sleepiness. A range of regulatory, technological, and therapeutic approaches are possible to ameliorate the problem of sleepiness among commercial drivers (Walsh et al., 2005). However, there has been limited study of the benefit of these strategies. Thus, before additional rules and regulations are developed, analysis of the effectiveness of the current regulations and statutory items is needed. This analysis will help the establishment of much-needed future rules and regulations pertaining to sleep loss and fatigue. Preplanned naps have been successfully tested in crew members on transmeridian flights; the findings show that safe and feasible rotations occurred as crew members took brief, 40-minute nap periods, and the naps improved alertness (Graeber et al., 1986a,b). Similarly, a study of Italian policemen who patrol highways found that prophylactic naps before a night shift can lower the risk of motor vehicle accidents during the shift, according to a combination of retrospective questionnaire, prospective analysis, and mathematical modeling (Garbarino et al., 2004)

The strongest evidence for the public health benefits of treatment comes from clinical trials and retrospective studies of the impact of CPAP therapy for sleep apnea. These studies also dispel any doubt of the causal relationship between sleep disorders and accidents. In a randomized, controlled clinical trial, 59 men with sleep apnea were assigned either to therapeutic CPAP or subtherapeutic CPAP. The latter does not deliver enough pressure to open the pharynx and achieve a therapeutic effect. One month later the men were placed in a steering simulator. Therapeutic CPAP significantly improved their steering performance and reaction time relative to subtherapeutic CPAP (Hack et al., 2000). Previous clinical trials had also shown CPAP to be effective in terms of reducing the rate of self-reported automobile crashes and performance on driving tests, but they were uncontrolled (Cassel et al., 1996; Krieger et al., 1997). A review and meta-analysis estimates that nearly 1,000 lives would be saved annually if all drivers with OSA were treated with CPAP (Sassani et al., 2004).

IMPACT ON FUNCTIONING AND QUALITY OF LIFE

Sleep problems, difficulty initiating and maintaining sleep, nonrestorative sleep, and excessive daytime sleepiness are associated with adverse effects on well-being, functioning, and quality of life, according to numerous studies covering the general population (Baldwin et al., 2001, 2004; Hasler et al., 2005; Strine and Chapman, 2005), working people (Kuppermann et al., 1995), and clinical populations (Simon and VonKorff, 1997), including pediatric samples (Rosen et al., 2002). Studies have used various measures of quality of life and functional status, the most common of which is a validated questionnaire known as the SF-36, a 36-item measure that asks about eight domains: (1) physical functioning; (2) role limitation due to physical health problems (role physical); (3) bodily pain; (4) general health perceptions; (5) vitality; (6) social functioning; (7) role limitations due to emotional health problems (role emotional); and (8) mental health. A similar measure is the health-related quality of life survey, which asks fewer questions. Individuals who suffer from primarily sleep apnea, narcolepsy, restless legs, primary parasomnias, and insomnia constantly report poorer quality of life compared to population norms (Reimer and Flemons, 2003).

Using health-related measures of quality of life, the functional impact of sleep loss was assessed by a large and nationally representative survey, the United States Behavioral Risk Factor Surveillance System (Strine and Chapman, 2005). The study focused on nocturnal sleep time in nearly 80,000 respondents. About 26 percent of the respondents reported obtaining insufficient sleep on a frequent basis (not enough sleep on 14 days or more over the past 30 days). This group was significantly more likely than those without frequent sleep insufficiency to report poorer functioning and quality of life on each of the eight items of the health-related quality of life.

Several studies have dealt with insomnia and its adverse impact on quality of life (Zammit et al., 1999; Leger et al., 2001; Katz and McHorney, 2002). People with severe insomnia reported lower quality of life on all eight domains of the SF-36 (Leger et al., 2001). Their low quality-of-life ratings were similar to ratings by patients with congestive heart failure and depression, according to a study of nearly 3,500 primary care patients (Katz and McHorney, 2002) (Figure 4-3). About 16 percent of the sample had severe insomnia, and the study adjusted for numerous factors including health habits, obesity, other chronic conditions, and severity of disease. A study of a large health maintenance organization population (n = 2,000) found that insomnia (versus no current insomnia) was associated with significantly greater impairment, as measured by the self-rated Social Disability Schedule and the interviewer-rated Brief Disability Questionnaire. Individuals with insomnia also had more days of restricted activity due to illness

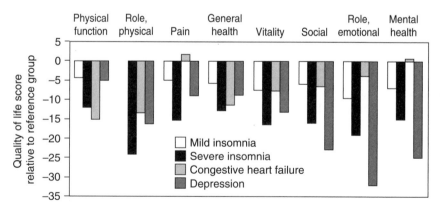

FIGURE 4-3 Severe insomnia affects quality of life.
SOURCE: Edinger and Means (2005).

and more days spent in bed (Simon and VonKorff, 1997). One study revealed a dose-response relationship, with higher levels of insomnia being associated with greater impairments in the ability to accomplish daily tasks and decreased enjoyment of interpersonal relationships (Roth and Ancoli-Israel, 1999).

Individuals with severe OSA also report significantly poorer quality of life, and mild OSA is also associated with reduced vitality (Baldwin et al., 2001). These effects are similar to those of other chronic diseases in the general population in the United States. Individuals with OSA who are compliant with CPAP treatment report improved changes in vitality and quality of life 2 months after the onset of CPAP treatment (Redline et al., 1998).

Symptoms of restless legs syndrome are associated with lower quality of life (Unruh et al., 2004), similar to the quality of life of individuals with type 2 diabetes mellitus and acute heart attack (Allen et al., 2003). Restless legs syndrome also affects marital relationships. Approximately one-third of couples sleep in separate beds due to the discomfort of their partner's repetitive leg movements (Montplaisir et al., 2005).

Approximately a quarter of children and adolescents report difficulty with sleep (Stein et al., 2001; Archbold et al., 2002). However, very few studies have assessed the association between sleep loss and sleep disorders and health-related quality of life in children. Analysis of a widely used parent report measure of children's physical, emotional, and social functional status and well being—the CHQ-PF50—found the quality of life of their children deteriorated with the severity of OSA (Rosen et al., 2002). This is consistent with a negative association between sleep difficulties and health-related quality of life that was observed a similar analysis of 80 parents of children referred to a pediatric sleep disorders clinic (Hart et al., 2005). Thus, sleep difficulties may broadly affect a child's development through its impact on children's social, emotional, and physical functioning.

Family and Community Function

The consequences of sleep loss and sleep disorders are not restricted to affected individuals; they also disrupt families and communities. Although relatively sparse, the research described in this section points to widespread impact on the health and well-being of sleep partners and/or other family members. Their sleep quality and health can be disrupted, as can their well-being, income, and capacity to care for children or ill family members. Adverse effects on family cohesiveness, in turn, can lead to severe family turmoil and divorce. Similarly, sleep disruption of family caregivers has broader societal effects by contributing to hospitalization or nursing home placement of ill family members for whom they provide care.

Most research on families and communities deals with bed partners of individuals with a sleep problem. Bed partners of individuals with sleep-disordered breathing report a lower quality of life, based on the SF-36 survey than the sleep-disordered breathing patients (Breugelmans et al., 2004). Further, in a large population-based sample of older individuals, bed partners report poor health, depressed mood, poor mental health, and marital unhappiness (Strawbridge et al., 2004).

Does CPAP therapy improve bed partners' sleep? At least four studies have addressed this question, with three showing improvement. Two of the studies that demonstrated a benefit were nonrandomized and used a *before* versus *after* study design. After approximately one month of CPAP therapy, partners experienced less daytime sleepiness as measured by the Epworth Sleepiness Scale and improved quality of life as measured by the SF-36 scale (Doherty et al., 2003; Parish and Lyng, 2003). A small, polysomnographic study of individuals using CPAP found that their partners show fewer arousals and greater sleep efficiency in the hours after CPAP's introduction versus the hours before (Beninati et al., 1999). The improvement in sleep efficiency (percentage of time asleep while in bed) translated to an extra hour of sleep per night. The only placebo-controlled study found that CPAP is associated with subjective improvement in bed partners' sleep (via the Pittsburgh Sleep Quality Inventory), but no objective improvement, as measured by polysomnography (McArdle et al., 2000).

Sleep-disordered breathing has also been found to heighten the rate of divorce and the use of paid personal leave, among other effects, according to a study of obese individuals with OSA. A team of Swedish researchers, studying a large registry of obese subjects, found that individuals with OSA (as defined by symptoms of snoring and daytime sleepiness) report about three times the rate of divorce of those without OSA and/or daytime sleepiness (Grunstein et al., 1995). The effects are even more pronounced among the women in the sample with OSA (n = 155). Men with OSA (n = 338) reported less income, and both genders reported more sick leave and disturbed work performance. These effects were independent of the effects of obesity and other health factors. In a separate study, 60 percent of bed partners reported that they slept apart versus 20 percent of controls. Although the partners' level of marital satisfaction was similar to controls', the partners reported greater dissatisfaction with the sleep behaviors of their apneic spouses (Billmann and Ware, 2002).

A common complaint of parents is being awakened by a young child with a sleep problem. Sleep loss is indeed reported more frequently by parents after the birth of a child than during pregnancy (Gay et al., 2004). Improvement in parents' sleep quality, as well as improvement of family well-being, occurs after the introduction of a behavioral intervention designed to train parents to overcome sleep problems in young children through a graduated conditioning program known as extinction (Eckerberg, 2004). Previously, controlled clinical trials had shown that parent training and extinction are effective for treating young children (Mindell, 1999; Ramchandani et al., 2000), but the trials had not measured the impact on sleep and well-being of parents and families.

Sleep disturbances in chronic illness, whether in the affected individual or in the caregiver, affect decisions about hospital or nursing home placement. This is especially true for patients with Alzheimer's disease, considering that up to 44 percent of them have sleep disturbances (Ritchie, 1996; McCurry et al., 1999). Indeed, sleep disturbance in Alzheimer's disease is a common risk factor for nursing home placement (Chenier, 1997; Hope et al., 1998). Sleep hygiene training, targeted at both Alzheimer's disease patients and the caregivers, can improve sleep quality in patients (McCurry et al., 1998, 2003, 2005). One area of future study is whether treating sleep problems (in either the patient or the caregiver) can delay institutionalization. Counseling of caregivers—although not explicitly targeted to their sleep disturbance or that of the patient—has been shown, in a separate randomized trial, to delay nursing home placement (Mittelman et al., 1996). Within nursing homes, behavioral and pharmacological therapies are effective at improving sleep problems (Alessi et al., 1999; Naylor et al., 2000).

ECONOMIC IMPACT OF SLEEP LOSS AND SLEEP DISORDERS

Although problems falling asleep or daytime sleepiness affect 35 to 40 percent of the population (Hossain and Shapiro, 2002), the full economic impact of sleep loss and sleep disorders on individuals and society is not known. There are limited data on the economic impact of insomnia, sleep-disordered breathing, and narcolepsy; the economic impact of other sleep disorders has not been analyzed. As will be discussed in further detail in Chapters 5 and 8, the lack of sufficient data result from inadequate reporting and surveillance mechanisms.

Increased Health Care Utilization

Daytime sleepiness, inadequate sleep time, insomnia, and other sleep disorders place a significant burden on the health care system through increased utilization of the health care system (see below). Patients in the highest quartile of the Epworth Sleepiness Scale are associated with an 11 percent increase in health care utilization, and individuals with sleep-disordered breathing or sleepiness and fatigue are associated with a 10 to 20 percent increase in utilization (Kapur et al., 2002b).

Insomnia

Individuals suffering from insomnia place an increased burden on the health care system (Ohayon and Roth, 2003). Their activity is more limited (Simon and VonKorff, 1997), and they are significantly more likely to access medical and psychiatric care than are individuals that do not have a sleep or psychiatric disorder (Weissman et al., 1997). Individuals with insomnia who also have an associated psychiatric disorder are more likely to seek treatment for emotional problems (14.9 percent versus 8 percent) (Weissman et al., 1997), have a greater number of physician visits, and be admitted to a hospital twice as often (Leger et al., 2002). The burden insomnia place on the health care system is long-term—the majority of individuals with either mild (59 percent) or severe (83 percent) insomnia continue to suffer symptoms of insomnia 2 years after initial diagnosis (Katz and McHorney, 1998). Consequently, individuals suffering from insomnia place a significant economic burden on society resulting in increased health care costs (see below).

Obstructive Sleep Apnea

Individuals with OSA also place a significant burden on the health care system. In the year prior to diagnosis, the medical expenses of individuals with OSA were almost two times as much as control individuals not diagnosed with OSA ($2,720 vs. $1,384) (Kapur et al., 1999). Around 80 to 90 percent of OSA cases remain undiagnosed and untreated, which increases the burden of this disorder (Young et al., 1997b; Kapur et al., 2002a). Analysis of health care utilization in Canadians with severe OSA found that during the year prior to diagnosis, individuals with severe OSA spent more than twice the number of days in the hospital compared to controls (251 versus 90). This was associated with an increase in cost of services—$49,000 to $99,000 (Kryger et al., 1996). This figure is likely greater in the United States, which also has 10 to 15 percent higher health care utilization associated with severe OSA (Kapur et al., 2002b)—due to higher health care costs compared to Canada. OSA also affects a child's health care utilization. A survey of 287 children with OSA found that in the year prior to diagnosis, children with OSA had a 226 percent increase in health care utilization and had significantly more visits to emergency departments (Reuveni et al., 2002).

A retrospective observational cohort study demonstrated that CPAP treatment reversed the trend of increasing health care utilization observed prior to OSA diagnosis (Bahammam et al., 1999; Albarrak et al., 2005). In a Canadian study, physician visits decreased during the 5 years following CPAP treatment, compared to the 5-year period prior to diagnosis, resulting in lower physician fees (Figure 4-4). After converting to American dol-

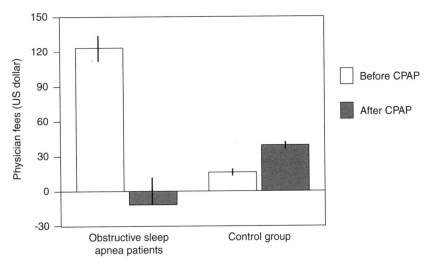

FIGURE 4-4 Effect of CPAP treatment on physician fees.
SOURCE: Albarrak et al. (2005).

lars, mean total fees were greater the year prior to OSA diagnosis ($179.09 ± $32.85) compared to the fifth year after diagnosis ($16.77 ± $33.66) in individuals who were compliant with CPAP treatment (Albarrak et al., 2005). The realized savings would likely be much larger in the United States due to higher associated health care costs.

Direct Costs of Sleep Loss and Sleep Disorders

Billions of dollars are spent each year in the United States on the direct costs of sleep loss and sleep disorders. These medical costs include expenses associated with doctor visits, hospital services, prescriptions and over-the-counter medications. In 1995 the direct cost of insomnia in the United States was estimated to be $13.9 billion (Walsh and Engelhardt, 1999). Further, based on the costs associated with a laboratory-based polysomnogram, it would cost over $17.5 billion to test and $3 billion to treat every person in the United States who has sleep apnea[1] (Sassani et al., 2004). Although it is predicted that the advent of more effective portable monitoring devices (Chapter 6) will decrease the costs associated with testing and diagnosis of sleep disorders, the total direct costs will still remain high and be a burden.

---

[1]Estimates based on a 5 percent prevalence and 2005 estimates of the United States population (295,734,134) and every individual receiving a type 4 polysomnography (CMS code 95810).

Indirect Costs of Sleep Loss and Sleep Disorders

The indirect costs associated with sleep loss and sleep disorders also result in billions of dollars of annual expenditures, including costs associated with illness-related morbidity and mortality, absenteeism, disability, reduction or loss of productivity, industrial and motor vehicle accidents, hospitalization, and increased alcohol consumption (Hossain and Shapiro, 2002). As is the case with direct costs, for each of these categories further analysis is required to determine the complete indirect costs of sleep loss and sleep disorders. The annual economic impact of sleep problems relating to workers inability to adjust to late shifts are estimated to be at minimum over $60 billion (Table 4-1) (Moore-Ede, 1993). In addition, it has been estimated that sleep-related fatigue costs businesses $150 billion a year in absenteeism, workplace accidents, and other lost productivity (Sleep Disorders Create Growing Opportunities for Hospitals, 2001).

A 1994 analysis of automobile accidents estimated the cost of accidents attributed to sleepiness to be between $29.2 to $37.9 billion (Leger, 1994). Over 50 percent of automobile crashes involving a truck, where a fatality occurred, were caused by sleep-related fatigue, costing approximately $2.7 million and 4,800 lives (NTSB, 1990a, 1990b; USDOT, 1991; Mitler et al., 2000). However, there is no standardized mechanism to record fatigue- and sleep-related accidents; therefore, these figures are likely underestimates of the total cost of automobile accidents.

Although the complete economic impact of sleep disorders and sleep loss is limited, the available data demonstrates the high burden that inadequate sleep has on the economy. With the average age of the population rising, incidence of sleep disorders is likely to rise, leading to increased costs (Phillips, 2005).

TABLE 4-1 Annual Economic Impact of Sleep Problems Due to Late Shifts

	Cost (billions $)
Reduced manufacturing productivity	50.0
Increased motor vehicle accidents	5.7
Increased industrial accidents	4.0
Increased accidents, injuries, and deaths at work	2.5
Increase in other medical and psychiatric illnesses	2.0
Personnel turnover and retraining	1.0
Total	65.2

SOURCE: Moore-Ede (1993).

Economic Impact of Insomnia

The total cost estimates of insomnia range from $30 billion (Walsh and Engelhardt, 1999) to $107.5 billion (Stoller, 1994). The large variation in the range is attributed to the underlying assumptions about the prevalence of insomnia in the United States, which range from 10 to 33 percent. However, it is evident that even using more conservative prevalence estimates the total annual costs in the United States exceeds tens of billions of dollars.

Direct Cost

In 1995 the direct costs of insomnia totaled approximately $13.96 billion (Table 4-2). However, this is an underestimate of the total costs, as approximately 12 percent of all physicians, including hospital-based or government employed physicians (including doctors in VA hospitals), were not included in these estimates. In 2002 it was estimated that in the United States 27 million prescriptions were filled for hypnotics, worth about $1.2 billion (Mendelson, 2005). Calculations based on medical claims showed that increased physician fees and medical expenses for elderly and non-elderly patients with insomnia were respectively $5,580 and $4,220 higher

TABLE 4-2 The Direct Costs of Insomnia in the United States for 1995

	Costs (millions $)
Substances used for insomnia	
Prescription medications	809.92
Nonprescription medications	325.80
Alcohol	780.39
Melatonin	50.00
Total Cost of Substances	**1,966.11**
Health care services for insomnia	
Outpatient physician visits	660.00
Psychologist visits	122.40
Social working visits	75.30
Sleep specialist visits	18.20
Mental health organizations	153.00
In-patient hospital care	30.80
Nursing home care	10,900.00
Total	**11,960.70**
Total direct costs	**13,926.11**

SOURCE: Walsh and Engelhardt (1999).

than match controls (Ozminkowski et al., 2004), demonstrating the expense incurred by individuals with insomnia.

In 1995 over 78 percent of direct costs associated with insomnia, $11.96 billion, was spent on nursing home care (Walsh and Engelhardt, 1999), a 132 percent increase since 1990 (Walsh et al., 1995). Although this proportion may seem high, almost half of the population over 65 years of age report difficulty with sleep (Mellinger et al., 1985), and 20.4 percent of admissions to a nursing home were attributed to sleep disturbances (Walsh and Engelhardt, 1999).

Two factors contribute to these higher costs associated with insomnia. First, the general population is typically reluctant to consult doctors about their sleep problems, and second, inadequate physician training prevents proper recognition, diagnosis, and treatment of patients with insomnia (see Chapters 5 and 7) (Walsh and Engelhardt, 1999; Benca, 2005; NIH, 2005).

Indirect Cost

To date there has not been a detailed analysis assessing the total indirect costs associated with insomnia. A 1988 study estimated that productivity loss resulting from insomnia cost $41.1 billion (Stoller, 1994). Absenteeism cost more than $57 billion (Walsh, 2004). Therefore, once the costs of industrial and motor vehicle collisions and related morbidities are included, the indirect cost of insomnia could top $100 billion.

Insomnia places a greater burden on individuals of lower socioeconomic status (Gellis et al., 2005), those who are less educated, and those who are more likely to be unemployed (Bixler et al., 1979; Karacan et al., 1983; Frisoni et al., 1993; Kim et al., 2000; Li et al., 2002). Falls caused by insomnia also contribute to its economic burden. A greater risk for falls was associated with both hypnotic use (29 percent, OR = 1.29) and insomnia (90 percent, OR = 1.90) (Avidan, 2005). Like other sleep disorders, insomnia is more prevalent in the elderly (Mellinger et al., 1985); therefore, as the United States population continues to age it is expected that the cost associated with falls caused by insomnia will also continue to rise.

Economic Impact of Obstructive Sleep Apnea

Direct Cost

Similar to other sleep disorders, there is very limited data on the direct costs associated with obstructive sleep apnea. Most of the analysis has explored the impact of OSA. The average costs of diagnosis and treatment over five years for an individual is over $4,000 (Table 4-3) (Chervin et al., 1999; Wittmann and Rodenstein, 2004). An analysis of 97 obese individuals with

TABLE 4-3 Cost of Diagnosis and Treatment of OSA

Polysomnogram	$1,190
CPAP titration	$1,190
CPAP equipment and setup	$1,290
Initial office visits	$210
Annual follow-up	$330
Total	**$4,210**

SOURCE: Chervin et al. (1999).

OSA in Canada found that over a 2-year period they had almost $30,000 in expenditures from physician claims and utilized $49,000 to $99,000 more in services than their control counterparts (Kryger et al., 1996).

Indirect Cost

There is also limited analysis of the total indirect costs associated with OSA. Based on estimates of from the Sleep Heart Health Study, only 10 to 20 percent of individuals with OSA are estimated to have been diagnosed (Kapur et al., 2002a). The annual medical costs resulting from untreated OSA was $3.4 billion (Kapur et al., 1999).

Automobile collisions attributed to OSA also contribute to the large economic burden of the syndrome. Sassani and colleagues performed a meta-analysis of PubMed from 1980 to 2003 and investigated the relationship between collisions and OSA (2004). This information was then combined with data from the National Safety Council to estimate OSA-related collisions, costs, and fatalities. Based on this analysis, it was estimated that in the year 2000 more than 800,000 drivers were involved in OSA-related motor vehicle collisions (Sassani et al., 2004). These collisions resulted in loss of life to 1,400 individuals and cost $15.9 billion. The authors calculated that annually it would cost $3.18 billion to provide CPAP treatment to all drivers who suffer from OSA, saving 980 lives and $11.1 billion to $7.9 billion if the cost of CPAP treatment is taken into account. For every dollar spent on CPAP, $3.49 would be saved in reduced collision costs. This savings does not include the presumed reduction in the number of accidents at work, decreased health care costs, or improved quality of life (Sassani et al., 2004).

Relationship Between Socioeconomic Status, Race, and Obstructive Sleep Apnea

The relationship between socioeconomic status, race, and obstructive sleep apnea is not well understood. There are limited data that suggest that the prevalence and severity of OSA is higher in African Americans compared to whites (Scharf et al., 2004), especially in adults under 25 years of age (Redline et al., 1994; Rosen et al., 2002). Compared to whites, African Americans with OSA are more likely to have a higher body mass index (Redline et al., 1994) and a lower mean income (Scharf et al., 2004). Analysis performed between Asians and whites found that OSA in Asians was significantly more severe compared to whites (Ong and Clerk, 1998). However, differences in age, gender, body mass index, or neck circumference did not account for these differences.

Economic Impact of Narcolepsy

The impact of narcolepsy on the economy is also not well understood. A review of the PubMed database through May of 2005 found only one relevant report. It examined narcolepsy's effect on 75 individuals in Germany (Dodel et al., 2004). After converting to American dollars the annual total costs to an individual were $15,410. The average direct costs accounted for 21 percent of the total expenditures ($3,310 total), $1,260 for hospital care, and $1,060 for medications. However, these figures have been extrapolated from a single German cohort and differences in the organization of their respective health care systems have not been taken into account. Therefore, improved surveillance data are needed to determine the actual economic impact of narcolepsy on the American population.

The socioeconomic status of an individual does not affect the prevalence and severity of narcolepsy; however, narcolepsy may worsen an individual's socioeconomic standing. In Germany individuals with narcolepsy have a significantly higher unemployment rate than average, 59 percent compared to the national average of 9 percent (Dodel et al., 2004). Similarly, studies performed in the United Kingdom (Daniels et al., 2001) and the United States (Goswami, 1998) found that 30 to 37 percent of respondents had lost their job due to narcolepsy.

Summary

Although the data are limited, the effect of sleep disorders, chronic sleep loss, and sleepiness on accident rates, performance deficits, and health care utilization on the American economy is significant. The high estimated costs to society of leaving the most prevalent sleep disorders untreated are far more than the costs that would be incurred by delivering adequate treatment. Hundreds of billions of dollars are spent and/or lost annually as a result of poor or limited sleep. However, greater surveillance and analysis are required to estimate the full economic implications of these problems.

REFERENCES

ACGME (Accreditation Council for Graduate Medical Education). 2003. *Common Program Requirements (Resident Duty Hours)*. [Online]. Available: http://www.acgme.org/dutyhours/dutyhourscommonpr.pdf [accessed May 13, 2005].

Adams N, Strauss M, Schluchter M, Redline S. 2001. Relation of measures of sleep-disordered breathing to neuropsychological functioning. *American Journal of Respiratory and Critical Care Medicine* 163(7):1626–1631.

Akerstedt T, Fredlund P, Gillberg M, Jansson B. 2002. A prospective study of fatal occupational accidents–relationship to sleeping difficulties and occupational factors. *Journal of Sleep Research* 11(1):69–71.

Albarrak M, Banno K, Sabbagh AA, Delaive K, Walld R, Manfreda J, Kryger MH. 2005. Utilization of healthcare resources in obstructive sleep apnea syndrome: A 5-year follow-up study in men using CPAP. *Sleep* 28(10):1306–1311.

Alessi CA, Yoon EJ, Schnelle JF, Al-Samarrai NR, Cruise PA. 1999. A randomized trial of a combined physical activity and environmental intervention in nursing home residents: Do sleep and agitation improve? *Journal of the American Geriatrics Society* 47(7):784–791.

Alexander BH, Rivara FP, Wolf ME. 1992. The cost and frequency of hospitalization for fall-related injuries in older adults. *American Journal of Public Health* 82(7):1020–1023.

Ali NJ, Pitson D, Stradling JR. 1996. Sleep-disordered breathing: Effects of adenotonsillectomy on behaviour and psychological functioning. *European Journal of Pediatrics* 155(1):56–62.

Allen RP, Picchietti D, Hening WA, Trenkwalder C, Walters AS, Montplaisir J, et al. 2003. Restless legs syndrome: Diagnostic criteria, special considerations, and epidemiology. A report from the restless legs syndrome diagnosis and epidemiology workshop at the National Institutes of Health. *Sleep Medicine* 4(2):101–119.

Archbold KH, Pituch KJ, Panahi P, Chervin RD. 2002. Symptoms of sleep disturbances among children at two general pediatric clinics. *Journal of Pediatrics* 140(1):97–102.

Avidan AY. 2005. Sleep in the geriatric patient population. *Seminars in Neurology* 25(1):52–63.

Avidan AY, Fries BE, James ML, Szafara KL, Wright GT, Chervin RD. 2005. Insomnia and hypnotic use, recorded in the minimum data set, as predictors of falls and hip fractures in Michigan nursing homes. *Journal of the American Geriatrics Society* 53(6):955–962.

Bahammam A, Delaive K, Ronald J, Manfreda J, Roos L, Kryger MH. 1999. Health care utilization in males with obstructive sleep apnea syndrome two years after diagnosis and treatment. *Sleep* 22(6):740–747.

Baldwin CM, Griffith KA, Nieto FJ, O'Connor GT, Walsleben JA, Redline S. 2001. The association of sleep-disordered breathing and sleep symptoms with quality of life in the Sleep Heart Health Study. *Sleep* 24(1):96–105.

Baldwin DC Jr, Daugherty SR. 2004. Sleep deprivation and fatigue in residency training: Results of a national survey of first- and second-year residents. *Sleep* 27(2):217–223.

Barger LK, Cade BE, Ayas NT, Cronin JW, Rosner B, Speizer FE, Czeisler CA, Harvard Work Hours HaS Group. 2005. Extended work shifts and the risk of motor vehicle crashes among interns. *New England Journal of Medicine* 352(2):125–134.

Bass JL, Corwin M, Gozal D, Moore C, Nishida H, Parker S, Schonwald A, Wilker RE, Stehle S, Kinane TB. 2004. The effect of chronic or intermittent hypoxia on cognition in childhood: A review of the evidence. *Pediatrics* 114(3):805–816.

Bedard MA, Montplaisir J, Richer F, Rouleau I, Malo J. 1991. Obstructive sleep apnea syndrome: Pathogenesis of neuropsychological deficits. *Journal of Clinical and Experimental Neuropsychology* 13(6):950–964.

Beebe DW, Gozal D. 2002. Obstructive sleep apnea and the prefrontal cortex: Towards a comprehensive model linking nocturnal upper airway obstruction to daytime cognitive and behavioral deficits. *Journal of Sleep Research* 11(1):1–16.

Belenky G, Wesensten NJ, Thorne DR, Thomas ML, Sing HC, Redmond DP, Russo MB, Balkin TJ. 2003. Patterns of performance degradation and restoration during sleep restriction and subsequent recovery: A sleep dose-response study. *Journal of Sleep Research* 12(1):1–12.

Benca RM. 2005. Diagnosis and treatment of chronic insomnia: A review. *Psychiatry Services* 56(3):332–343.

Beninati W, Harris CD, Herold DL, Shepard JW Jr. 1999. The effect of snoring and obstructive sleep apnea on the sleep quality of bed partners. *Mayo Clinic Proceedings* 74(10): 955–958.

Billmann SJ, Ware JC. 2002. Marital satisfaction of wives of untreated sleep apneic men. *Sleep Medicine* 3(1):55–59.

Bixler EO, Kales A, Soldatos CR, Kales JD, Healey S. 1979. Prevalence of sleep disorders in the Los Angeles metropolitan area. *American Journal of Psychiatry* 136(10):1257–1262.

Blunden S, Lushington K, Kennedy D, Martin J, Dawson D. 2000. Behavior and neurocognitive performance in children aged 5-10 years who snore compared to controls. *Journal of Clinical and Experimental Neuropsychology* 22(5):554–568.

Brassington GS, King AC, Bliwise DL. 2000. Sleep problems as a risk factor for falls in a sample of community-dwelling adults aged 64-99 years. *Journal of the American Geriatrics Society* 48(10):1234–1240.

Breugelmans JG, Ford DE, Smith PL, Punjabi NM. 2004. Differences in patient and bed partner-assessed quality of life in sleep–disordered breathing. *American Journal of Respiratory and Critical Care Medicine* 170(5):547–552.

Carskadon MA. 2004. Sleep deprivation: Health consequences and societal impact. *Medical Clinics of North America* 88(3):767–776.

Cassel W, Ploch T, Becker C, Dugnus D, Peter JH, von Wichert P. 1996. Risk of traffic accidents in patients with sleep-disordered breathing: Reduction with nasal CPAP. *European Respiratory Journal* 9(12):2606–2611.

Chenier MC. 1997. Review and analysis of caregiver burden and nursing home placement. *Geriatric Nursing (London)* 18(3):121–126.

Chervin RD, Dillon JE, Bassetti C, Ganoczy DA, Pituch KJ. 1997. Symptoms of sleep disorders, inattention, and hyperactivity in children. *Sleep* 20(12):1185–1192.

Chervin RD, Murman DL, Malow BA, Totten V. 1999. Cost-utility of three approaches to the diagnosis of sleep apnea: Polysomnography, home testing, and empirical therapy. *Annals of Internal Medicine* 130(6):496–505.

Chervin RD, Clarke DF, Huffman JL, Szymanski E, Ruzicka DL, Miller V, Nettles AL, Sowers MR, Giordani BJ. 2003. School performance, race, and other correlates of sleep-disordered breathing in children. *Sleep Medicine* 4(1):21–27.

CNTS (Center for National Truck Statistics). 1996. *Truck and Bus Accident Factbook—1994.* UMTRI-96-40. Washington, DC: Federal Highway Administration Office of Motor Carriers.

Connor J, Norton R, Ameratunga S, Robinson E, Civil I, Dunn R, Bailey J, Jackson R. 2002. Driver sleepiness and risk of serious injury to car occupants: Population-based case control study. *British Medical Journal* 324(7346):1125.

Daniels E, King MA, Smith IE, Shneerson JM. 2001. Health-related quality of life in narcolepsy. *Journal of Sleep Research* 10(1):75–81.

Dinges DF, Graeber RC, Carskadon MA, Czeisler CA, Dement WC. 1989. Attending to inattention. *Science* 245(4916):342.

Dinges D, Rogers N, Baynard MD. 2005. Chronic sleep deprivation. In: Kryger MH, Roth T, Dement WC, eds. *Principles and Practice of Sleep Medicine.* 4th ed. Philadelphia: Elsevier/ Saunders. Pp. 67–76.

Dodel R, Peter H, Walbert T, Spottke A, Noelker C, Berger K, Siebert U, Oertel WH, Kesper K, Becker HF, Mayer G. 2004. The socioeconomic impact of narcolepsy. *Sleep* 27(6):1123–1128.

Doherty LS, Kiely JL, Lawless G, McNicholas WT. 2003. Impact of nasal continuous positive airway pressure therapy on the quality of life of bed partners of patients with obstructive sleep apnea syndrome. *Chest* 124(6):2209–2214.

Drake CL, Roehrs T, Roth T. 2003. Insomnia causes, consequences, and therapeutics: An overview. *Depression and Anxiety* 18(4):163–176.

Drake CL, Roehrs T, Richardson G, Walsh JK, Roth T. 2004. Shift work sleep disorder: Prevalence and consequences beyond that of symptomatic day workers. *Sleep* 27(8):1453–1462.

Durmer JS, Dinges DF. 2005. Neurocognitive consequences of sleep deprivation. *Seminars in Neurology* 25(1):117–129.

Eastridge BJ, Hamilton EC, O'Keefe GE, Rege RV, Valentine RJ, Jones DJ, Tesfay S, Thal ER. 2003. Effect of sleep deprivation on the performance of simulated laparoscopic surgical skill. *American Journal of Surgery* 186(2):169–174.

Eckerberg B. 2004. Treatment of sleep problems in families with young children: Effects of treatment on family well-being. *Acta Paediatrica* 93(1):126–134.

Edinger JD, Means MK. 2005. Overview of insomnia: Definitions, epidemiology, differential diagnosis, and assessment. In: Kryger MH, Roth T, Dement WC, eds. *Principles and Practice of Sleep Medicine.* 4th ed. Philadelphia: Elsevier/Saunders. Pp. 702–713.

Emancipator JL, Storfer-Isser A, Taylor HG, Rosen CL, Kirchner HL, Johnson NL, Zambito AM, Redline SR. 2006. Variation of cognition and achievement with sleep-disordered breathing in full-term and preterm children. *Archives of Pediatrics and Adolescent Medicine* 160(2):203–210.

Engleman HM, Kingshott RN, Martin SE, Douglas NJ. 2000. Cognitive function in the sleep apnea/hypopnea syndrome (SAHS). *Sleep* 23(suppl 4):S102–S108.

Fairclough SH, Graham R. 1999. Impairment of driving performance caused by sleep deprivation or alcohol: A comparative study. *Human Factors* 41(1):118–128.

Federal Motor Carrier Safety Administration. 1996. *Commercial Motor Vehicle/Driver Fatigue and Alertness Study.* Washington, DC: Office of Research and Technology.

Fitzpatrick P, Kirke PN, Daly L, Van Rooij I, Dinn E, Burke H, Heneghan J, Bourke G, Masterson J. 2001. Predictors of first hip fracture and mortality post fracture in older women. *Irish Journal of Medical Science* 170(1):49–53.

Fletcher KE, Davis SQ, Underwood W, Mangrulkar RS, McMahon LF Jr, Saint S. 2004. Systematic review: Effects of resident work hours on patient safety. *Annals of Internal Medicine* 141(11):851–857.

Fredriksen K, Rhodes J, Reddy R, Way N. 2004. Sleepless in Chicago: Tracking the effects of adolescent sleep loss during the middle school years. *Child Development* 75(1):84–95.

Friedman BC, Hendeles-Amitai A, Kozminsky E, Leiberman A, Friger M, Tarasiuk A, Tal A. 2003. Adenotonsillectomy improves neurocognitive function in children with obstructive sleep apnea syndrome. *Sleep* 26(8):999–1005.

Frisoni GB, De Leo D, Rozzini R, Bernardini M, Buono MD, Trabucchi M. 1993. Night sleep symptoms in an elderly population and their relation with age, gender, and education. *Clinical Gerontology* 13(1):51–68.

Garbarino S, Mascialino B, Penco MA, Squarcia S, De Carli F, Nobili L, Beelke M, Cuomo G, Ferrillo F. 2004. Professional shift-work drivers who adopt prophylactic naps can reduce the risk of car accidents during night work. *Sleep* 27(2):1295–1302.

Gay CL, Lee KA, Lee SY. 2004. Sleep patterns and fatigue in new mothers and fathers. *Biological Research for Nursing* 5(4):311–318.

Gellis LA, Lichstein KL, Scarinci IC, Durrence HH, Taylor DJ, Bush AJ, Riedel BW. 2005. Socioeconomic status and insomnia. *Journal of Abnormal Psychology* 114(1):111–118.

Goswami M. 1998. The influence of clinical symptoms on quality of life in patients with narcolepsy. *Neurology* 50(2 suppl 1):S31–S36.

Gottlieb DJ, Chase C, Vezina RM, Heeren TC, Corwin MJ, Auerbach SH, Weese-Mayer DE, Lesko SM. 2004. Sleep-disordered breathing symptoms are associated with poorer cognitive function in 5-year-old children. *Journal of Pediatrics* 145(4):458–464.

Gozal D. 1998. Sleep-disordered breathing and school performance in children. *Pediatrics* 102(3 Pt 1):616–620.

Graeber RC, Dement WC, Nicholson AN, Sasaki M, Wegmann HM. 1986a. International cooperative study of aircrew layover sleep: Operational summary. *Aviation Space and Environmental Medicine* 57(12 Pt 2):B10–B13.

Graeber RC, Lauber JK, Connell LJ, Gander PH. 1986b. International aircrew sleep and wakefulness after multiple time zone flights: A cooperative study. *Aviation Space and Environmental Medicine* 57(12 Pt 2):B3–B9.

Grantcharov TP, Bardram L, Funch-Jensen P, Rosenberg J. 2001. Laparoscopic performance after one night on call in a surgical department: Prospective study. *British Medical Journal* 323(7323):1222–1223.

Greenberg GD, Watson RK, Deptula D. 1987. Neuropsychological dysfunction in sleep apnea. *Sleep* 10(3):254–262.

Grunstein RR, Stenlof K, Hedner JA, Sjostrom L. 1995. Impact of self-reported sleep-breathing disturbances on psychosocial performance in the Swedish Obese Subjects (SOS) study. *Sleep* 18(8):635–643.

Gurubhagavatula I, Maislin G, Nkwuo JE, Pack AI. 2004. Occupational screening for obstructive sleep apnea in commercial drivers. *American Journal of Respiratory and Critical Care Medicine* 170(4):371–376.

Hack M, Davies RJ, Mullins R, Choi SJ, Ramdassingh-Dow S, Jenkinson C, Stradling JR. 2000. Randomised prospective parallel trial of therapeutic versus subtherapeutic nasal continuous positive airway pressure on simulated steering performance in patients with obstructive sleep apnoea. *Thorax* 55(3):224–231.

Hack MA, Choi SJ, Vijayapalan P, Davies RJO, Stradling JR. 2001. Comparison of the effects of sleep deprivation, alcohol and obstructive sleep apnoea (OSA) on simulated steering performance. *Respiratory Medicine* 95(7):594–601.

Hart CN, Palermo TM, Rosen CL. 2005. Health-related quality of life among children presenting to a pediatric sleep disorders clinic. *Behavioral Sleep Medicine* 3(1):4–17.

Hasler G, Buysse DJ, Gamma A, Ajdacic V, Eich D, Rossler W, Angst J. 2005. Excessive daytime sleepiness in young adults: A 20-year prospective community study. *Journal of Clinical Psychiatry* 66(4):521–529.

Hausdorff JM, Rios DA, Edelberg HK. 2001. Gait variability and fall risk in community-living older adults: A 1-year prospective study. *Archives of Physical Medicine and Rehabilitation* 82(8):1050–1056.

Hope T, Keene J, Gedling K, Fairburn CG, Jacoby R. 1998. Predictors of institutionalization for people with dementia living at home with a carer. *International Journal of Geriatric Psychiatry* 13(10):682–690.

Horne JA, Reyner LA. 1995. Sleep-related vehicle accidents. *British Medicine Journal* 310(6979):565–567.

Hossain JL, Shapiro CM. 2002. The prevalence, cost implications, and management of sleep disorders: An overview. *Sleep and Breathing* 6(2):85–102.

Howard ME, Desai AV, Grunstein RR, Hukins C, Armstrong JG, Joffe D, Swann P, Campbell DA, Pierce RJ. 2004. Sleepiness, sleep-disordered breathing, and accident risk factors in commercial vehicle drivers. *American Journal of Respiratory and Critical Care Medicine* 170(9):1014–1021.

Howell AJ, Jahrig JC, Powell RA. 2004. Sleep quality, sleep propensity and academic performance. *Perceptual and Motor Skills* 99(2):525–535.

IOM (Institute of Medicine). 2000. *To Err Is Human: Building a Safer Health System.* Washington, DC: National Academy Press.

Kapur V, Blough DK, Sandblom RE, Hert R, de Maine JB, Sullivan SD, Psaty BM. 1999. The medical cost of undiagnosed sleep apnea. *Sleep* 22(6):749–755.

Kapur V, Strohl KP, Redline S, Iber C, O'Connor G, Nieto J. 2002a. Underdiagnosis of sleep apnea syndrome in U.S. communities. *Sleep and Breathing* 6(2):49–54.

Kapur VK, Redline S, Nieto F, Young TB, Newman AB, Henderson JA. 2002b. The relationship between chronically disrupted sleep and healthcare use. *Sleep* 25(3):289–296.

Karacan I, Thornby J, Williams R. 1983. Sleep disturbance: A community survey. In: Guilleminault C, Lugaresi E, eds. *Sleep/Wake Disorders: Natural History, Epidemiology, and Long-Term Evolution.* New York: Raven Press. Pp. 37–60.

Katz DA, McHorney CA. 1998. Clinical correlates of insomnia in patients with chronic illness. *Archives of Internal Medicine* 158(10):1099–1107.

Katz DA, McHorney CA. 2002. The relationship between insomnia and health-related quality of life in patients with chronic illness. *Journal of Family Practice* 51(3):229–235.

Kennedy JD, Blunden S, Hirte C, Parsons DW, Martin AJ, Crowe E, Williams D, Pamula Y, Lushington K. 2004. Reduced neurocognition in children who snore. *Pediatric Pulmonology* 37(4):330–337.

Kim HC, Young T, Matthews CG, Weber SM, Woodard AR, Palta M. 1997. Sleep-disordered breathing and neuropsychological deficits: A population-based study. *American Journal of Respiratory and Critical Care Medicine* 156(6):1813–1819.

Kim K, Uchiyama M, Okawa M, Liu X, Ogihara R. 2000. An epidemiological study of insomnia among the Japanese general population. *Sleep* 23(1):41–47.

Krieger J, Meslier N, Lebrun T, Levy P, Phillip-Joet F, Sailly J-C, Racineux JL. 1997. Accidents in obstructive sleep apnea patients treated with nasal continuous positive airway pressure: A prospective study. *Chest* 112(6):1561–1566.

Kryger MH, Roos L, Delaive K, Walld R, Horrocks J. 1996. Utilization of health care services in patients with severe obstructive sleep apnea. *Sleep* 19(9 suppl):S111–S116.

Kuppermann M, Lubeck DP, Mazonson PD, Patrick DL, Stewart AL, Buesching DP, Fifer SK. 1995. Sleep problems and their correlates in a working population. *Journal of General Internal Medicine* 10(1):25–32.

Landrigan CP, Rothschild JM, Cronin JW, Kaushal R, Burdick E, Katz JT, Lilly CM, Stone PH, Lockley SW, Bates DW, Czeisler CA. 2004. Effect of reducing interns' work hours on serious medical errors in intensive care units. *New England Journal of Medicine* 351(18):1838–1848.

Leger D. 1994. The cost of sleep-related accidents: A report for the National Commission on Sleep Disorders Research. *Sleep* 17(1):84–93.

Leger D, Scheuermaier K, Philip P, Paillard M, Guilleminault C. 2001. SF-36: evaluation of quality of life in severe and mild insomniacs compared with good sleepers. *Psychosomatic Medicine* 63(1):49–55.

Leger D, Guilleminault C, Bader G, Levy E, Paillard M. 2002. Medical and socio-professional impact of insomnia. *Sleep* 25(6):625–629.

Li RHY, Wing YK, Ho SC, Fong SYY. 2002. Gender differences in insomnia—A study in the Hong Kong Chinese population. *Journal of Psychosomatic Research* 53(1):601–609.

Lindberg E, Carter N, Gislason T, Janson C. 2001. Role of snoring and daytime sleepiness in occupational accidents. *American Journal of Respiratory and Critical Care Medicine* 164(11):2031–2035.

Lockley SW, Cronin JW, Evans EE, Cade BE, Lee CJ, Landrigan CP, Rothschild JM, Katz JT, Lilly CM, Stone PH, Aeschbach D, Czeisler CA, Harvard Work Hours HaS Group. 2004. Effect of reducing interns' weekly work hours on sleep and attentional failures. *New England Journal of Medicine* 351(18):1829–1837.

Marcus CL, Loughlin GM. 1996. Effect of sleep deprivation on driving safety in house staff. *Sleep* 19(10):763–766.

McArdle N, Grove A, Devereux G, Mackay-Brown L, Mackay T, Douglas NJ. 2000. Split-night versus full-night studies for sleep apnoea/hypopnoea syndrome. *European Respiratory Journal* 15(4):670–675.

McCurry SM, Logsdon RG, Vitiello MV, Teri L. 1998. Successful behavioral treatment for reported sleep problems in elderly caregivers of dementia patients: A controlled study. *Journals of Gerontology Series B-Psychological Sciences and Social Sciences* 53(2):122–129.

McCurry SM, Logsdon RG, Teri L, Gibbons LE, Kukull WA, Bowen JD, McCormick WC, Larson EB. 1999. Characteristics of sleep disturbance in community-dwelling Alzheimer's disease patients. *Journal of Geriatric Psychiatry and Neurology* 12(2):53–59.

McCurry SM, Gibbons LE, Logsdon RG, Vitiello M, Teri L. 2003. Training caregivers to change the sleep hygiene practices of patients with dementia: The NITE-AD project. *Journal of American Geriatrics Society* 51(10):1455–1460.

McCurry SM, Gibbons LE, Logsdon RG, Vitiello MV, Teri L. 2005. Nighttime insomnia treatment and education for Alzheimer's disease: A randomized, controlled trial. *Journal of American Geriatrics Society* 53(5):793–802.

Mellinger GD, Balter MB, Uhlenhuth EH. 1985. Insomnia and its treatment: Prevalence and correlates. *Archives of General Psychiatry* 42(3):225–232.

Mendelson WB. 2005. Hypnotic medications: Mechanisms of action and pharmacologic effects. In: Kryger MH, Roth T, Dement WC, eds. *Principles and Practice of Sleep Medicine.* 4th ed. Philadelphia: Elsevier/Saunders. Pp. 444–451.

Millman RP, Working Group on Sleepiness in Adolescents/Young Adults, and AAP Committee on Adolescence. 2005. Excessive sleepiness in adolescents and young adults: Causes, consequences, and treatment strategies. *Pediatrics* 115(6):1774–1786.

Mindell JA. 1999. Empirically supported treatments in pediatric psychology: Bedtime refusal and night wakings in young children. *Journal of Pediatric Psychology* 24(6):465–481.

Mitler M, Dement WC, Dinges DF. 2000. Sleep medicine, public policy, and public health. In: Kryger MH, Roth T, Dement WC, eds. *Principles and Practice of Sleep Medicine.* 3rd ed. Philadelphia: Elsevier/Saunders. Pp. 580–588.

Mittelman MS, Ferris SH, Shulman E, Steinberg G, Levin B. 1996. A family intervention to delay nursing home placement of patients with Alzheimer disease: A randomized controlled trial. *Journal of the American Medical Association* 276(21):1725–1731.

Montplaisir J, Allen RP, Walters AD, Lerini-Strambi L. 2005. Restless legs syndrome and periodic limb movements during sleep. In: Kryger MH, Roth T, Dement WC, eds. *Principles and Practice of Sleep Medicine.* 4th ed. Philadelphia: Elsevier/Saunders. Pp. 839–852.

Moore-Ede MC. 1993. *The Twenty-Four-Hour Society: Understanding Human Limits in a World That Never Stops.* Reading, MA: Addison-Wesley.

Moss TH, Sills DL. 1981. *The Three Mile Island Nuclear Accident: Lessons and Implications.* New York: New York Academy of Sciences.

Murphy SL. 2000. Deaths: Final data for 1998. *National Vital Statistics Report* 48(11):1–105.

Naegele B, Thouvard V, Pepin JL, Levy P, Bonnet C, Perret JE, Pellat J, Feuerstein C. 1995. Deficits of cognitive executive functions in patients with sleep apnea syndrome. *Sleep* 18(1):43–52.

Naylor E, Penev PD, Orbeta L, Janssen I, Ortiz R, Colecchia EF, Keng M, Finkel S, Zee PC. 2000. Daily social and physical activity increases slow-wave sleep and daytime neuropsychological performance in the elderly. *Sleep* 23(1):87–95.

NCSDS (National Commission on Sleep Disorders Research). 1994. *Wake Up America: A National Sleep Alert. Volume II: Working Group Reports.* 331-355/30683. Washington, DC: Government Printing Office.

NHTSA (National Highway Traffic Safety Administration). 1994. *Crashes and Fatalities Related to Driver Drowsiness/Fatigue.* Washington, DC: United States Department of Transportation.

NIH (National Institutes of Health). 2005. NIH State of the Science Conference Statement on Manifestations and Management of Chronic Insomnia in Adults Statement: Manifestations and Management of Chronic Insomnia in Adults. *Journal of Clinical Sleep Medicine* 1(4):412–421.

NSF (National Sleep Foundation). 2005. *2005 Sleep in America Poll.* [Online]. Available: http://www.sleepfoundation.org/_content/hottopics/2005_summary_of_findings.pdf [accessed June 7, 2005].

NTSB (National Transportation Safety Board). 1990a. *Safety Study: Fatigue, Alcohol, Other Drugs, and Medical Factors in Fatal-to-the-Driver Heavy Truck Crashes (Volume I).* Washington, DC: National Transportation Safety Board.

NTSB. 1990b. *Safety Study: Fatigue, Alcohol, Other Drugs, and Medical Factors in Fatal-to-the-Driver Heavy Truck Crashes (Volume II).* Washington, DC: National Transportation Safety Board.

NTSB. 1997. *Grounding of the Liberian Passenger Ship Star Princess on Poundstone Rock, Lynn Canal, Alaska June 23, 1995: Marine Accident Report.* Washington, DC: National Transportation Safety Board [Online] Available: http://www.ntsb.gov/publictn/1997/MAR9702.pdf [accessed March 6, 2006].

O'Brien LM, Holbrook CR, Mervis CB, Klaus CJ, Bruner JL, Raffield TJ, Rutherford J, Mehl RC, Wang M, Tuell A, Hume BC, Gozal D. 2003. Sleep and neurobehavioral characteristics of 5- to 7-year-old children with parentally reported symptoms of attention-deficit/hyperactivity disorder. *Pediatrics* 111(3):554–563.

O'Brien LM, Mervis CB, Holbrook CR, Bruner JL, Smith NH, McNally N, McClimment MC, Gozal D. 2004. Neurobehavioral correlates of sleep-disordered breathing in children. *Journal of Sleep Research* 13(2):165–172.

O'Hara R, Schroder CM, Kraemer HC, Kryla N, Cao C, Miller E, Schatzberg AF, Yesavage JA, Murphy GM Jr. 2005. Nocturnal sleep apnea/hypopnea is associated with lower memory performance in APOE epsilon4 carriers. *Neurology* 65(4):642–644.

Ohayon MM, Roth T. 2003. Place of chronic insomnia in the course of depressive and anxiety disorders. *Journal of Psychiatric Research* 37(1):9–15.

Ohayon MM, Lemoine P, Arnaud-Briant V, Dreyfus M. 2002. Prevalence and consequences of sleep disorders in a shift worker population. *Journal of Psychosomatic Research* 53(1):577–583.

Ong KC, Clerk AA. 1998. Comparison of the severity of sleep-disordered breathing in Asian and Caucasian patients seen at a sleep disorders center. *Respiratory Medicine* 92(6):843–848.

Ozminkowski R, Wang S, Trautman H, Orsini L. 2004. Estimating the cost burden of insomnia for health plans. *Journal of Managed Care Pharmacy* 10(5):467.

Pack AI, Pack AM, Rodgman E, Cucchiara A, Dinges DF, Schwab CW. 1995. Characteristics of crashes attributed to the driver having fallen asleep. *Accident Analysis and Prevention* 27(6):769–775.

Parish JM, Lyng PJ. 2003. Quality of life in bed partners of patients with obstructive sleep apnea or hypopnea after treatment with continuous positive airway pressure. *Chest* 124(3):942–947.

Phillips B. 2005. *The Future of Sleep Medicine*. Northbrook, IL: American College of Chest Physicians.

Powell NB, Schechtman KB, Riley RW, Li K, Troell R, Guilleminault C. 2001. The road to danger: The comparative risks of driving while sleepy. *Laryngoscope* 111(5):887–893.

Ramchandani P, Wiggs L, Webb V, Stores G. 2000. A systematic review of treatments for settling problems and night waking in young children. *British Medical Journal* 320(7229): 209–213.

Randazzo AC, Muehlbach MJ, Schweitzer PK, Walsh JK. 1998. Cognitive function following acute sleep restriction in children ages 10-14. *Sleep* 21(8):861–868.

Redline S, Kump K, Tishler PV, Browner I, Ferrette V. 1994. Gender differences in sleep-disordered breathing in a community-based sample. *American Journal of Respiratory and Critical Care Medicine* 149(3 Pt 1):722–726.

Redline S, Strauss ME, Adams N, Winters M, Roebuck T, Spry K, Rosenberg C, Adams K. 1997. Neuropsychological function in mild sleep-disordered breathing. *Sleep* 20(2):160–167.

Redline S, Adams N, Strauss ME, Roebuck T, Winters M, Rosenberg C. 1998. Improvement of mild sleep-disordered breathing with CPAP compared with conservative therapy. *American Journal of Respiratory and Critical Care Medicine* 157(3 Pt 1):858–865.

Reimer MA, Flemons WW. 2003. Quality of life in sleep disorders. *Sleep Medicine Review* 7(4):335–349.

Reuveni H, Simon T, Tal A, Elhayany A, Tarasiuk A. 2002. Health care services utilization in children with obstructive sleep apnea syndrome. *Pediatrics* 110(1 Pt 1):68–72.

Rhodes SK, Shimoda KC, Waid LR, O'Neil PM, Oexmann MJ, Collop NA, Willi SM. 1995. Neurocognitive deficits in morbidly obese children with obstructive sleep apnea. *Journal of Pediatrics* 127(5):741–744.

Ritchie K. 1996. Behavioral disturbances of dementia in ambulatory care settings. *International Psychogeriatrics* 8(suppl 3):439–442.

Roehrs T, Greenwald M, Roth T. 2004. Risk-taking behavior: Effects of ethanol, caffeine, and basal sleepiness. *Sleep* 27(5):887-893.

Rogers AE, Hwang WT, Scott LD, Aiken LH, Dinges DF. 2004. The working hours of hospital staff nurses and patient safety. *Health Affairs (Millwood)* 23(4):202–212.

Rosen CL, Palermo TM, Larkin EK, Redline S. 2002. Health-related quality of life and sleep-disordered breathing in children. *Sleep* 25(6):657–666.

Rosen CL, Storfer-Isser A, Taylor HG, Kirchner HL, Emancipator JL, Redline S. 2004. Increased behavioral morbidity in school-aged children with sleep-disordered breathing. *Pediatrics* 114(6):1640–1648.

Roth T, Ancoli-Israel S. 1999. Daytime consequences and correlates of insomnia in the United States: Results of the 1991 National Sleep Foundation survey. II. *Sleep* 22(suppl 2):S354–S358.

Sassani A, Findley LJ, Kryger M, Goldlust E, George C, Davidson TM. 2004. Reducing motor-vehicle collisions, costs, and fatalities by treating obstructive sleep apnea syndrome. *Sleep* 27(3):453–458.

Scharf SM, Seiden L, DeMore J, Carter-Pokras O. 2004. Racial differences in clinical presentation of patients with sleep-disordered breathing. *Sleep and Breathing* 8(4):173–183.

Schechter MS. 2002. Technical report: Diagnosis and management of childhood obstructive sleep apnea syndrome. *Pediatrics* 109(4):e69.

Shin C, Kim J, Lee S, Ahn Y, Joo S. 2003. Sleep habits, excessive daytime sleepiness and school performance in high school students. *Psychiatry and Clinical Neurosciences* 57(4):451–453.

Simon GE, VonKorff M. 1997. Prevalence, burden, and treatment of insomnia in primary care. *American Journal of Psychiatry* 154(10):1417–1423.

Sleep Disorders Create Growing Opportunities for Hospitals. 2001. *Health Care Strategy Management* 19(2):16–17.

Spilsbury JC, Storfer-Isser A, Drotar D, Rosen CL, Kirchner LH, Benham H, Redline S. 2004. Sleep behavior in an urban U.S. sample of school-aged children. *Archives of Pediatrics and Adolescent Medicine* 158(10):988–994.

Stein MA, Mendelsohn J. Obermeyer WH, Amromin J, Benca R. 2001. Sleep and behavior problems in school-aged children. *Pediatrics* 107(4):E60.

Steinbrook R. 2002. The debate over residents' work hours. *New England Journal of Medicine* 347(16):1296–1302.

Stoller MK. 1994. Economic effects of insomnia. *Clinical Therapeutics: The International Peer-Reviewed Journal of Drug Therapy* 16(5):873–897.

Stone KL, Schneider JL, Blackwell T, Ancoli-Israel S, Redline S, Claman D, Cauley JA, Ensrud KE, Hillier TA, Cummings SR. 2004. Impaired sleep increases the risk of falls in older women: A prospective atigraphy study. *Sleep* 27(276 abstract supplement):A125.

Stoohs RA, Bingham L, Itoi A, Guilleminault C, Dement WC. 1995. Sleep and sleep-disordered breathing in commercial long-haul truck drivers. *Chest* 107(5):1275–1282.

Stradling JR, Thomas G, Warley AR, Williams P, Freeland A. 1990. Effect of adenotonsillectomy on nocturnal hypoxaemia, sleep disturbance, and symptoms in snoring children. *Lancet* 335(8684):249–253.

Strawbridge WJ, Shema SJ, Roberts RE. 2004. Impact of spouses' sleep problems on partners. *Sleep* 27(3):527–531.

Strine TW, Chapman DP. 2005. Associations of frequent sleep insufficiency with health-related quality of life and health behaviors. *Sleep Medicine* 6(1):23–27.

Stutts JC, Wilkins JW, Scott OJ, Vaughn BV. 2003. Driver risk factors for sleep-related crashes. *Accident Analysis and Prevention* 35(3):321–331.

Swaen GMH, Van Amelsvoort LGPM, Bultmann U, Kant IJ. 2003. Fatigue as a risk factor for being injured in an occupational accident: Results from the Maastricht Cohort Study. *Occupational and Environmental Medicine* 60(suppl 1):88–92.

Teran-Santos J, Jimenez-Gomez A, Cordero-Guevara J. 1999. The association between sleep apnea and the risk of traffic accidents. Cooperative group Burgos-Santander. *New England Journal of Medicine* 340(11):847–851.

Thomas M, Sing H, Belenky G, Holcomb H, Mayberg H, Dannals R, Wagner H, Thorne D, Popp K, Rowland L, Welsh A, Balwinski S, Redmond D. 2000. Neural basis of alertness and cognitive performance impairments during sleepiness. I. Effects of 24 h of sleep deprivation on waking human regional brain activity. *Journal of Sleep Research* 9(4):335–352.

Ulfberg J, Carter N, Talback M, Edling C. 1996. Excessive daytime sleepiness at work and subjective work performance in the general population and among heavy snorers and patients with obstructive sleep apnea. *Chest* 110(3):659–663.

United States Senate Committee on Energy and National Resources. 1986. *The Chernobyl Accident.* Washington, DC: Government Printing Office.

Unruh ML, Levey AS, D'Ambrosio C, Fink NE, Powe NR, Meyer KB. 2004. Restless legs symptoms among incident dialysis patients: Association with lower quality of life and shorter survival. *American Journal of Kidney Disease* 43(5):900–909.

Urschitz MS, Wolff J, Sokollik C, Eggebrecht E, Urschitz-Duprat PM, Schlaud M, Poets CF. 2005. Nocturnal arterial oxygen saturation and academic performance in a community sample of children. *Pediatrics* 115(2):204–209.

USDOT (United States Department of Transportation). 1991. *The Costs of Highway Crashes.* Washington, DC: Federal Highway Administration.

USNRC (United States Nuclear Regulatory Commission). 1987. *Report on the Accident at the Chernobyl Nuclear Power Station.* NU-REG 1250. Washington, DC: Government Printing Office.

Van Dongen HP, Maislin G, Mullington JM, Dinges DF. 2003. The cumulative cost of additional wakefulness: Dose-response effects on neurobehavioral functions and sleep physiology from chronic sleep restriction and total sleep deprivation. *Sleep* 26(2):117–126.

Wahlstrom KL, Davison ML, Choi J, Rossm JN. 2001. *Minneapolis Public Schools Start Time Study: Executive Summary—August 2001.* Twin Cities, MN: University of Minnesota.

Walsh JK. 2004. Clinical and socioeconomic correlates of insomnia. *Journal of Clinical Psychiatry* 65(suppl 8):13–19.

Walsh JK, Engelhardt CL. 1999. The direct economic costs of insomnia in the United States for 1995. *Sleep* 22(suppl 2):S386–S393.

Walsh JK, Engelhardt CL, Hartman PG. 1995. The direct economic cost of insomnia. In: Nutt DJ, Mendelson WB, eds. *Hypnotics and Anxiolytics.* London: Bailliere Tindall.

Walsh JK, Dement WC, Dinges DF. 2005. Sleep medicine, public policy, and public health. In: Kryger MH, Roth T, Dement WC, eds. *Principles and Practice of Sleep Medicine.* 4th ed. Philadelphia: Elsevier/Saunders. Pp. 648–656.

Weaver TE, George CFP. 2005. Cognition and performance in patients with obstructive sleep apnea. In: Kryger MH, Roth T, Dement WC, eds. *Principles and Practice of Sleep Medicine.* 4th ed. Philadelphia: Elsevier/Saunders. Pp. 1023–1033.

Weissbluth M, Liu K. 1983. Sleep patterns, attention span, and infant temperament. *Journal of Developmental and Behavioral Pediatrics* 4(1):34–36.

Weissman MM, Greenwald S, Nino-Murcia G, Dement WC. 1997. The morbidity of insomnia uncomplicated by psychiatric disorders. *General Hospital Psychiatry* 19(4):245–250.

Wittmann V, Rodenstein DO. 2004. Health care costs and the sleep apnea syndrome. *Sleep Medicine Reviews* 8(4):269–279.

Wolfson AR, Carskadon MA. 1998. Sleep schedules and daytime functioning in adolescents. *Child Development* 69(4):875–887.

Wolfson AR, Carskadon MA. 2003. Understanding adolescents' sleep patterns and school performance: A critical appraisal. *Sleep Medicine Reviews* 7(6):491–506.

Young T, Blustein J, Finn L, Palta M. 1997a. Sleep-disordered breathing and motor vehicle accidents in a population-based sample of employed adults. *Sleep: Journal of Sleep Research and Sleep Medicine* 20(8):608–613.

Young T, Evans L, Finn L, Palta M. 1997b. Estimation of the clinically diagnosed proportion of sleep apnea syndrome in middle-aged men and women. *Sleep* 20(9):705–706.

Zammit GK, Weiner J, Damato N, Sillup GP, McMillan CA. 1999. Quality of life in people with insomnia. *Sleep* 22 (suppl 2):S379–S385.

5

Improving Awareness, Diagnosis, and Treatment of Sleep Disorders

CHAPTER SUMMARY   *The public health burden of chronic sleep loss and sleep disorders coupled with the low awareness among the general population, health care professionals, and policy makers requires a well-coordinated strategy to improve sleep-related health care. Increasing the awareness and improving the diagnosis and treatment of sleep disorders necessitates a multipronged effort that includes three key components: public education, training for health professionals, and surveillance and monitoring. First, a public health campaign is required to increase awareness among the general population. Second, specific education and training strategies are needed to increase awareness among health care professionals, including improved curriculum content and certification requirements. There are a number of surveillance and monitoring tools, but very few examine issues pertaining to sleep loss and sleep disorders. Thus, third, improved surveillance and monitoring of the general population is needed. The preeminent goal of this strategy is to create and sustain a broad societal commitment to engaging in proper sleep habits as a primary tenet of health. Such a commitment will involve participation by those individuals and organizations in a position to educate the public at national, state, local, and community levels—including K–12 education, colleges and universities, medical schools and other health profession education programs, hospitals, community clinics, local health departments, private industry (e.g., transportation, manufacturing facilities, nursing homes), and entertainment media. It will also require simultaneous investment in public education cam-*

paigns for all age groups as well as a sustained effort to integrate sleep-related content into curricula of undergraduate health science programs all the way through continuing education programs for health professionals.

CHALLENGES FACING INDIVIDUALS WITH SLEEP DISORDERS

Sleep is often viewed by the general public as a "perceptual hole in time"—during which nothing productive occurs (Dement and Vaughn, 1999). One only has to examine common colloquialisms such as "don't get caught napping," "if you snooze you loose," or "time is money" to gain a sense of the prevailing attitude that sleep is either optional, a luxury, or unimportant. In fact, being able to "get by on 4 hours of sleep" (and thus being able to increase productivity) is often considered an enviable trait.

Daily sleeping and waking patterns are no longer driven by the light and dark cycle but, rather, by work schedules, economic interests, and increasing globalization. Unfortunately, the resulting "24/7" schedules are typically not optimal in terms of filling physiological requirements for sleep. Thus, daytime sleepiness and its consequences are becoming increasingly common problems affecting up to 15 percent of the population (Punjabi et al., 2003). For some, sleep disruption and constant sleepiness are often deemed an inevitable part of their social roles as spouses, workers, caregivers, and so on. Although improving diet and exercise as a part of a healthy lifestyle program is acceptable, sleep continues to be considered an expendable luxury (Dzaja et al., 2005). Thus, performance and social responsibilities may often take precedence over sleep, largely because of multiple role demands and expectations.

Stigma is a problem that often complicates chronic illness. Acceptable standards for roles and activities are socially determined, and individuals who deviate from these expectations because of chronic illness are often labeled as "different" and are thus stigmatized (Falvo, 2005). Similarly, individuals with certain sleep disorders, which are often chronic in nature, may also be stigmatized because of the inability to fulfill role expectations. An additional factor that may underlie this stigma is that sleep is typically misperceived as an "asocial" activity. However, sleep is actually a very important type of social interaction—an activity that is negotiated with self, family, friends, employers, lawmakers, fellow drivers on the road, and so on (Meadows, 2005). When, where, and how sleep occurs is an extremely important sociocultural matter (Taylor, 1993; Williams, 2002), and there can be considerable negative sociocultural consequences when the sleep behavior, either intentionally or unintentionally, is unacceptable (Mehlman,

2001; Moore et al., 2002). Obesity also presents another challenge to some individuals with sleep disorders. Obesity engenders negative feelings among caregivers, which may affect an individual's health care (Banno and Kryger, 2004).

The lack of awareness among the general public that results from the absence of sleep content in public health education programs causes patients to be hesitant about discussing sleep problems with their health care providers. In addition, fear of being labeled as having a psychiatric problem or exhibiting drug-seeking behaviors are also deterrents (Culpepper, 2002). In the case of insomnia, the most common of all sleep-related complaints, patients typically do not seek help because they believe either that nothing can be done or that the health care providers will do nothing to address the problem (Engstrom et al., 1999).

Patients with excessive daytime sleepiness represent the largest group seeking help at sleep laboratories but often only after they have encountered numerous problems that interfere with performance of normal activities of daily living, their ability to hold a job and maintain a marriage, interact socially, or have had an accident. All too often, these individuals have been labeled lazy or unmotivated. For children with narcolepsy, for example, the stigma associated with their increased daytime sleep tendency can affect social acceptance owing to unusual behavior as well as future risk of increased psychiatric disorders, potential obesity, and depressive symptoms (Dahl et al., 1994; Guilleminault and Pelayo, 1998). Thus, individuals may have to overcome a stigma attached to having a sleep disorder, and seeking appropriate treatment is a very serious issue.

Somnology Public Health Education Campaigns

A review of the National Center on Sleep Disorders Research (NCSDR), Centers for Disease Control and Prevention (CDC), and private foundations demonstrate a limited investment in education and awareness campaigns directed toward increasing the general public's knowledge of the health implications associated with chronic sleep loss and sleep disorders.

National Center on Sleep Disorders Research Public Education Campaigns

The NCSDR was established within the National Heart, Lung, and Blood Institute (NHLBI), partially in response to the previous experience and success the NHLBI had in public education campaigns (see below). As directed by the congressional authorization language, the NCSDR is responsible for coordinating the "disseminat[ion of] public information concerning the impact of sleep disorders and sleep deprivation" (Appendix D)

(U.S. Congress, Senate, 1993). It has also developed a variety of education materials; however, resources have not been devoted to an in-depth evaluation of the effectiveness of these materials. The primary education programs that the NCSDR have initiated include the following:

• *Sleep, Sleep Disorders, and Biological Rhythms* is a curriculum supplement developed for grades 9 through 12 (NHLBI, 2003b). Approximately 12,000 copies of the curriculum supplement have been sent to teachers. There have been more than 11,000 visitors to the sleep curriculum website and 10,000 downloads. More than 2,000 students entered sleep diary data on the Internet.

• The Garfield Star Sleeper Campaign was designed to educate children, parents, educators, and health care providers about the importance of nighttime sleep during childhood (NHLBI, 2005b).

• *Time For Kids* is a magazine on sleep that was developed and distributed by the NCSDR to 30,000 third-grade teachers and the 750,000 children in their classes in connection with National Sleep Awareness Week (NHLBI, 2004).

• The *Healthy Sleep Handbook* is a booklet that will be available to the general public and provide an overview of sleep disorders with signs and symptoms, consequences, and potential treatments. It will explain why sleep is needed, what happens if you don't get enough sleep, and tips on how to obtain enough sleep (NHLBI, 2006).

As these examples demonstrate, apart from campaigns directed toward children and adolescents, which have been inadequately evaluated, the NCSDR has not engaged in widespread multimedia public education campaigns directed toward other susceptible populations, including college students, adults (especially shift workers), elderly people, and high-risk minority populations. This is in part owing to the limited resources of the NCSDR for public education (see Chapter 7). A potential strategy to strengthen these activities is to collaborate with other federal agencies including the CDC, as was directed by the congressional authorization; however, there has been limited involvement of the CDC and other federal agencies in these activities.

Private Foundations Education and Awareness Campaigns

Although limited, private foundations and professional societies, and to a lesser extent patient advocacy organizations, have developed a number of public education programs. A highly successful example is the National Sleep Foundation's (NSF) National Sleep Awareness Week campaign. This campaign coincides annually with the start of daylight savings time and brings together over 750 sleep centers and 100 government agencies and other nonprofit organizations to plan and implement several public awareness and education projects. Activities have included sleep health fairs, lectures, and a public policy and sleep leadership forum. The NSF also conducts the *Sleep in America* poll, an annual telephone survey that gauges how and when Americans sleep, and created a multimedia educational tool called *Cycles of Sleeping and Waking with the Doze Family* that illustrates information about sleep and includes a website, print materials, and CD-ROM.

Although the Sleep Research Society (SRS) and the American Academy of Sleep Medicine (AASM) are primarily professional societies, they also have contributed to increasing the awareness among researchers, health care providers, and the general public. For example the SRS is a cosponsor of the Trainee Day at annual meeting of Associated Professional Sleep Societies, recently published the Basics of Sleep Research guide, and established the Sleep Research Society Foundation, which annually supports up to six $20,000 grants. The AASM professional initiatives and public education efforts include among others, the CPAP (continuous positive airway pressure) Compliance Campaign, establishing accreditation programs for sleep technologists and behavioral sleep medicine training programs, and assisting in the development of new clinical practice guidelines. Other private organizations such as the American Sleep Apnea Association, Restless Legs Syndrome Foundation, and Academy of Dental Sleep Medicine have also created smaller public education tools such as patient education brochures, support groups, and online videos.

Educational Activities of the Centers for Disease Control and Prevention

The public education efforts coordinated by the CDC provide additional models that could be used to increase awareness about the health implications of chronic sleep loss and disorders. The CDC has extensive experience in health education and has developed very effective programs in such diverse areas as obesity, colorectal cancer screening, and adolescent health.

The CDC's public information campaign to encourage physical activity includes a website that covers the importance of physical fitness including the health benefits, how much exercise is needed, how to overcome barriers to exercise, and specific tips for becoming more active. The website includes references to documents and other organizations that are resources for individuals interested in this topic (CDC, 2006).

The CDC also partners with other related government and private entities to make these public health campaigns even more effective. For example, the Screen for Life campaign is a successful multimedia colorectal cancer screening education program in which the CDC has partnered with other organizations including state departments of health, the National Colorectal Cancer Research Alliance, and the Entertainment Industry Foundation. This program targets the general public as well as health professionals and encourages colorectal cancer screening for every person after age 50. In addition to the education and awareness campaign, the CDC also developed a nationwide surveillance program to assess the capacity to perform colorectal cancer screening tests and follow-up for the United States population aged 50 years or older.

One advantage of working with an organization such as the CDC is its credibility and connections to individuals and organizations that can increase program effectiveness. For example, Katie Couric, NBC *Today Show* host, and Academy Award-winning actor Morgan Freeman have served as spokespersons for different campaigns.

Given that chronic sleep loss and sleep disorders are a major public health problem, a public and professional campaign on sleep conditions would fit in well with existing CDC mission and programs.

PUBLIC EDUCATION

Sleep loss and daytime sleepiness affect 30 to 40 percent of the general population (Hossain and Shapiro, 2002); however, millions of individuals suffering from sleep disorders remain undiagnosed and untreated. For example, 80 to 90 percent of obstructive sleep apnea cases remain undiagnosed, which increases the burden of this disorder (Young et al., 1997; Kapur et al., 2002). Most large-scale public health education programs and campaigns to date have focused primarily on diet and exercise and have not included adequate information about sleep. However, the time is right for the development of a sleep campaign. There is a beginning public awareness of the importance of sleep owing to recent articles in the popular press and television programs. Two concurrent strategies are required to increase awareness among the general public: a multimedia public education and awareness campaign, and improved education and training programs to increase awareness among health care professionals.

National Sleep Public Education and Awareness Campaign

Considering the burden that chronic sleep loss and sleep disorders have on all age groups, a multifocal campaign is required to improve awareness among children, adolescents, adults, elderly people, and high-risk populations. The primary role of a campaign would be to improve recognition of the health and economic benefits of proper sleep, as well as educating parents and adults of the consequences associated with not receiving adequate sleep. In this regard it will be important to inform the public and policy makers of the negative consequences of chronic sleep loss and sleep disorders. The campaign could argue that by taking specific personal actions to improve sleep hygiene, by recommending specific behaviors for all age groups, the adverse health and economic consequences could be reduced. The need for such a campaign rests on the following assumptions:

- The general public does not recognize the prevalence of, or the consequence associated with chronic sleep loss and/or sleep disorders.
- Most health care providers neither recognize the prevalence of, nor the many risks associated with, chronic sleep loss and/or sleep disorders.
- Many of the technological advances made in the previous century (e.g., television, Internet) serve to deprive people, especially children and adolescents, of needed sleep.
- Sleep loss and sleep disorders are associated with numerous other health complications
- Increased understanding will lead to better sleep behaviors and thus improved health and function.

Treatment of sleep problems, even if only behavioral and educational in nature, has the potential to increase an individual's well-being and productivity. Such a campaign would offer new information to both the general population and health care providers. In addition, the activities of a broad sleep awareness campaign could be linked to all stakeholders—government agencies, private industry, foundations, professional societies, patient advocacy organizations, educators, colleges and universities, and community organizations.

The committee envisions that wherever possible, a national campaign would coordinate activities with local needs and provide for the tailoring of its messages for different communities, including specific age groups, minority groups, and shift workers. In addition, the committee envisions that the campaign should be developed in coordination with the NCSDR, CDC, the proposed National Somnology and Sleep Medicine Research and Clinical Network (see Chapter 8), the Department of Transportation, the Department of Labor, the Department of Education, other relevant federal departments and agencies, with input from private organizations such as the NSF and the AASM. Rigorous evaluation is a critical component. Further, this campaign could be integrated and coordinated with other public health campaigns, including those on obesity and heart disease, with the purpose of increasing the awareness among all Americans of the importance of sleep and the adverse health and social consequences of poor sleep. Further, reinforcing messages should be provided in diverse media and effectively coordinated with other events and dissemination activities.

In proposing the National Sleep Public Education and Awareness Campaign, this committee considered and recognized the associated costs and challenges. These include the following:

• Educating and convincing leaders in the public health field that the health and economic burden associated with chronic sleep loss and sleep disorders requires a national campaign.
• The expenses associated with developing and operating a large nationwide public education and awareness program.
• Coordinating federal, state, and local government agencies that would be involved in a campaign.
• Coordinating the activities of foundations, professional societies, and private companies.
• The large number of individuals experiencing sleep loss or sleep disorders span all age groups, each of which will require a specific strategy.

In summary, although evidence is limited, previously coordinated health education campaigns demonstrate the potential value of efforts designed to increase the awareness of both the prevalence and consequences of chronic sleep loss and sleep disorders. For example, broad coordinated national campaigns such as the NHLBI's National High Blood Pressure Campaign (Roccella, 2002), the National Institute of Child Health and Human Development's (NICHD) Back to Sleep Campaign, the CDC's Screen for Life colorectal cancer campaign, the antitobacco efforts of the late 1960s and early 1970s and the late 1990s and early 2000s (Warner, 1981; Siegel, 2002), and the antidrug campaigns of the middle 1980s (IOM, 2002) have had corresponding reductions in risky behavior.

Back to Sleep Campaign

The Back to Sleep program offers an example of a very successful public education awareness campaign that arose from a strong associative discovery between infant sleeping position and the risk of sudden infant death syndrome (SIDS) (Willinger, 1995; Kemp et al., 1998). In 1993, the American Academy of Pediatrics released its first policy statement on reducing the risk of SIDS that recommended that infants be placed on their backs while sleeping. The following year, the NICHD spearheaded the Back to Sleep campaign. Cosponsors included the Maternal and Child Health Bureau, the American Academy of Pediatrics, the SIDS Alliance, and the Association of SIDS and Infant Mortality Programs. The NCSDR was involved in planning and developing communication materials for the campaign.

Before it was instituted, the death rate for SIDS was approximately 1.3 per 1,000 live births (CDC, 1996). Postsurveillance analysis showed a 50 percent reduction in SIDS rates since the Back to Sleep campaign began (NICHD, 2003). The campaign increased public awareness of SIDS risks and safety through a series of radio and television public service announcements and distribution of more than 20 million pieces of literature to health care professionals and the public.

National High Blood Pressure Education Campaign

Another successful public education program is the National High Blood Pressure Education Program. It was established by the NHLBI in 1972 "to reduce death and disability related to high blood pressure through programs of professional, patient, and public education" (NHLBI, 2005a). The NHLBI coordinates a group of federal agencies, voluntary and professional organizations, state health departments, and numerous community-based programs. At the core of the education activities is the program's coordinating committee, which follows a consensus-building process to identify major issues of concern and to develop program activities. Each representative from the coordinating committee member organizations work together to provide program guidance and to develop and promote educational activities through their own constituencies. The National High Blood Pressure Education Program is responsible for the five following areas: information collection and dissemination; public, patient, and professional education; community program development; evaluation and data analysis; and technology transfer and electronic distribution of materials.

The education campaign does not depend greatly on advertising, but rather relies heavily on actions by other institutions: campaign organizers working with physicians' organizations to encourage physicians to provide advice about high blood pressure consistent with national guidelines; proposing stories to newspapers and television and radio that convey the priority messages; and developing affiliations with, and providing materials to, grassroots organizations interested in hypertension (Roccella, 2002). When the program began there was very little awareness and treatment for hypertension. Less than one-fourth of the American population understood the relationship between hypertension and stroke and hypertension and heart disease and only 31 percent sought treatment. Today, more than three-fourths of the population recognizes that relationship and over 53 percent seek treatment (NHLBI, 2005a).

Recommendation 5.1: The National Center on Sleep Disorders Research and the Centers for Disease Control and Prevention should establish a multimedia public education campaign.

The National Center on Sleep Disorders Research—working with the Centers for Disease Control and Prevention, the proposed National Somnology and Sleep Medicine Research Network, private organizations and foundations, entertainment and news media, and private industry—should develop, implement, and evaluate a long-term national multimedia and public awareness campaign directed to targeted segments of the population (e.g., children, their parents, and teachers in preschool and elementary school; adolescents; college students and young adults; middle-aged adults; and elderly people) and specific high-risk populations (e.g., minorities).

To implement this recommendation, the following should be done:
* This campaign should be developed in coordination with appropriate federal departments and agencies and with input from independent experts to focus on building support for policy changes.
* This campaign should be built upon and integrated within existing public health campaigns, including those focused on diet and exercise (e.g., obesity and heart disease).
* Reinforcing messages disseminated through multiple media should be effectively coordinated with events targeting providers of health information such as physicians, nurses, and teachers.

PROFESSIONAL TRAINING AND AWARENESS IS REQUIRED

Societal misperceptions also stem from a lack of professional knowledge about the benefits and impact of sleep. Therefore, the success of the proposed National Sleep Public Education Awareness Campaign particularly relies on increased awareness and more sleep-oriented curricula for the health care providers. Further, underutilization of sleep centers in the United States to assist in diagnosing and treating sleep disorders partly stems from both the lack of public and professional awareness and insufficient training of primary caregivers (Wyatt, 2004). Without widespread recognition of the importance of sleep on the part of both the public and health care providers, society is at significant risk for sleep-related health problems. If health care providers are unaware of the symptoms and problems that occur as a result of compromised sleep, they simply will not pursue the topic with patients. Thus, patient contacts with the health care system are often major sources of "missed opportunities" to diagnose sleep problems and share important information about sleep. In addition, increasing the awareness of health care providers also offers an opportunity to attract health care professionals into the field (see Chapter 7 for detailed discussion). Those who receive sleep-related education are more likely to ask individuals about past or current sleep problems (Haponik and Camp, 1994).

Some progress is being made in developing strategies to improve education and awareness among health care professionals. For example, competency-based goals and teaching strategies for sleep and chronobiology in undergraduate medical education have recently been proposed (Harding and Berner, 2002; Federman, 2003). Similar curricula content has also been developed for undergraduate and graduate nursing programs (Lee et al., 2004). A survey conducted in 1992 revealed that minimal, if any, didactic content on sleep was included in medical and nursing programs (Buysse et al., 2003; Rosen et al., 1998; NHLBI, 2003a). Although curricula in medical and nursing school have been updated since 1992, and there are no recent surveys, anecdotal evidence suggests that sleep-related content is still not adequately addressed. Considerable progress remains to be made.

Treatment of Sleep Disorders Requires Interdisciplinary Training

Sleep disorders vary widely in their complexity, their comorbidities, the risks they represent, and the scope of their manifestations (Chapter 3). They may be a symptom of a behavioral or social change, a secondary manifestation associated with a primary disease, or may be the primary problem. Examination of the disorders associated with each of these categories demonstrates the requirement for educated multidisciplinary health care specialists who have the capacity to recognize, diagnose, and treat chronic sleep loss and sleep disorders. At minimum, there are 13 different health care specialties and subspecialties that are involved in diagnosis and treatment—anesthesiology, cardiology, dentistry, endocrinology, immunology, neurology, nursing, nutrition, otolaryngology, pediatrics, psychiatry, psychology, and pulmonology. For example, individuals with obstructive sleep apnea (OSA) typically require recognition by a primary care physician, and diagnosis and treatment from a sleep specialist who is a pulmonologist, neurologist, psychiatrist, or otolaryngologist. Following, or concurrent with, diagnosis and treatment, the chronic nature of a sleep disorder also may require being seen by a specialist (e.g., endocrinologist for diabetes and obesity, cardiologist for hypertension). Patient and family education, primary care, follow-up and support are often provided by nurses with expertise in the field. Therefore, proper treatment of chronic sleep loss and sleep disorders requires multidisciplinary care. However, as discussed below, there has been very little education of health care professionals about the pathology, etiology, or treatment of chronic sleep loss and sleep disorders.

Undergraduate Sleep-Related Education

Education at the undergraduate level provides a unique opportunity to share important health information when readiness to learn has transcended adolescent levels. It also provides an important opportunity to expose students to the topics and potentially increase the number of individuals interested in this area of medicine. In fact, curricula that include sleep-related material at the undergraduate level may be particularly appropriate and effective for a number of reasons.

First, leaving home to attend college is often the first time that young adults are totally responsible for self-care. Numerous studies have demonstrated that one of the most common difficulties undergrads experience is sleep disturbance. For example, in a survey of 191 college students, most reported that they had developed some form of sleep disturbance (Buboltz et al., 2001). Further, a recent study of 964 undergraduate residence hall students found that sleep problems were among the list of significant predictors of stress (Dusselier et al., 2005). A study of 1,300 students in the United States Military Academy found that incoming cadets were significantly sleep deprived, receiving only about 4 hours and 50 minutes of sleep per night during the week in their first fall semester (Miller and Shattuck, 2005). The reasons for the high prevalence of these sleep problems in undergraduate students are likely related to a variety of factors including poor sleep hygiene, stress associated with changes in lifestyle, study demands, socializing, use of stimulants, and in some cases a feeling of the need to demonstrate mental and physical toughness.

Undergraduates also experience the consequences of poor sleep habits and require the necessary health information to make appropriate lifestyle changes. Earlier studies demonstrated that students' poor sleep quality was associated with increased tension, irritability, depression, confusion, and lower life satisfaction as well as increases use of marijuana and alcohol (Pilcher et al., 1997). In addition, poor sleep has been associated with impaired academic performance and deficits in learning and memory (Lack, 1986; Gais et al., 2000; Stickgold et al., 2000; Walker et al., 2003; Fenn et al., 2003). Unfortunately, many students who experience academic problems do not realize that poor sleep may be a crucial contributing factor (Buboltz et al., 2001).

Chronic Sleep Loss and Sleep Disorders Awareness
Programs for Undergraduates

Although some sleep-related public health educational activities have been developed (see previous section), their impact appears to be minimal. Thus, new ways to incorporate sleep education into undergraduate student life are needed. First and foremost, university administrators need to recognize and acknowledge that students' sleep habits and problems are an important component of campus life. Including content regarding sleep in orientation programs, even in the form of a simple informational flier, may provide a forum for further discussions in other types of programs and activities. Advisors might ask basic questions regarding overall sleep patterns and make recommendations regarding class times that are more compatible with a student's normal sleep patterns. Further, university and college administrators should examine how campus and community environments, such as activities, schedules, sports, and work routines, contribute to sleep disruption (Buboltz et al., 2001) and encourage academic departments to educate their faculty regarding the sleep-related problems of students (Miller and Shattuck, 2005). In addition, awareness campaigns should be developed to target undergraduate students in dormitories and academic health centers. Similar effective programs have been developed for public health campaigns concerning sexually transmitted disease, alcohol abuse, nutrition, and suicide. For example, the American College Athletic Association and the National Association of Student Personnel Administrators have helped design and integrate a number of public health campaigns for college students, such as the Health Education and Leadership Program.

Undergraduate Somnology and Sleep Medicine Curriculum Development

Colleges and universities can both educate students and stimulate interest in the field by making simple cost-effective changes in curriculum. For example, at the United States Military Academy, the general psychology course that is taken by all freshmen now includes information on acute and chronic sleep loss (Miller and Shattuck, 2005). Numerous other types of freshman courses, such as general health, biology, and sports education, might include similar content and easily incorporate it with other health-related information such as nutrition, alcohol and drug abuse, and suicide prevention (Miller and Shattuck, 2005). Offering an elective course, perhaps in collaboration with an academic sleep center, might also help recruit future clinicians and scientists to the field. Curriculum recommendations for both nursing and undergraduate medical students have recently been proposed (Strohl et al., 2003; Lee et al., 2004). Other types of novel activities might include the following:

- Develop undergraduate research experiences in sleep to increase the interactions of these students with graduate students in this area (Box 5-1).
- Develop sleep consortiums among two or more universities and educational programs that could be shared using advanced technology, as the

BOX 5-1
Summer Sleep and Chronobiology Research Apprenticeship

The Summer Sleep and Chronobiology Research Apprenticeship is a unique undergraduate training program in the behavioral sciences at Brown University, which fosters behavioral science research education primarily for undergraduate students, but also for young pre- and post-doctoral scientists. The program provides undergraduate students an intensive research and academic experience in a human sleep and chronobiology research laboratory. It spans 13 weeks, including 2.5 weeks of intensive laboratory skills training, a week attending the annual meeting of the sleep professional societies (APSS), and a 10-week research apprenticeship in an ongoing study of sleep and circadian rhythms in adolescents. The program also supports one or two graduate student teaching assistants, providing role models to the apprentices, additional teaching experience, time for research projects, and full summer stipend. Each year the program concludes with a 2-day "retreat" colloquium. At this retreat, every apprentice is responsible for preparing and presenting a brief talk at the APSS meeting on a research theme they began to examine and researched through the summer.

The National Institute of Mental Health (NIMH) should be commended for funding the training program for 8 years. This brought an unprecedented level of fiscal stability, focus, and opportunity for young trainees. Unfortunately, the NIMH no longer supports undergraduate training programs. The Trans-NIH Sleep Research Coordinating Committee should be encouraged to continue to support similar undergraduate mentorship programs.

Because the program is largely designed for undergraduate students, its success is somewhat difficult to measure. Not every student has gone on to behavioral science research; some are in medicine, others in such disparate fields as law or business. Others, however, have followed the route to graduate study. One former student is working with a noted sleep and chronobiology scientist. Another student is performing research on sleep in birds. A third is a graduate student in neurobiology using electroencephalograms (EEG) and magnetic resource imaging (MRI) as methods to investigate the relationship between thalamic activation and cortical activation during sleep spindles. Another individual recently received a young investigator award from the European Sleep Research Society (2004, Prague ESRS meeting) for research on adolescent sleep patterns.

numbers of faculty qualified to teach information about sleep may be limited in particular settings.

Students in the clinical health science majors, such as those in nursing and premedicine, should have didactic and associated clinical work in sleep medicine that include specific content in the following:

- Interactions between sleep and health.
- The neurobiology and functions of sleep.
- Effects of restricted or reduced sleep on pathophysiology of diseases.
- Mechanisms that lead to sleep disorders across the life span and across genders.
- Normal sleep processes across ages, genders, and socioeconomic groups.
- Effective sleep interventions for sleep disorders (Strohl et al., 2003).

GRADUATE RESEARCH TRAINING IN SOMNOLOGY AND SLEEP DISORDERS

Graduate school is traditionally a time of focused concentration on a specific area of investigation, and the curricular requirements for graduate degrees in biological sciences are typically highly variable among disciplines, programs, and universities. Exposure to research on sleep-related topics is probably most applicable to interdisciplinary programs in neuroscience, as well as to single-discipline programs (e.g., pharmacology, physiology, biochemistry, anatomy, and cell biology). Although the content of these curricula typically depend on the research interests of the local faculty, it is in the interest of the students to have a broad exposure to neuroscience that is usually accomplished via a graduate level survey course in the field, and for that course, or other relevant courses, to include some exposure to sleep-related research. Although there are limited data, it appears that this exposure does not occur. For example, one of the top neuroscience and sleep programs, the neuroscience graduate course in the health sciences and technology program at Harvard University and Massachusetts Institute of Technology, includes only a single lecture on the molecular biology of circadian rhythms and no exposure to sleep-related research (personal communication, C.B. Saper, Harvard University, December 1, 2005).

OVERVIEW OF MEDICAL SCHOOL SOMNOLOGY EDUCATION

The inadequacy of somnology education in medical curricula has been a long-standing issue. As far back as 1978, a survey by the American Sleep Disorders Association (now the AASM) revealed that 46 percent of medical schools provided no sleep-related education and 38 percent sponsored minimal instruction (Orr et al., 1980). Although the percentage of medical schools that include sleep disorders in their curricula has risen modestly from 54 percent in 1978 (Orr et al., 1980) to 63 percent in 1993, the time devoted averages only 2.11 hours (Rosen et al., 1998). Eighty-nine percent of medical students never performed a clinical evaluation of an individual with a sleep disorder (Rosen et al., 1993).

The situation has slowly improved. A survey performed by a special subcommittee of the AASM, called Taskforce 2000, in 1995 indicated a growth in time devoted to somnology content to 4 hours in the preclinical basic sciences and 2 hours in the clinical clerkships (Rosen et al., 1998). However, structured learning experience in the sleep laboratory and clinical evaluation of individuals with sleep disorder remain limited. Major barriers continue to be lack of time in the medical curriculum, the need for better resources and teaching facilities, and the need for leadership and effective advocacy.

Barriers to Implementation of Sleep-Related Medical Curriculum

Efforts to enhance the training and education in somnology and sleep medicine at all levels of medical education continue to face important challenges. These include the following:

• Somnology and sleep medicine is still a relatively new field, cutting across many traditional disciplinary boundaries. Therefore, there is a need to implement a cohesive, interdisciplinary, and centrally organized sleep medicine curriculum.
• The importance of sleep to good health is often poorly appreciated; hence, it is underrepresented in the medical curriculum.
• Somnology and sleep medicine is a budding interdisciplinary field; sleep and circadian rhythms interact and influence nearly every organ system. A coordinated curriculum that includes content related to somnology and sleep disorders is needed in every related teaching block.
• Limited availability of faculty and mentors with appropriate scientific and clinical expertise creates a need for "content champions" to push the educational agenda in a centrally organized way.
• A paucity of local educational resources, including clinical infrastructure, exists (Orr et al., 1980; Rosen et al., 1993, 1998; Owens, 2005). As described below, the NIH and AASM have contributed significant resources to the development and establishment of somnology medicine curricula in the past. However, there has been limited evaluation of these efforts.

Sleep Academic Award

From 1996 to 2003 the NCSDR and the NHLBI cosponsored the Sleep Academic Award program. Its primary objective was to develop and evaluate model curricula in somnology and sleep medicine for adaptation into academic institutions. In tandem with curricular development, the Sleep Academic Award program also sought to promote interdisciplinary learning environments and faculty development in somnology and sleep medicine. The model curriculum for medical schools encompassed these four basic core competencies:

- Explain the nature and causation of sleep.
- Discuss the impact of sleep and circadian disorders.
- Perform a sleep history.
- Initiate measures to improve sleep and to reduce sleepiness.

Other Sleep Academic Award professional education initiatives included the addition of sleep questions to board examinations in psychiatry, pediatrics, otolaryngology, and pulmonary medicine; the creation of a sleep clinical case vignette bank for use in objective structured clinical examinations and problem-based learning seminars; the development of continuing medical education lectures and courses; and the implementation of faculty development workshops.

The Sleep Academic Award program also undertook initiatives in graduate medical training related to the effects of sleep loss and fatigue. These initiatives included collaboration with the American Medical Association and the Accreditation Council for Graduate Medical Education (ACGME) on work hours for residents. The MedSleep dissemination initiative distributes educational resources and products for free, including web-based materials, slide sets, videotaped case histories, and curriculum outlines (AASM, 2005). In addition, the AASM Medical Education Committee has established a network of sleep-related education advocates in over 100 of the nation's medical schools to continue the development and implementation of educational materials and to provide evaluation.

Effectiveness of the Sleep Academic Award Program

Although the overall impact and durability of Sleep Academic Award program initiatives have not been measured, they have provided time and money for academic career development in somnology (research and scholarship), training in educational methodology, opportunity for mentorship, and access to leadership positions in professional organizations. Similarly, the durability of institutional impact, while difficult to predict precisely, has included: provision of teaching, educational support, and materials; increases in the knowledge base of graduates; research opportunities; and engagement of multiple disciplines in somnology and sleep medicine education. Several empirical studies regarding somnology medical education supported by the Sleep Academic Award program have been published in a special section of the January 2005 edition of *Sleep Medicine*. These studies have shown the following:

• The efficacy of a pediatric screening tool (the BEARS) to increase the amount of sleep information recorded in primary health care settings (Owens and Dalzell, 2005).
• The development and validation of a tool (the Dartmouth Sleep Knowledge and Attitude Survey) in assessing outcomes of educational interventions in sleep medicine (Sateia et al., 2005).
• The impact of education in improving the recognition of sleep disorders in a community-based setting (Zozula et al., 2005).
• The positive impact of lecture and case-based discussion on the performance of medical students in an objective structured clinical examination (Papp and Strohl, 2005).
• The use of the objective structured clinical examination for sleep medicine to gain access to the medical school curriculum by providing objective structured clinical examinations on sleep problems such as obstructive sleep apnea and chronic insomnia (Rosen et al., 2005).

One important outcome of the Sleep Academic Award has been an improvement in the number of somnology and sleep disorders questions on board exams; however, the representation is still low, given the public health burden. For example, the content outline of the board exam for internal medicine indicates zero to two sleep-related questions. The American Board of Otolaryngology lists corrective sleep surgery as 1 of 22 surgical concepts that is covered in the exam, where surgical concepts represents 15 percent of the exam content (American Board of Otolaryngology, 2006). The American Board of Psychiatry and Neurology mentions somnology and sleep disorders as 1 of 20 areas covered in the exam's physiology section—physiology also constitutes 15 percent of the exam (American Board of Psychiatry and Neurology, 2006). The content specifications for the American Board of Pediatrics mentions somnology and sleep disorders 19 times (American Board of Pediatrics, 2006).

Nurses as Care Managers

Another key group of health care providers that could play an especially significant role in advocating healthy sleep and promoting the diagnosis and management of sleep problems are nurses—the largest number of health care providers in the United States. Nurses are in a unique position to contribute to new knowledge about sleep and health promotion, provide primary care, as well as monitor sleep habits and disseminate information to patients, and enhance patient compliance with treatment (Lee et al., 2004). Unfortunately, nursing education faces many of the same challenges as other health care provider educational programs regarding the incorporation of sufficient sleep content in its programs. Recently, curriculum recommendations for somnology and chronobiology education for nursing at the undergraduate and graduate level programs have been developed (Lee et al., 2004). These guidelines have been integrated into a limited number of nursing programs; however, greater integration of sleep-related material is required in nursing education programs.

OVERVIEW OF SOMNOLOGY IN MEDICAL RESIDENCY TRAINING CURRICULA

To ensure a high degree of recognition and the most effective clinical care, it is important that more training programs educate residents about the need for early detection and, whenever possible, the prevention of chronic sleep loss and sleep disorders. Primary care providers are largely responsible for this surveillance in the medical system. Therefore, it is imperative that internists, family medicine doctors, and pediatricians are sufficiently trained to assume the surveillance role. As many individuals are referred to pulmonologists, neurologists, psychiatrists, and otolaryngologists for disorders that are related to sleep problems, extensive training in sleep medicine also should be integrated into those program curricula.

The current ACGME program requirements for residency training in internal medicine, family medicine, pediatrics, and psychiatry do not mention chronic sleep loss or sleep disorders. Program requirements for residency in neurology list sleep disorders as one of 22 subjects to be addressed in seminars and conferences. However, except for residency programs in otolaryngology, none of the other four residency program requirements address clinical experiences in sleep medicine (ACGME, 2005a).

Curricula should be designed to ensure that knowledge and skills required to detect the broad range of sleep disorders and to manage those that are not complex should be a component of general competency in each of the five relevant specialty areas of medicine. General competency in somnology and sleep medicine should be certified and recertified by the respective boards of the American Board of Medical Specialties (ABMS). With guidance from the residency review committee of the ACGME, each training program in these five specialty areas must develop curriculum content for somnology and sleep medicine. Departments sponsoring these training programs have a responsibility to have in place, or alternatively, to identify faculty-level expertise in somnology and sleep medicine, and ensure availability of these individuals for learners in the residency training program. As a result of the multidisciplinary nature of sleep medicine, interdepartmental sharing of expertise for training should be required in many settings. Clinical experience with diagnosis and management of patients with sleep disorders is preferred to didactic experiences. For this reason, the presence of an institutional sleep disorders clinic, laboratory, or center should be a key component of the educational infrastructure. Exposure of residents to the multidisciplinary nature of sleep evaluation and treatment will best prepare them for roles as primary caregivers, particularly for identification, treatment of simple sleep problems, and triage of more complicated patients to appropriate subspecialists.

Residents should become aware of the general health consequences of sleep disorders, such as the relationship between sleep deprivation and obesity, cardiovascular disease, and behavioral disorders. In addition, subspecialists in internal medicine and pediatric prevention, diagnosis, and treatment should be fully familiar with the sleep-related consequences of chronic disease and incorporate this awareness into their practices and subspecialty fellow training. Providing generalists with sleep-related education would enable them to be competent to care for a substantial number of sleep problems and refer individuals to sleep specialists as needed.

In view of the workforce shortage in the field (see Chapter 7) and the small number of both training programs and individuals enrolled in somnology and or sleep medicine training programs (see below), exposure of residents to this area of medicine will enhance awareness of career opportunities in this discipline and improve clinical care. Thus, the goal of embedding somnology and sleep medicine exposure and experiences in core residency training is to prepare a wide range of individuals to participate as frontline caregivers, and also to ensure that somnology and sleep medicine is visible to learners early in their training process and possibly foster their consideration of somnology or sleep medicine as a career focus. Exposure of residents to discovery and translational research related to sleep medicine might also enhance the attractiveness of the field. Therefore, somnology and sleep medicine investigators should participate, wherever possible, in the residency training process.

OVERVIEW OF SLEEP MEDICINE FELLOWSHIP TRAINING

AASM-Accredited Fellowship Training Programs

Until recently fellowship training programs in sleep medicine were rare, with a small number of academic institutions, hospitals, and other facilities hosting programs that were not standardized. To address this, a formal accreditation program for fellowship training programs in sleep medicine was established by the AASM. The number of fellowships has grown progressively, particularly over the last decade. There are now 53 fellowship training programs (Table 5-1). Reflecting the multidisciplinary roots of sleep medicine, these training programs are housed in various departments within these institutions.

TABLE 5-1 Accredited Programs for Fellowship Training in Somnology and Sleep Medicine

Date Accredited	Name of Institution	Department Affiliation
1980	Stanford University	Psychiatry and Behavioral Sciences
1989	Center for the Study of Sleep and Waking	Psychiatry and Behavioral Sciences
1991	Detroit Veterans Affairs Medicinal Center	Neurology
1991	Henry Ford Hospital	Pulmonary Division
1992	Mount Sinai Sleep Disorders Center	Pulmonary Division
1993	Michael S. Aldrich Sleep Disorders Laboratory	Neurology and Psychiatry
1993	Newark Beth Israel Sleep Disorders Center	Department of Pulmonary Medicine
1993	University of Pittsburgh School of Medicine	Psychiatry and Medicine, Pulmonary Division
1994	Cleveland Clinic Foundation	Neurology
1995	Mayo Sleep Disorders Center	Pulmonary and Critical Care
1996	Rush University Medical Center	Departments of Psychology and Medicine
1997	Wayne State University	Pulmonary Division
1998	University of Kentucky	Internal Medicine
1998	University of Mississippi Medical Center	Psychiatry
1998	Intermountain Sleep Disorders Center	Pulmonary Division
1999	Children's Memorial Hospital	Pediatrics
2000	Brigham and Women's Hospital	Medicine
2000	Duke University Medical Center	Pulmonary, Clinical Neurology, and Clinical Neuropathology

continued

TABLE 5-1 continued

Date Accredited	Name of Institution	Department Affiliation
2001	Sleep Medicine and Circadian Biology Program/ Indiana University School of Medicine	Pulmonary, Allergy, Critical Care, and Occupational Medicine
2001	State University of New York at Buffalo School of Medicine	Medicine
2001	University of Nebraska Medical Center	Pulmonary Critical Care Section of the Department of Internal Medicine
2001	Rush University Medical Center	Department of Psychology
2001	Northwestern University Medical School	Department of Neurology
2001	Worcester Medical Center Campus at St. Vincent Hospital	Department of Neurology
2001	Scott and White Memorial Hospital and Clinic	Department of Pulmonary/Critical Care
2001	Lahey Clinic	Pulmonology
2001	University of Pennsylvania	Pulmonary, Critical Care, and Sleep Section
2001	Case Western Reserve University	Departments of Medicine, Pediatrics, and Neurology
2002	Southwestern Medical Center	Department of Psychiatry
2002	Seton Hall University School of Graduate Medical Education	
2002	St. Elizabeth's Medical Center	Pulmonary Division, Department of Medicine
2002	Long Island Jewish Medical Center	Department of Medicine
2002	New Mexico Center for Sleep Medicine	
2002	University of Iowa Hospitals and Clinics Sleep Disorder Center	Neurology
2002	Hackensack University Medical Center Institute of Sleep-Wake Disorders	
2002	Dartmouth Hitchcock Medical Center	Department of Psychiatry
2003	Mayo Clinic/Mayo Graduate School of Medicine, Jacksonville	Division of Education Services
2003	Johns Hopkins University Sleep Disorders Center	Pulmonary/Critical Care

TABLE 5-1 continued

Date Accredited	Name of Institution	Department Affiliation
2003	Tulane University Health Science Center	Comprehensive Sleep Medicine Center
2003	Wake Forest University Health Sciences	Department of Psychiatry
2003	Beth Israel Deaconess Medical Center	Department of Neurology
2003	Beth Israel Deaconess Medical Center	Division of Pulmonary, Critical Care, Sleep Medicine
2003	University of Texas Health Science Center, Houston	Division of Pulmonary, Critical Care, Sleep Medicine
2003	Center for Sleep Disorders at Johnson City Medical Center	Pulmonary/Critical Care/Internal Medicine
2003	University of Wisconsin-Madison	Department of Medicine
2003	Clinilabs, Inc. (Sleep Disorders Institute)	
2003	State University of New York at Buffalo	Department of Neurology
2004	St. Mary's Medical Center/Ultimate Health Services	Regional Sleep Center
2004	University of Washington	Medicine and Neurology
2004	Norwalk Hospital Sleep Disorders Center	Department of Medicine
2004	Temple University Health System Sleep Disorders Center	Department of Internal Medicine, Division of Pulmonary and Critical Care
2004	Washington University School of Medicine	Department of Neurology
2004	University of Louisville/Kosair Children's Hospital	Department of Pediatrics

SOURCE: Personal communication, J. Barrett, AASM, December 12, 2005.

With the complex nature of sleep medicine in mind, the guidelines for accreditation allowed programs to design fellowship training in two ways. The first design allowed for the sleep medicine fellowship to be a minimum of 12 months of training in comprehensive sleep medicine that could be done during or after specialty fellowship training. The second design allowed for the sleep medicine fellowship to be of a combined nature, in which a substantial portion of the sleep medicine training is embedded within the primary specialty training.

The guidelines for accreditation of fellowship training required that programs provide graduates with clinical, technical, and research experience that promotes sound clinical judgment and a high level of knowledge about the diagnosis, treatment, and prevention of sleep disorders. The guidelines emphasized education in specific content areas, including basic neurological sleep mechanisms; chronobiological mechanisms; cardiovascular, pulmonary, endocrine, and gastrointestinal sleep physiology; specific disorders of sleep; and the psychopharmacology of sleep, as well as the operation of polysomnographic equipment, polysomnographic interpretation, and troubleshooting.

Eligibility requirements for an accredited program include at least one year of training preceded by the completion of an accredited residency program, and sponsorship by an institution that meets fellowship training requirements set forth by the ACGME. The director of the program must be a physician who is a diplomate of the American Board of Sleep Medicine (ABSM), and the program has to be associated with a sleep disorders center accredited by the AASM.

Completion of training in an accredited program satisfies requirements for eligibility to sit for the sleep medicine certification examination administered by the ABSM.

ACGME Sleep Medicine Fellowship Training Programs

In 2002, the AASM submitted an application to ACGME for accreditation of fellowship training programs in sleep medicine. ACGME approved the program requirements for sleep medicine fellowship training programs in June 2004. Accreditation of fellowship training programs by the ACGME now provides a framework for the continued expansion of specialized clinical training in sleep medicine and draws greater attention to the necessity of training programs.

The ACGME fellowship requires 1 year of clinical sleep medicine. Trainees can enter the sleep medicine fellowship if they have been trained in one of the following: general internal medicine (3 years of postgraduate training); neurology (4 years of postgraduate training); psychiatry (4 years of postgraduate training); general pediatrics (3 years of postgraduate training); otolaryngology (5 years of postgraduate training).

In June 2004, ACGME convened a Sleep Medicine Working Group to develop requirements for fellowship training in sleep medicine and formalize the accreditation process. The working group created a comprehensive program guideline that included requirements to ensure competence in core areas, including facility and resources for training, faculty, assignment of rotation and duty, curriculum, program content, and clinical experience (ACGME, 2005b). The first round of program accreditation was effective July 1, 2005, and 25 programs have received accreditation from ACGME for fellowship training.

DEMONSTRATION OF KNOWLEDGE: BOARD CERTIFICATION

ABSM Certification

In response to increasing recognition and awareness of the importance of sleep and sleep disorders, professional certification in sleep medicine has been administered for physicians and practitioners to demonstrate skill and competence.

The American Sleep Disorders Association (now the AASM) in 1978 established an examination committee. That same year, the committee held the inaugural clinical polysomnography examination; 21 candidates passed the exam. Each year the examination committee received an increasing number of applications, which led to discussions regarding the future of certification. In 1989, the AASM voted to create an independent entity, and in 1991 the ABSM was incorporated and assumed all the activities and responsibilities of the former examination committee.

The ABSM is an independent nonprofit organization and has a board of directors that oversees all aspects of exam administration and governance. The ABSM was self-designated and was not recognized by the ABMS.

Until 2005, the ABSM certification examination consisted of two parts. The part I examination consisted of multiple choice questions covering the basic sciences of sleep, clinical sleep medicine, and interpretation of polysomnogram fragments and other material. Part II was computer-based and consisted of a series of clinical cases with partial polysomnograms, Multiple Sleep Latency Tests, and other relevant data, with candidates typing short answers to questions. The ABSM decided to fuse the two parts of the examination in 2005 and offer a single-day, one-part examination that incorporates the format of both former parts.

Eligibility for the examination is dependent on a candidate fulfilling five requirements as well as possessing acceptable experience in the evaluation of sleep disorders patients. These eligibility requirements ensure adequate and proper education and training—either through an accredited fellowship program or through a combination of training and experience—and competency evaluation through certification of a primary board. Professionals from other clinical disciplines, such as doctoral psychologists and nurses who met all criteria, were also eligible to sit for the examination.

Over the past 14 years, the ABSM certification examination has developed a strong reputation in the medical community and experienced tremendous growth in terms of applicants. The number of candidates applying for the certification examination as well as the number of diplomates (Figure 5-1) has increased dramatically each year; however, as will be discussed in detail in Chapter 6, the capacity is still not sufficient to diagnose and treat all individuals with sleep disorders.

Establishment of the ABMS in Sleep Medicine

Despite its growth in reputation and numbers of diplomates, it became evident by the late 1990s that the ABSM as a freestanding board would not be recognized as fully legitimate by organized medicine. Because sleep medicine requires only 1 year of postresidency fellowship training, the ABSM was ineligible to join the ABMS as an independent board.

In 2002, the ABSM met with several specialty societies and professional organizations to discuss the necessity for certification examination in sleep medicine and the best design for such an examination. A consensus plan was developed for the establishment of a new subspecialty examination in sleep medicine to be jointly offered by the American Board of Internal Medicine, the American Board of Psychiatry and Neurology, and the American Board of Pediatrics; the American Board of Otolaryngology joined later as a sponsoring board. Following further successful negotiations, a plan for this examination was submitted to the ABMS in early 2004. In March 2005, the ABMS announced approval of the certification examination in sleep medicine. A specific time frame for the new examination has not been set; it is expected, however, that the first examination cycle will begin in 2007.

There are three pathways that qualify physicians to sit for the new examination: (1) certification by one of the primary sponsoring boards and

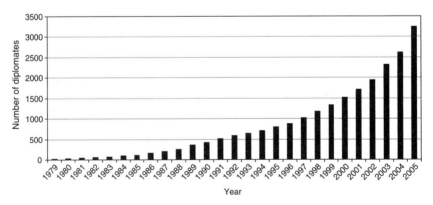

FIGURE 5-1 Total number of diplomates of the ABSM (1979–2005).
SOURCE: Personal communication, J. Barrett, AASM, December 15, 2005.

the current ABSM; (2) certification by one of the primary sponsoring boards and completion of training in a 1-year sleep medicine fellowship program, not overlapping with any other residency or fellowship; and (3) clinical practice experience. This clinical practice experience pathway may consist of a 5-year "grandfathering" period open to physicians who are board certified in one of the sponsoring specialty boards and who can attest that he or she has the equivalent of 1 year of clinical practice experience in sleep medicine during the prior 5 years. This experience could, for example, be gained by an individual practitioner who has devoted one-third of his or her practice to sleep medicine over 3 years. Physicians in the clinical practice pathway will also have to attest to a specified minimum number of patients seen and polysomnograms and Multiple Sleep Latency Tests read. At the end of this initial 5-year period, the only route to board eligibility will be through an ACGME accredited fellowship training program. This creates a one-time, unprecedented opportunity for pulmonologists, neurologists, otolaryngologists, psychiatrists, and other physicians already working in the field to sit for the board examination. However, not all sleep clinicians will be eligible for this accreditation. The ACGME only permits accreditation of doctors, thus nurses, dentists, and doctorally prepared sleep specialists (e.g. psychologists and behavioral health specialists) in other fields are no longer eligible to sit for the examination. As a consequence, there is the potential that in the future particular bodies of knowledge will not be represented in sleep medicine.

Representatives from all four boards are developing and setting standards for the new examination. The American Board of Internal Medicine has administrative responsibility for examination development, and the participating/sponsoring boards have responsibility for setting admission criteria for their own diplomates. These standards and criteria are expected to be announced in 2006.

Although this new structure is based on sleep medicine becoming recognized as an independent specialty, it is too early to tell how well this new approach will work in developing the needed workforce of practitioners for sleep medicine and the next generation of physician-scientists. The fellowship is somewhat unusual in that there is only the requirement for 1 year of training beyond completion of residency. It is unclear whether pulmonologists, who have until now formed the majority of the clinical workforce in sleep medicine (60 percent of diplomates in 2005), will continue to be attracted to the field (Figure 5-2). Clinical requirements for pulmonary medicine involve 18 months of training beyond residency. It appears that this will not count to training in sleep medicine even though there is now a defined curriculum for sleep medicine in pulmonary medicine (American Thoracic Society, 2005) and 10 to 15 percent of the board examination for pulmonary medicine is about sleep disorders. An additional clinical year of train-

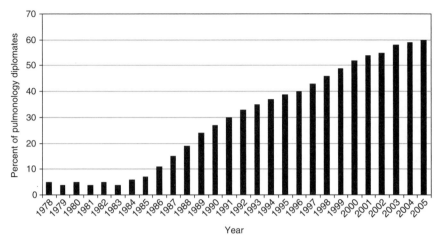

FIGURE 5-2 Percent of pulmonology diplomates of ABSM.
SOURCE: Personal communication, J. Barrett, AASM, December 15, 2006.

ing above and beyond that for pulmonary medicine may represent a barrier to pulmonologists entering this discipline. It is hoped that this issue is addressed, as pulmonologists encompass a significant percentage of the clinical workforce of practitioners in sleep medicine.

Another area of uncertainty is funding for these new sleep fellowships. Previously, when the fellowship was not ACGME-approved, fellows could obtain reimbursements for their clinical activities, including sleep study interpretation. In some other programs, sleep medicine training was incorporated into multiyear research training supported by training grants from the National Institutes of Health (NIH). Neither of these options is available in the new format.

Unfortunately, the rules introduced by the ACGME are not flexible and require 1 complete year of clinical training even in programs that are multiyear and committed to research training. This may have a negative impact on the already fragile pipeline of physician-scientists in this new discipline as outlined elsewhere in this report (see Chapter 7). As described in detail in Chapter 8, the committee encourages the proposed Type II comprehensive academic sleep centers to incorporate research training into their sleep medicine fellowships, while for Type III centers this is considered an essential component.

A final potential limitation of this new examination structure is that it is open exclusively to physicians. Other clinician scientists in fields such as psychology, neuroscience, and nursing will not be eligible to sit for the examination as was the case in prior years. Currently, there are 154 ABSM

PhDs board-certified by the AASM (personal communication, J. Barrett, AASM, January 13, 2006). Excluding these individuals may have an important negative effect on patient access, interdisciplinary nature of sleep programs, and the decision of talented potential scientists and clinicians to pursue the study of somnology.

NEXT STEPS

Medical, nursing, and pharmacy students along with individuals in graduate training, residency, and fellowship training programs require greater exposure to the public health burden of sleep loss and disorders; they also must understand the relationship between sleep problems and the proper diagnosis and treatment of a wide range of medical problems throughout an individual's life span. Although the data are limited, they suggest that focused training about sleep can positively influence the performance of medical students (Haponik and Camp, 1994), residents (Owens and Dalzell, 2005), physicians (Haponik et al., 1996; Rosen et al., 2005; Papp and Strohl, 2005), and primary care clinical staff (Zozula et al., 2005). For example, interns who had previous instruction about sleep-related material often asked patients about past or current sleep problems (82 percent of the time), while sleep histories were rarely obtained by interns who did not have any previous instruction (13 percent of the time) (Haponik et al., 1996).

The challenges that lie ahead, outlined below, are many:

• Sustaining educational initiatives begun by the Sleep Academic Award program.
• Monitoring progress and developing new and updated educational materials, such as sleep objective structured clinical examinations.
• Coordinating efforts across institutions.
• Identifying remaining gaps by assessing the impact of sleep education on physician knowledge, skills, and attitudes; clinical practice; and public health.
• Assessing the relative value and effectiveness of sleep curricula that are integrated across other areas versus those that are stand-alone units.
• Developing means of credentialing nurses, psychologists, and other clinicians who will not qualify for American Board of Medical Specialties certification.
• Integrating sleep-related content into continuing education requirements.

To these ends, educational outcomes research grants and partnerships with appropriate medical subspecialty groups for development and dissemination of educational programs is essential. Further, many health care-related programs are actively embracing new technologies for teaching (e.g., computer simulations of office practices) that provide an opportunity to ensure that sleep-related materials are incorporated into evolving curricula.

Most important, however, somnology health care providers need to be engaged in curriculum development and implementation. This will enable more effective curricular time and resources necessary for addressing basic educational goals in sleep disorders medicine and for integrating sleep materials into other academic areas. A coordinated curriculum—one that is not departmentally based—offers many advantages to encouraging more rational allocation of time and resources to critical areas of public health, including sleep and its disorders (Reynolds et al., 1995). This could be critical to a new integrative approach to teaching and learning about somnology and sleep disorders for the rest of the medical curriculum.

> **Recommendation 5.2: Academic health centers should integrate the teaching of somnology and sleep medicine into baccalaureate and doctoral health sciences programs, as well as residency and fellowship training and continuing professional development programs.**

The subjects of sleep loss and sleep disorders should be included in the curricula of relevant baccalaureate and graduate educational and research programs of all the health sciences. Similarly, postgraduate, residency, and fellowship training programs, as well as continuing professional development programs, must include this content. The curriculum should expose students in the fields of medicine and allied health fields to the etiology, pathophysiology, diagnosis, treatment, prevention, and public health burden of sleep loss and sleep disorders. Relevant accrediting bodies and licensing boards ought to define sleep-related curriculum requirements and expectations for knowledge and competency (e.g., Liaison Committee on Medical Education, Accreditation Council for Graduate Medical Education, American Board of Medical Specialties, the National League for Nursing, the Commission on Collegiate Nursing Education, and the Council on Education for Public Health). Further, a means for credentialing nonphysicians should be maintained by the American Board of Sleep Medicine, or new mechanisms should be developed by relevant organizations.

DATA SYSTEMS FOR SURVEYING SLEEP
AND SLEEP DISORDERS

Adequate public health education not only requires informing public and health care practitioners, but also adequate monitoring of the public health burden. The development of adequate surveillance and monitoring systems is important for informing policy makers, health care providers, researchers, and the public about the effectiveness of health care services, programs, and policies. However, there is currently very little ongoing nationwide surveillance. A number of existing national and statewide databases that can be used for surveillance and monitoring of disease burden in the United States population are available. The CDC manages and coordinates many of the large national surveys. Two of these databases, the National Health and Nutrition Examination Survey (NHANES) and the National Health Interview Survey (NHIS), have readily available information relevant to chronic sleep patterns and sleep disorders. Other data systems would need to add new components that incorporate sleep-related measures to be of use to researchers in the field. However, not only is it important for new criteria to be added to surveillance and monitoring systems, but researchers must also be encouraged to make use of these datasets.

National Center for Health Statistics

The National Center for Health Statistics (NCHS) is one of the centers of the CDC, and its primary goal is to monitor health trends throughout the nation and to guide actions and policies to improve the health of Americans. The NCHS has permanent surveillance systems of health and disease outcomes (e.g., vital statistics); it also conducts permanently ongoing nationwide studies and surveys. In addition, it conducts special studies as need arises (e.g., supplemental components to national surveys on a limited time basis). As described below, data relevant to sleep research are currently available from some of these systems, but the possibility of additional data collection to fill current knowledge gaps should be carefully considered.

There are a number of major health statistics sources in the United States, stratified according to the local, state, and national nature of their frame. Some sources are purely national (e.g., NHANES, the National Health Care Survey, and the Medical Expenditure Panel Survey); others are state (e.g., Behavioral Risk Factor Surveillance System, the State and Local Area Integrated Telephone Survey) or local (e.g., the National Immunization Survey); yet, the frame for other sources span across all levels of government (e.g., vital statistics, Medicare, and Medicaid).

National Health and Nutrition Examination Survey (NHANES)

Since 1959, a series of health examination surveys of the United States population have been conducted by the CDC and the NCHS. NHANES protocol is designed to monitor the health and nutritional status of Americans. In 1999 NHANES was changed from a periodic survey to an annual survey with public data files released in 2-year periods to protect confidentiality and increase statistical reliability. As in previous national health examination surveys, participants are interviewed in their homes followed by a complete health examination, part of which includes biological specimen collection. The examinations are conducted in a mobile examination center. Each mobile examination center consists of four interconnected specially designed trailers, which house biomedical equipment and laboratory capabilities. An examination team composed of 16 specially trained health professionals and support staff, including a licensed dentist, physician, interviewers, health technicians, and an x-ray technician, operates each mobile examination center.

NHANES monitors the prevalence of diseases and risk factors, nutritional habits and anthropometry status, growth and development, and environmental exposures. Because of its cyclical nature, in addition to its core components, NHANES temporarily adds components (either additional questionnaires or exam procedures). Starting in 2005, and scheduled to end in 2008, a sleep section was added to the household questionnaire. This was done with cosponsorship from the NHLBI and targeted participants in the survey older than 16 years. The NHANES sleep questionnaire is based on instruments previously used in epidemiological studies and includes questions on sleep habits as well as questions on functional outcomes of sleep disorders (Table 5-2).

National Health Interview Survey

The NHIS is the core survey of the Department of Health and Human Services, and since its establishment in 1957 it has been the principal source of information on the health of the civilian noninstitutionalized population of the United States (excluding patients in long-term care facilities, Armed Forces personnel on active duty, and U.S. nationals living abroad). Its main objective is to monitor the health of the U.S. population through the collection and analysis of data on a broad range of health topics. It is designed as a cross-sectional household interview continuously running throughout each year. The current sampling plan was redesigned in 1995, and it is based on a multistage area probability sample that permits the selection of a nationwide representative sample of households on a weekly basis. Approximately 43,000 households (including about 106,000 persons) are successfully re-

TABLE 5-2 NHANES Sleep Questionnaire, 2005–2008

How often do you experience:
  Trouble falling asleep
  Wake up during night/difficulty getting back to sleep
  Wake up too early/difficulty getting back to sleep
  Feel unrested during the day
  Feel excessively sleepy during the day
  Do not get enough sleep
  Take sleeping pills
  Nasal stuffiness, etc., at night
  Leg cramps and leg jerks
Have you ever been told you have a sleep disorder?
  What sleep disorder?
  Sleep apnea?
  Insomnia?
  Restless legs syndrome?
Have you ever snored?
How long does it take for you to fall asleep?
Do you have difficulty carrying out following activities because you are too tired or sleepy:
  Concentrating
  Remembering
  Working on a hobby
  Performing employed or volunteer work
  Operating a motor vehicle

cruited each year. Since 1995, both African American and Hispanic persons are oversampled, and samples are drawn for each state.

The core content of the survey questionnaire (the "basic module") remains largely unchanged from year to year, thus allowing for trend analyses and for data from more than 1 year to be pooled to increase sample size for analytical purposes. However, survey content is updated every 10 to 15 years. The latest significant revision was put in place in 1997. It includes the Family Core, the Sample Adult Core, and the Sample Child Core. The Family Core includes information on household composition, sociodemographic characteristics, information for matches to administrative databases, and basic indicators of health status and utilization of health care services; it is the sampling frame for additional integrated surveys such as the Medical Expenditure Panel Survey (see below). From each family, one sample adult and one sample child (if any) are randomly selected and given the corresponding core interviews that cover the individual's health status, disability, health behaviors, use of health care services, and immunizations. In addition to the Basic Module, the NHIS includes a Periodic Module and a Topical Module that contain supplemental sections to respond to new public health data needs as they arise.

The NHIS has only one question related to sleep: "On average how many hours of sleep do you get a night (24-hour period)?". This question was included in the supplemental surveys administered in 1977, 1985, and 1990, and was added to the core survey in 2004. Based on these data, the percentage of adults who reported sleeping 6 hours or less jumped from approximately 20 percent of the population in 1985 (Schoenborn, 1986) to 25 percent in 2004 (National Center for Health Statistics, National Health Interview Survey, 2004) across all age groups.

One important feature of the NHIS is its use as a sampling frame for other national surveys such as the National Survey of Family Growth and the Medical Expenditure Panel Survey. Because of its relevance for this report, the latter is described in more detail below.

Vital Statistics and the National Death Index

Vital statistics include data on all births and deaths. The latter are based on information contained in the death certificate and include identifying information (name and social security number), demographic data, and data on underlying and contributing causes of death. NCHS's National Death Index is a resource available to investigators seeking information surrounding the death of individual participants in prospective cohort studies. This is useful for investigators exploring the association between sleep disorders identified in study participants and risk of mortality from certain causes (e.g., cardiovascular, disease, hypertension, depressive disorders, and injuries). It also provides the opportunity to conduct aggregate analyses of distribution and trends of mortality directly attributable to sleep problems.

National Health Care Survey

The National Health Care Survey is a collection of health care provider surveys that obtains information about the facilities that supply health care, the services rendered, and the characteristics of the patients served (Table 5-3). Each survey is based on a multistage sampling design that includes health care facilities or providers and patient records. Data are collected directly from the establishments and/or their records, rather than from the patients. The participating surveys identify health care events—such as hospitalizations, surgeries, and long-term stays—and offer the most accurate and detailed data on diagnosis and treatment, as well as on the characteristics of the institutions. These data are used by policy makers, planners, researchers, and others in the health community to monitor changes in the use of health care resources, to monitor specific diseases, and to examine the impact of new medical technologies, to mention a few.

TABLE 5-3 Surveys Included in the National Health Care Survey's System

National Ambulatory Medical Care Survey
National Employer Health Insurance Survey
National Health Provider Inventory
National Home and Hospice Care Survey
National Hospital Ambulatory Medical Care Survey
National Hospital Discharge Survey
National Nursing Home Survey
National Survey of Ambulatory Surgery

Two of the participating surveys are of particular relevance for the study of health care resources utilization in relation to sleep disorders: the National Ambulatory Medical Care Survey and the National Hospital Discharge Survey.

The National Ambulatory Medical Care Survey

The National Ambulatory Medical Care Survey, which has been conducted annually since 1989, is a national survey designed to meet the need for objective, reliable information about the provision and use of ambulatory medical care services in the United States. Findings are based on a sample of visits to non-federally employed office-based physicians who are primarily engaged in direct patient care. Specially trained interviewers visit the physicians prior to their participation in the survey in order to provide them with survey materials and instruct them on how to complete the forms. Data collection from the physician, rather than from the patient, provides an analytic base that expands information on ambulatory care collected through other NCHS surveys. Each physician is randomly assigned to a 1-week reporting period. During this period, data for a systematic random sample of visits are recorded by the physician or office staff on an encounter form provided for that purpose. Data are obtained on patients' symptoms, physicians' diagnoses, and medications ordered or provided. The survey also provides statistics on the demographic characteristics of patients and services provided, including information on diagnostic procedures, patient management, and planned future treatment.

The National Hospital Discharge Survey

The National Hospital Discharge Survey (NHDS), which has been conducted annually since 1965, is a national probability survey designed to provide information on characteristics of inpatients discharged from nonfederal short-stay hospitals in the United States. The NHDS collects data from a sample of approximately 270,000 inpatient records acquired from a national sample of about 500 hospitals. Only hospitals with an average length of stay of fewer than 30 days for all patients, general hospitals, or children's general hospitals are included in the survey. However, the NHDS excludes data from a number of hospitals, including federal, military, and Veterans Affairs (VA) hospitals; hospital units of institutions (such as prison hospitals); and hospitals with fewer than six beds staffed for patient use. The data includes information related to the personal characteristics of the patient—age, sex, race, ethnicity, marital status, expected sources of payment, and diagnoses and procedures coded to the *International Classification of Diseases, 9th Revision, Clinical Modification*. It also includes administrative items such as admission and discharge dates (which allow calculation of length of stay). Annually, data from the NHDS are made available to the public. As an example of the amount of data available in this survey, the estimated number of all listed sleep disorders diagnoses in NHDS in 2003 was 322,000. Although the NHDS excludes information obtained through VA hospitals, there is a similar database provided by the VA that has been used to examine the association of psychiatric disorders and sleep apnea (Sharafkhaneh et al., 2005).

Data from these surveys could be used to monitor prevalence of complaints related to sleep disorders; trends in sleep-related diagnosis and services; characteristics of patients, characteristics of health care providers; use of medical technology and how use differs according to region or patients' access to care; emergence of alternative care sites; and medication use in ambulatory care settings.

Behavioral Risk Factor Surveillance System

Funded by CDC, the Behavioral Risk Factor Surveillance System complements the NCHS national surveys by providing state-specific data on prevalence of the major behavioral risks among adults associated with premature morbidity and mortality. The main objective is to collect data on actual behaviors, rather than on attitudes or knowledge, that would be especially useful for planning, initiating, supporting, and evaluating health promotion and disease prevention programs at the state and local levels.

The Behavioral Risk Factor Surveillance System is an annual telephone survey (based on random digit dialing) in each participating state. The telephone surveys methodology was chosen not only because of cost advantages but also because telephone surveys were considered especially desirable at the state and local level, where the necessary expertise and resources for conducting area probability sampling for in-person household interviews were not likely to be available.

The survey started in 1984 with 15 participating states. By 1994, all states, the District of Columbia, and three territories were participating. Although the survey was designed to collect state-level data, a number of states from the outset stratified their samples to allow them to estimate prevalence for regions within their respective states. The CDC developed a standard core questionnaire for states to use to provide data that could be compared across states.

The emergence of telemarketing and increasing use of mobile phones and automatic answering systems resulted in dwindling response rates over the last few years. However it remains as the only state-specific source of health-related data nationwide. There are currently no sleep-related questions in Behavioral Risk Factor Surveillance System.

Medical Expenditure Panel Survey

Funded by the Agency for Healthcare Research and Quality, the Medical Expenditure Panel Survey is a national probability survey designed to continually provide policy makers, health care administrators, businesses, and others with timely, comprehensive information about health care use and costs in the United States, and to improve the accuracy of their economic projections. The survey began in 1977 and comprises three component surveys: the Household Component, the Medical Provider Component, and the Insurance Component. The Household Component provides a variety of measures of health status, health insurance coverage, health care use and expenditures, and sources of payment for health services. The Medical Provider Component covers hospitals, physicians, and home health care providers and is meant to estimate the expenses of people enrolled in health maintenance organizations and other types of managed care plans. Finally the Insurance Component is used to analyze the behavior and choices made with respect to health care use and spending, as well as the amount, types, and costs of health insurance available to Americans through their workplace.

Medicare Current Beneficiary Survey

Funded by Centers for Medicare and Medicaid Services, the Medicare Current Beneficiary Survey is a continuous, multipurpose survey of a nationally representative sample of aged, disabled, and institutionalized Medicare beneficiaries. The Medicare Current Beneficiary Survey is the only comprehensive source of information on the health status, health care use and expenditures, health insurance coverage, and socioeconomic and demographic characteristics of the entire spectrum of Medicare beneficiaries. The purpose of the survey is to determine expenditures and sources of payment for all services used by Medicare beneficiaries; to establish all types of health insurance coverage and relate coverage to sources of payment; and to trace changes over time, such as health status, and the impacts of programmatic changes. It includes survey data on measures of health status and access to care that are linked to the physicians and hospital claims data. The survey was initiated in 1991 and is designed to support both cross-sectional and longitudinal analysis. Data are collected through interviews that take place over 4-month intervals. Each interview includes questions regarding the household composition; an accounting of the individual's health insurance coverage; a review of an individual's health care utilization in the period since the last interview; details about each type of service, provider characteristics, and medicines prescribed; and a detailed account of charges and payments associated with these health care events. The interview data are linked to Medicare claims.

Youth Risk and Behavior Survey

The Youth Risk Behavior Surveillance System includes national, state, and local school-based surveys of representative samples of 9th- through 12th-grade students (National Center for Chronic Disease Prevention and Health Promotion, 2005). These surveys are conducted every 2 years, usually during the spring semester. The national survey, conducted by CDC, provides data representative of high school students in public and private schools in the United States. The state and local surveys, conducted by departments of health and education, provide data representative of the state or local school district. The Risk Behavior Surveillance System was developed in 1990 to monitor priority health risk behaviors that contribute markedly to the leading causes of death, disability, and social problems among youth and adults in the United States. These behaviors, often established during childhood and early adolescence, include: tobacco use, dietary behaviors, physical activity, alcohol and other drug use, sexual behaviors, and behaviors that contribute to unintentional injuries and violence. Despite the importance of sleep deprivation and other sleep disorders in young adolescents (see Chapter 3), no questions on sleep and sleep behaviors have ever been included in the survey.

Process for Inclusion of New Components in Surveys

One impediment for the addition of greater sleep-related content in surveillance and monitoring instruments is the process required to have new components added. In addition to a high standard of scientific merit, inclusion of new components also often requires specific sponsorship. The following is a description of the criteria for adding components or questions to NHANES. Other surveys and monitoring instruments have similar requirements.

Criteria for Adding Components to NHANES

Criteria for adding components or questions to NHANES and the NHIS are based on scientific merit, public health importance, costs, sponsorship, lead time, feasibility and logistics in the context of the rest of the survey components, priority ranking in relation to competing components, and survey burden.

NHANES runs in 2-year cycles and is governed by an internal committee formed by NCHS leadership, epidemiologists, statisticians, and physicians. Every 2 years, this committee requests proposals for adding components to the upcoming 2-year cycle, including both questionnaire components and mobile examination center exams. Proposals are received through a competitive bidding process and are expected to include detailed rationale for the public health relevance of the proposal, eligibility criteria (e.g., age, gender eligibility), detailed estimates of costs, personnel needs, amount of time required to do the exam, needs for laboratory or other type of equipment, statistical power estimates, quality assurance/quality control procedures, and the availability of external funds to subsidize the additional component. The committee then makes a preliminary determination as to its suitability before it reviews the proposal. Proposals under consideration are then examined by a team of NCHS personnel and proponents to carefully study and work out all the details and logistics of the implementation of the new exam.

New components to the exam are typically introduced for a single 2-year cycle, sometimes for multiple cycles (e.g., the sleep questionnaire is introduced for two cycles from 2005 to 2008). Eventually components are rotated off when sufficient data and sample size are acquired; some exams may be rescheduled at a later date in order to monitor changes and trends overtime. Other NCHS surveys follow similar procedures for review of added components with a few differences.

Both public and private organizations are eligible to propose new components to add to the NHANES and other NCHS surveys. Federal, state, or local government agencies can provide funds to the NCHS to cofinance the costs of the proposed additions. For example, the sleep questions on NHANES are sponsored by the NHLBI. Nonprofit organizations and private companies can also make proposals but cannot provide funds to the NCHS; cosponsorship from private industry, however, can occur through money deposited in the CDC foundation.

Recommendation 5.3: The Centers for Disease Control and Prevention and National Center on Sleep Disorders Research should support additional surveillance and monitoring of sleep patterns and sleep disorders.

The Centers for Disease Control and Prevention, working with the National Center on Sleep Disorders Research, should support the development and expansion of adequate surveillance and monitoring instruments designed to examine the American population's sleep patterns and the prevalence and health outcomes associated with sleep disorders.

REFERENCES

AASM (American Academy of Sleep Medicine). 2005. *MedSleep*. [Online]. Available: http://www.aasmnet.org/MedSleep_Home.aspx [accessed December 17, 2005].

ACGME (Accreditation Council of Graduate Medical Education). 2005a. *Program Requirements for Residency Education in Neurology*. [Online]. Available: http://www.acgme.org/acWebsite/downloads/RRC_progReq/180pr105.pdf [accessed March 22, 2006].

ACGME. 2005b. *Residency Review Committees for Sleep Medicine*. [Online]. Available: http://www.acgme.org/acWebsite/downloads/RRC_PIF/520pif2_0405.doc [accessed December 16, 2005].

American Board of Otolaryngology. 2006. *Otolaryngology Training Exam*. [Online]. Available: http://www.aboto.org/blueprint.pdf [accessed January 10, 2006].

American Board of Pediatrics. 2006. *General Pediatrics Examination*. [Online]. Available: http://www.abp.org/ [accessed January 10, 2006].

American Board of Psychiatry and Neurology. 2006. *Psychiatry and Neurology Examination*. [Online]. Available: http://www.abpn.com/certification/neuro-neuro_items.html [accessed January 10, 2006].

American Thoracic Society. 2005. Curriculum and competency assessment tools for sleep disorders in pulmonary fellowship training programs. *American Journal of Respiratory and Critical Care Medicine* 172(3):391–397.

Banno K, Kryger MH. 2004. Factors limiting access to services for sleep apnea patients. *Sleep Medicine Reviews* 8(4):253–255.

Buboltz WC, Brown F, Soper B. 2001. Sleep habits and patterns of college students: A preliminary study. *Journal of the American College of Health* 50(3):131–135.

Buysse DJ, Barzansky B, Dinges D, Hogan E, Hunt CE, Owens J, Rosekind M, Rosen R, Simon F, Veasey S, Wiest F. 2003. Sleep, fatigue, and medical training: Setting an agenda for optimal learning and patient care. *Sleep* 26(2):218–225.

CDC (Centers for Disease Control and Prevention). 1996. *Sudden Infant Death Syndrome—United States, 1983-1994*. [Online]. Available: http://www.cdc.gov/mmwr/preview/mmwrhtml/00043987.htm [accessed November 29, 2005].

CDC. 2006. *Physical Activity for Everyone*. [Online]. Available: http://www.cdc.gov/nccdphp/dnpa/physical/index.htm [accessed January 6, 2006].

Culpepper L. 2002. Generalized anxiety disorder in primary care: Emerging issues in management and treatment. *Journal of Clinical Psychiatry* 63(suppl 8):35–42.

Dahl RE, Holttum J, Trubnick L. 1994. A clinical picture of child and adolescent narcolepsy. *Journal of the American Academy of Child and Adolescent Psychiatry* 33(6):834–841.

Dement WC, Vaughn C. 1999. *The Promise of Sleep: The Scientific Connection Between Health, Happiness, and a Good Nights Sleep.* London: Macmillian.

Dusselier L, Dunn B, Wang Y, Shelley MC II, Whalen DF. 2005. Personal, health, academic, and environmental predictors of stress for residence hall students. *Journal of the American College of Health* 54(1):15–24.

Dzaja A, Arber S, Hislop J, Kerkhofs M, Kopp C, Pollmacher T, Polo-Kantola P, Skene DJ, Stenuit P, Tobler I, Porkka-Heiskanen T. 2005. Women's sleep in health and disease. *Journal of Psychiatric Research* 39(1):55–76.

Engstrom CA, Strohl RA, Rose L, Lewandowski L, Stefanek ME. 1999. Sleep alterations in cancer patients. *Cancer Nursing* 22(2):143–148.

Falvo D. 2005. *Medical and Psychosocial Aspects of Chronic Illness and Disability.* 3rd ed. Sudbury, MA: Jones and Bartlett.

Federman DD. 2003. Competency-based goals for sleep and chronobiology in undergraduate medical education. *Sleep* 26(3):251.

Fenn KM, Nusbaum HC, Margoliash D. 2003. Consolidation during sleep of perceptual learning of spoken language. *Nature* 425(6958):614–616.

Gais S, Plihal W, Wagner U, Born J. 2000. Early sleep triggers memory for early visual discrimination skills. *Nature Neuroscience* 3(12):1335–1339.

Guilleminault C, Pelayo R. 1998. Narcolepsy in prepubertal children. *Annals of Neurology* 43(1):135–142.

Haponik E, Camp G. 1994. I snored: A simple sleep history for clinicians. *American Journal of Respiratory and Critical Care Medicine* 149(A53).

Haponik EF, Frye AW, Richards B, Wymer A, Hinds A, Pearce K, McCall V, Konen J. 1996. Sleep history is neglected diagnostic information. Challenges for primary care physicians. *Journal of General Internal Medicine* 11(12):759–761.

Harding SM, Berner ES. 2002. Developing an action plan for integrating sleep topics into the medical school curriculum. *Sleep and Breathing* 6(4):155–160.

Hossain JL, Shapiro CM. 2002. The prevalence, cost implications, and management of sleep disorders: An overview. *Sleep and Breathing* 6(2):85–102.

IOM (Institute of Medicine). 2002. *Speaking of Health: Assessing Health Communication Strategies for Diverse Populations.* Washington, DC: The National Academies Press.

Kapur V, Strohl KP, Redline S, Iber C, O'Connor G, Nieto J. 2002. Underdiagnosis of sleep apnea syndrome in U.S. communities. *Sleep and Breathing* 6(2):49–54.

Kemp JS, Livne M, White DK, Arfken CL. 1998. Softness and potential to cause rebreathing: Differences in bedding used by infants at high and low risk for sudden infant death syndrome. *Journal of Pediatrics* 132(2):234–239.

Lack LC. 1986. Delayed sleep and sleep loss in university students. *Journal of the American College of Health* 35(3):105–110.

Lee KA, Landis C, Chasens ER, Dowling G, Merritt S, Parker KP, Redeker N, Richards KC, Rogers AE, Shaver JF, Umlauf MG, Weaver TE. 2004. Sleep and chronobiology: Recommendations for nursing education. *Nursing Outlook* 52(3):126–133.

Meadows R. 2005. *The "Negotiated Night:" An Embodied Conceptual Framework for the Sociological Study of Sleep.* Oxford: Blackwell.

Mehlman M. 2001. Employee/employer interactions and responsibilities with special reference to genetically related sleep disorders. *Sleep and Breathing* 5(3):153–161.

Miller NL, Shattuck LG. 2005. Sleep patterns of young men and women enrolled at the United States Military Academy: Results from year 1 of a 4-year longitudinal study. *Sleep* 28(7):837–841.

Moore PJ, Adler NE, Williams DR, Jackson JS. 2002. Socioeconomic status and health: The role of sleep. *Psychosomatic Medicine* 64(2):337–344.

National Center for Chronic Disease Prevention and Health Promotion. 2005. *YRBSS: Youth Risk Behavior Surveillance System.* [Online]. Available: http://www.cdc.gov/Healthy Youth/yrbs/index.htm [accessed December 18, 2005].

National Center for Health Statistics, National Health Interview Survey. 2004. *Percentage of Adults Who Reported an Average of <6 Hours of Sleep per 24-Hour Period, by Sex and Age Group.* [Online]. Available: http://www.cdc.gov/mmwr/preview/mmwrhtml/mm 5437a7.htm [accessed November 14, 2005].

NHLBI (National Heart, Lung, and Blood Institute). 2003a. *National Sleep Disorders Research Plan, 2003.* Bethesda, MD: National Institutes of Health.

NHLBI. 2003b. *Sleep, Sleep Disorders, and Biological Rhythms: NIH Curriculum Supplement Series, Grades 9-12.* Colorado Springs, CO: Biological Sciences Curriculum Study.

NHLBI. 2004. Be a Star Sleep (Student and Teacher Guide Supplement). New York: Time, Inc.

NHLBI. 2005a. *National High Blood Pressure Education Program.* [Online]. Available: http:// www.nhlbi.nih.gov/about/nhbpep/nhbp_pd.htm [accessed November 22, 2005].

NHLBI. 2005b. *Garfield Star Sleeper.* [Online]. Available: http://www.nhlbi.nih.gov/health/ public/sleep/starslp/ [accessed December, 2005].

NHLBI. 2006. *Your Guide to Healthy Sleep.* [Online]. Available: http://www.nhlbi.nih.gov/ health/public/sleep/healthy_sleep.htm [accessed May 27, 2006].

NICHD (National Institute of Child Health and Human Development). 2003. *SIDS rate and sleep position 1998-2003.* [Online]. Available: http://www.nichd.nih.gov/sids/SIDS_ rate_backsleep_03.pdf [accessed November 18, 2005].

Orr WC, Stahl ML, Dement WC, Reddington D. 1980. Physician education in sleep disorders. *Journal of Medical Education* 55(4):367-369.

Owens J. 2005. Introduction to special section: NIH Sleep Academic Award program. *Sleep Medicine* 6(1):45-46.

Owens JA, Dalzell V. 2005. Use of the "BEARS" sleep screening tool in a pediatric residents' continuity clinic: A pilot study. *Sleep Medicine* 6(1):63-69.

Papp KK, Strohl KP. 2005. The effects of an intervention to teach medical students about obstructive sleep apnea. *Sleep Medicine* 6(1):71-73.

Pilcher JJ, Ginter DR, Sadowsky B. 1997. Sleep quality versus sleep quantity: Relationships between sleep and measures of health, well-being and sleepiness in college students. *Journal of Psychosomatic Research* 42(6):583-596.

Punjabi NM, Bandeen-Roche K, Young T. 2003. Predictors of objective sleep tendency in the general population. *Sleep* 26(6):678-683.

Reynolds CF III, Adler S, Kanter SL, Horn JP, Harvey J, Bernier GM Jr. 1995. The undergraduate medical curriculum: Centralized versus departmentalized. *Academy of Medicine* 70(8):671-675.

Roccella E. 2002. The contributions of public health education toward reduction of cardiovascular disease mortality: Experiences from the National High Blood Pressure Education Program. In: Hornik R, ed. *Public Health Communication: Evidence for Behavior Change.* Mahwah, NJ: Lawrence Erlbaum. Pp. 73-84.

Rosen GM, Harris I, Mahowald MW. 2005. Objective structured clinical examinations (OSCE) for sleep. *Sleep Medicine* 6(1):75-80.

Rosen RC, Rosekind M, Rosevear C, Cole WE, Dement WC. 1993. Physician education in sleep and sleep disorders: A national survey of U.S. medical schools. *Sleep* 16(3):249-254.

Rosen R, Mahowald M, Chesson A, Doghramji K, Goldberg R, Moline M, Millman R, Zammit G, Mark B, Dement W. 1998. The Taskforce 2000 Survey on Medical Education in Sleep and Sleep Disorders. *Sleep* 21(3):235-238.

Sateia MJ, Reed VA, Christian JG. 2005. The Dartmouth Sleep Knowledge and Attitude Survey: Development and validation. *Sleep Medicine* 6(1):47-54.

Schoenborn CA. 1986. Health habits of U.S. adults, 1985: the "Alameda 7" revisited. *Public Health Report* 101(6):571–580.

Sharafkhaneh A, Giray N, Richardson P, Young T, Hirshkowitz M. 2005. Association of psychiatric disorders and sleep apnea in a large cohort. *Sleep* 28(11):1405–1411.

Siegel M. 2002. The effectiveness of state-level tobacco control interventions: A review of program implementation and behavioral outcomes. *Annual Review of Public Health* 23:45–71.

Stickgold R, James L, Hobson JA. 2000. Visual discrimination learning requires sleep after training. *Nature Neuroscience* 3(12):1237–1238.

Strohl KP, Veasey S, Harding S, Skatrud J, Berger HA, Papp KK, Dunagan D, Guilleminault C. 2003. Competency-based goals for sleep and chronobiology in undergraduate medical education. *Sleep* 26(3):333–336.

Taylor B. 1993. Unconsciousness and society: The sociology of sleep. *International Journal of Politics, Culture, and Society* 6(3):463–474.

U.S. Congress, Senate. 1993. *National Institutes of Health Revitalization Act of 1993.* 103rd Cong., S.104:285b-7.

Walker MP, Brakefield T, Hobson JA, Stickgold R. 2003. Dissociable stages of human memory consolidation and reconsolidation. *Nature* 425(6958):616–620.

Warner KE. 1981. Cigarette smoking in the 1970s: The impact of the antismoking campaign on consumption. *Science* 211(4483):729–731.

Williams SJ. 2002. Sleep and health: Sociological reflections on the dormant society. *Health (N Y)* 6(2):173–200.

Willinger M. 1995. SIDS prevention. *Pediatric Annals* 24(7):358–364.

Wyatt JK. 2004. Delayed sleep phase syndrome: Pathophysiology and treatment options. *Sleep* 27(6):1195–1203.

Zozula R, Rosen RC, Jahn EG. 2005. Recognition of sleep disorders in a community-based setting following an educational intervention. *Sleep Medicine* 6(1):55–61.

6

Ensuring Adequate Diagnosis and Treatment: Access, Capacity, and Technology Development

CHAPTER SUMMARY   *Millions of individuals suffering from sleep disorders remain undiagnosed and untreated. Most American communities do not have adequate health care resources to meet the clinical demands. Further, the current diagnostic and therapeutic capacity is not sufficient for the present demand, let alone the predicted increase in demand arising from the proposed public education campaign. Thus, additional technology development is required. Based on estimates of the prevalence of sleep disorders, millions of individuals are undiagnosed and untreated. As awareness increases, greater investment in the development and validation of new diagnostic and therapeutic technologies will be required to meet the anticipated demand. Numerous technological advances have enhanced the feasibility of portable diagnosis and treatment, but they have not been fully evaluated and validated. Therefore, the committee urges the evaluation and validation of existing diagnostic and therapeutic technologies, as well as the development of new technologies.*

Increased awareness among the general public and health care practitioners will present numerous challenges to existing health care providers and researchers who are already stretched too thin. Therefore, as described in the following sections, development and improved capacity through technology development is required.

An increased recognition of sleep disorders has resulted in an increase in demand. In a 3-year period over the late 1990s, demand for a sleep test doubled in the United States (Pack and Gurubhagavatula, 1999). In France the number of patients diagnosed and receiving continuous positive airway pressure (CPAP) treatment is annually increasing by 20 percent (Gagnadoux et al., 2002). Demand has been accompanied by improved patient access to physicians and other clinicians trained in sleep medicine and to facilities where clinical sleep tests, polysomnograms, can be performed. There are currently an estimated 1,292 sleep centers or laboratories in the United States, 39 percent of which were accredited by the American Academy of Sleep Medicine (AASM) (Tachibana et al., 2005). However, resources have not kept up with demand. For example, 80 to 90 percent of obstructive sleep apnea (OSA) cases remain undiagnosed and untreated, which increases the burden of this disorder (Kapur et al., 2002). Narcolepsy, too, is infrequently detected (Singh et al., 2005), but precise rates of under diagnosis are not available because this condition is less common. Similarly, there is poor recognition and treatment of insomnia (Benca, 2005), as well as poor communication between patient and physician. Thus, even with a growth in resources, this issue is of significant importance to the millions of individuals suffering from sleep disorders.

DEVELOPING PORTABLE DIAGNOSTIC TOOLS

Polysomnography, the "gold standard" procedure for the diagnosis of most sleep disorders, is not readily available for everyone who needs it. These procedures employ simultaneous monitoring of numerous physiological parameters including brain wave activity, eye movements, muscle activity (chin and legs), heart rate, body position, and respiratory variables, including oxygen saturation. The test is typically performed overnight in a sleep laboratory with a technician in attendance, requiring an individual to sleep in the laboratory. Thus, this procedure necessitates facilities that accommodate overnight testing (beds and monitoring areas), highly sophisticated equipment, trained staff who are willing to work night shifts, and physicians trained in sleep medicine.

Although there may currently be cost-effective ways to manage sleep disorder, the capacity does not currently exist to diagnose and treat all individuals. Most American communities do not have adequate health care resources to meet the clinical demands of treating the large number of patients with sleep disorders (Banno and Kryger, 2004; Tachibana et al., 2005). In many health care systems and communities, waiting lists may be as long as 10 weeks (Rodsutti et al., 2004), with even longer waiting times in certain systems such as Veterans Affairs Medical Centers (Sharafkhaneh et al., 2004). Although this is not a problem that is unique to the field, long wait lists cause significant delays in diagnosing and treating individuals (Banno and Kryger, 2004). This is of particular concern for individuals with sleep disorders that lead to increased chance of injury. For example, undiagnosed severe OSA can lead to death or serious harm of self or others due to crashes (George, 2001). Further, long wait times contribute to high no-show rates that in turn increases the length of the wait-lists (Callahan and Redmon, 1987; Olivares, 1990). This also may decrease market share (Christl, 1973; Antle and Reid, 1988). It has been estimated that sleep apnea alone, a diagnosis that necessitates polysomnography to meet current criteria set out by third-party payers, annually requires at least 2,310 polysomnograms per 100,000 population to address the demand for diagnosis and treatment (Flemons et al., 2004). However, on average, only 427 polysomnograms per 100,000 population are performed each year in the United States, a level far below the need. In fact, 32 states annually perform less than 500 polysomnograms (Tachibana et al., 2005). Only Maryland annually performs more than 1,000. This large geographic variability in levels of sleep services is not explained by Medicare reimbursement rates, race, or distribution of OSA risk factors in these areas (Tachibana et al., 2005). Further, such geographical variability suggests the need for more standardized approaches for diagnosis and disease management.

Limitations in providing overnight diagnostic sleep laboratory services are attributed to a number of factors. Direct costs associated with having a polysomnogram performed (Chapter 4) are high. In addition, there are high expenses to sleep laboratories, including costs related to the initial investment in equipment (hardware and software) and information technology needed to manage large amounts of digital data. There are considerable personnel costs related to dedicating one to two trained technicians to each patient for a 10- to 12-hour period (for orientation, hookup, and minute-by-minute monitoring) and for scoring of studies (2 to 3 hours per study), overhead for space (which traditionally has used in-patient hospital space and more recently has used space in upscale hotels that contract with health care organizations to provide rooms or floors that serve as "community-based sleep laboratories"), and costs related to consumable supplies used for monitoring. Most insurers require sleep laboratories to be supervised by physicians or other clinicians certified by the American Academy of Sleep Medicine. In addition, many patients are reluctant to undergo somewhat intrusive monitoring and to spend one or more nights away from home. The latter is of special concern to individuals with home care (of their children or parents) responsibilities. These factors have contributed to an interest in developing portable, and perhaps simpler, less costly and less intrusive devices that can be used in a patient's own home, with the goals of improving access and decreasing the cost of sleep studies.

The Potential of Developing Portable Sleep Monitoring

Numerous technological advances have enhanced the feasibility of portable monitoring. These include miniaturization of recording components, efficiencies of digital data storage, remote monitoring capabilities (allowing centrally based technicians to monitor signals at home via wireless or modem communications), and development of new physiological sensors. Advances have been such that essentially the same data that are collected using full polysomnography in the laboratory can be collected in the home with monitors that weigh less than 300 grams. Large-scale epidemiological studies have demonstrated the feasibility of such multichannel recordings done in children and in middle-aged and elderly individuals (Goodwin et al., 2003; Redline et al., 1998). Recent experience in a community sample of almost 3,000 older men, a large percentage of whom had OSA and periodic limb movements, indicates that this approach can yield high quality data in 97 percent of studies performed (personal communication, S. Redline, Case Western Reserve University School of Medicine, December 15, 2005). The improvement in the high quality of data in this study compared to previous studies is largely due to technological advances. A study comparing the quality of data obtained from an in-home to an in-laboratory study demonstrates comparable quality and evidence of slightly less stage 1 sleep (i.e., lighter sleep) in the home, suggesting that patients may sleep better and have more representative sleep at home (Iber et al., 2004). The apnea-hypopnea index (AHI) determined using the two methods were highly correlated; however, a Bland Altman plot showed that at lower AHIs, the AHI tended to be lower in the laboratory than at home, and at higher AHIs, the AHI was higher in the laboratory than home. The latter phenomenon was thought to relate to positional differences in apnea severity, with severely affected patients probably spending more time on their back when sleeping in the typical hospital bed than when studied at home. However, although recent studies suggest low failure rates, there may be significant differences in the failure rates of unattended monitoring in less controlled settings. Thus examination of the efficacy of such technologies should be performed in less controlled settings, as may occur in clinical practice.

Despite the promise of this technology, such comprehensive monitoring, even at home, is probably as burdensome to patients as when performed in the laboratory, requires a technician to travel to the patient's home to set up and retrieve the units, and has a higher failure rate due to all the vagaries of using many sensors in an unattended manner. Failure rates between 5 to 20 percent have been reported for ambulatory diagnostic devices (Redline et al., 1998; Whitney et al., 1998; Fry et al., 1998; Mykytyn et al., 1999; Portier et al., 2000); however, since these reports were released there have been many technological improvements. A formal cost-benefit analysis of 12 to 14 multichannel in-home monitoring compared to in-laboratory monitoring has not been performed. Thus, there is interest in use of simpler technology with sufficient predictive value to be used in decision making.

Technological advances also have led to the incorporation and packaging of various groups of sensors, many novel, designed to provide simpler means for quantifying airflow limitation or breathing effort, oxygen desaturation, snoring sounds, movement, heart rate, blood pressure, and vascular tone variability.

Several of these devices are designed to primarily provide estimates of sleep and wake time over 24-hour periods, such as wrist actigraphs (i.e., a movement detector coupled with software that uses movement patterns to provide estimated sleep and wake times) (Ancoli-Israel et al., 1997). These are used more often in research than in clinical settings, although clinically they have been used to enhance evaluation of sleep-wake disorders. These devices provide estimates of sleep time that correlate moderately well to polysomnography-based estimates; however, in certain high-risk subgroups, such as children with attention-deficit/hyperactivity disorder or sleep apnea, they may perform less well (Bader et al., 2003).

A detailed review of different ambulatory technologies for sleep apnea measurement was recently performed (Flemons et al., 2003; Tice, 2005). Most devices have been designed to screen or diagnose sleep apnea. Several novel portable devices that have been informed by a growing knowledge of physiological correlates of sleep apnea have been developed. A recent review by the AASM has identified the utility of measuring nasal pressure from a sensor placed in the outer nares, which accurately detects airflow limitation (Krieger et al., 2002), the sine qua non of OSA. Several devices combine this sensor with sensors that measure oxygen saturation, snoring, and other sleep apnea correlates. For example, a relatively simple device has been designed to measure nasal pressure, oximetry, head movement, and snoring with a head band containing these sensors that is placed around the forehead and can be self-applied without glue or skin preparation (Westbrook et al., 2005). The AHI derived using an early version of this device tested in both in-home and in-laboratory settings in a large sample showed sensitivities of 92 to 98 percent and specificities of 86 to 100 percent for identification of sleep apnea. An advantage of such technology includes its potential to easily measure sleep over two or more nights (enhancing reliability) and its potential reduced cost (estimated at 30 to 50 percent of that of in-laboratory polysomnography). There has also been great interest in the use of completely novel sensors that have not been traditionally used in the sleep laboratory, but which are based on growing interests in the autonomic sequelae of sleep apnea. One such device measures peripheral artery tone from a sensor placed on the finger and has been shown to provide estimates of vascular flow, a measure that reflects variations in breathing and sleep-related arousals (Lavie et al., 2000). One wrist-worn device that uses this sensor in combination with sensors measuring oxygen saturation, heart rate, and movement has shown promising utility for sleep apnea detection. Preliminary data from one study showed a 95 percent sensitivity and 100 percent specificity (Pittman et al., 2004). Other studies have also supported this approach (Ayas et al., 2003), including results from a study of almost 100 individuals (Zou et al., 2006). Another exciting advance is the development of oximeters that are relatively resistant to movement artifact, thus improving the accuracy of such data in unattended settings (Barker, 2002).

CHALLENGES TO DEVELOPING AMBULATORY TECHNOLOGIES

Despite the promise of this technology, use of portable monitoring for diagnosis or management of sleep disorders has not yet been endorsed by any professional organization. Dozens of studies have been conducted that evaluate different aspects of technology use (ranging from evaluation of the accuracy of individual sensors to use in epidemiological studies to use in case identification); however, very few studies have met rigorous criteria for endorsement of a new diagnostic test, including comparison to a reference standard, blinded assessments, and use of large samples (Tice, 2005). Although development and evaluation of new and improved sleep monitors are much needed, the industry has failed to invest in conducting such rigorous studies. The National Institutes of Health (NIH) has invested in such assessments mostly through Small Business Innovation Research (SBIR) grants; however, between 2002 to 2005, only 17 SBIR grants were awarded to develop and evaluate new sleep technology, and many of these studies were designed to test feasibility (phase I) rather than efficacy.

There are several challenges to technology development and evaluation that may be fairly specific to sleep medicine. Challenges relate to the underlying uncertainty over: (1) which physiological signals best capture the stresses associated with sleep apnea and thus would most optimally identify patients who are either at increased risk for sleep apnea-related morbidity or who are most likely to require and respond to therapy; and (2) what threshold values, if any, for quantitative data derived from physiological monitoring best identify patients at risk or likely to respond to therapy. The collection of 12 or more channels of physiological data on sleep architecture, cardiovascular responses, and disordered breathing potentially provides the clinician a comprehensive panel of data from which to make treatment decisions. The influences of reducing this panel of data on clinical decisions and short- and long-term disease management are unclear. Emerging data suggest that different sleep apnea-related outcomes may be differentially predicted by alternative indexes of physiological stress captured by polysomnography. One recent cross-sectional study, for example, showed that while indexes of overnight hypoxemia were most strongly associated with glucose impairment, the arousal index best predicted hypertension (Sulit et al., 2006). Thus, monitors that selectively record one set of physiological disturbances may be well suited for predicting some, but not all outcomes. Threshold values may also differ according to the physiological outcome of interest. For example, data from the Sleep Heart Health Study suggest that an increased prevalence of hypertension may be observed at a threshold AHI that is higher than the threshold associated with other cardiovascular manifestations (Nieto et al., 2000; Shahar et al., 2001). Such uncertainties hamper technological efforts at choosing sensor "packages" that are most clinically relevant and evaluation procedures that require clear consensus over affection status to determine sensitivity and specificity.

Implicit in the challenges noted above are the very limited available data that address the clinical utility of the most commonly considered reference standard of polysomnography, coupled with current practice that focuses on specific numbers obtained from this test to make specific diagnoses. However, the latter practice is actually not well supported by evidence, and there is much debate over which threshold levels define "disease" and what combinations of data should be used to construct each metric (Ryan et al., 1988; Redline and Sanders, 1999). Little available research has evaluated the specific contribution of polysomnography over information obtained by other clinical assessments, including history and examination. As mentioned, although multiple physiological variables are captured, there is no clear consensus on how these data are most optimally combined for case identification or for disease assessment. Historically, the field (including third-party insurers) have used a single metric such as the AHI for defining sleep apnea, or the periodic limb movement index (PLMI) for periodic limb movement disorder, defining disease by using a single cutoff value for each (e.g., AHI greater than 5 for sleep apnea or PLMI greater than 5 for periodic limb movement disorder). However, this approach, which emphasizes the centrality of a single number—and which is known to vary from night to night (Quan et al., 2002)—differs from that in other fields where data from physiological tests are used as one of many indices to gauge disease severity and to follow treatment responses, but are not used as the sole diagnostic instrument. For example, asthma, a common chronic inflammatory disease of the airways, is diagnosed predominantly using a careful history; lung function tests are used to gauge disease severity and treatment responses and sometimes to help differentiate asthma from other respiratory conditions. The issues that plague equipment development and laboratory access in the sleep laboratory have not impeded the development of lung function laboratories. Rather, the development and accreditation of lung function laboratories and lung function equipment (including portable spirometers) are based on collecting reproducible data that meet physiological criteria for accuracy, independent of the role of such equipment as tools evaluated on their ability to independently classify disease status. It is recognized that the latter requires consideration of multiple factors, including symptoms, level of impairment, response to allergic and irritant triggers, and often empiric responses to therapeutic trials.

Other challenges relate to designing studies that specifically address a number of distinct potential applications of portable sleep monitoring. These include screening—which is often population-based, and intended to detect cases independent of symptoms; clinical case definition—identification of cases among patients referred because of health concerns; disease management in which sleep monitoring provides quantitative data on progression or regression of disease severity; and epidemiological studies—in which sleep monitoring is used to provide a quantitative assessment of a physiological exposure or outcome. It is important that any given evaluation study of new technologies be designed to address a specific question or related series of questions.

Scoring and Processing of Sleep Studies

Current scoring approaches use a system of epoch by epoch scoring (30 seconds per epoch) developed over 40 years ago when polysomnography used only paper-based systems based on analog data. This approach is recognized to be both labor-intensive and time-consuming. Further, reliance on human scorers using visual pattern recognition requires intensive and ongoing training to achieve high reliability (Whitney et al., 1998), which may be lower than that potentially attained by automated methods (which also have their limitations). Visual scoring also may not maximally utilize the spectral components of the electrophysiological data, which may provide useful information on sleep architecture. Furthermore, there is a shortage of trained sleep technicians. Currently there are only 2,198 certified technicians to monitor and score sleep tests, far below the need (Association of Polysomnographic Technologists, 1999). Recognizing these issues, the AASM convened a task force in 2004 to reassess current scoring approaches, critically evaluate both sensors and scoring algorithms, and update scoring approaches as appropriate to include digital analysis of electrophysiological data. This report, scheduled for release in 2006, should provide important advances for the diagnosis of chronic sleep loss and sleep disorders.

Summary of Formal Evaluation Reviews

Three recent in-depth reviews have been performed to examine the effectiveness of portable monitoring devices (Ross et al., 2000; ATS, 2004; Tice, 2005). As described above, these reports were largely aimed at evaluating the literature regarding the accuracy of clinical diagnosis relative to reference in lab polysomnography, with some attempt at also evaluating the literature relative to cost-effectiveness and clinical prediction. In 1998, the Agency for Healthcare Research and Quality performed a literature review and meta-analysis on studies of portable monitoring for OSA. The review concluded that at the time there was insufficient evidence to make firm recommendations for use of portable monitoring for the diagnosis of sleep apnea (Ross et al., 2000).

An executive summary on the systematic review and practice parameters for portable monitoring in the investigation of suspected sleep apnea in adults was published in 2004 by an evidence review committee consisting of members from the American Thoracic Society, the American College of Chest Physicians, and the American Academy of Sleep Medicine (ATS, 2004; Flemons and Littner, 2003). In that summary, the following recommendations were made:

• Given the available data, the use of portable device was not recommended for general screening.

• The use of portable devices was not recommended in patients with comorbid conditions or secondary sleep complaints.

• The use of portable devices should require review of raw data by trained sleep specialists.

The review committee also recognized the need for further development of portable devices and suggested several goals for future research. It was found that most studies on portable monitoring were performed primarily on white males with OSA who had few comorbidities. The evidence review committee recommended that future studies should include more diverse populations, other than patients with sleep apnea, that are not subject to selection bias. Additional recommendations were that future studies should address clinical predictive algorithms in combination with portable monitoring in the diagnosis of sleep apnea, and study design should assess the cost-effectiveness and outcomes associated with different diagnostic and management strategies.

The California Technology Assessment Forum most recently evaluated the evidence that supported use of ambulatory devices over in-laboratory procedures for the purposes of diagnosing sleep apnea (Tice, 2005). The following five technology assessment criteria were identified:

• The technology must have final approval from government regulatory bodies.
• The scientific evidence must permit conclusions concerning the effectiveness of the technology regarding health outcomes.
• The technology must improve health outcomes.
• The technical must be as beneficial as any established alternatives.
• The technology must be attainable outside of the investigational setting.

They determined that only the first two criteria had been met, but the last three were not. This review also identified the paucity of data regarding the "reference standard" (laboratory polysomnography) as improving health outcomes and suggested that a therapeutic trial of CPAP therapy may be a more efficient and clinically relevant approach than use of either in-home or in-laboratory sleep monitoring.

Evaluating Daytime Sleepiness

There is also a need to improve diagnostic procedures aiming at the quantification of excessive daytime sleepiness and the diagnosis of narcolepsy and hypersomnia. The current gold standard is the clinical Multiple Sleep Latency Test (MSLT), conducted after nocturnal polysomnography is performed (Littner et al., 2005). Sleepiness is considered consistent with hypersomnia or narcolepsy when a mean sleep latency less or equal to 8 minutes is observed (AASM, 2005). The observation of multiple sleep onset rapid eye movement (REM) periods (SOREMPs) during five naps is considered diagnostic for narcolepsy (see Chapter 3). Problematically however, the MSLT is sensitive to sleep deprivation and sleep-disordered breathing; thus, the test is often difficult to interpret. Population-based studies with the experimental MSLT, a modified version of the MSLT where mean sleep latency, but not SOREMP are measured, suggest that a large portion of the population has a short sleep latency (Kim and Young, 2005) and that the test correlates only partially with subjective measures of excessive daytime sleepiness. This has led to the revised diagnostic criteria that suggest that the MSLT should only be interpreted in the absence of sleep apnea and sufficient sleep prior to the MSLT (total sleep time equal to or greater than 6 hours) (AASM, 2005). Very limited clinical MSLT data are available in population samples, but data to date suggest that 3.9 percent of individuals may be positive for SOREMPs independent of daytime sleepiness (Singh et al., 2005). Similarly, the Maintenance of Wakefulness Test (MWT), a test in which the subject is asked to try not to fall asleep in naps and sleep latency is measured, has been used to objectively measure alertness in drug trials but is not validated to demonstrate an ability to stay awake for patients at risk, for example in medicolegal cases and the evaluation of driving abilities (Littner et al., 2005).

As conducted, the MSLT and the MWT are time-consuming and expensive, and validation in the general population sample is lacking. How sleep apnea and prior sleep time in and outside the laboratory affects the occurrence of SOREMPs in MSLTs is not established. It is also unknown whether these tests may not be more valid after a night at home and verification of sleep with actigraphy or other procedures, a modification that would reduce cost in some cases. Finally, performance tests such as the psychomotor vigilance task, used commonly to evaluate performance after sleep deprivation, may have applications in this area (Dauvilliers and Buguet, 2005), especially if those tests can be adjusted to be used in ambulatory situations. Biochemical and imaging research aiming at discovering biomarkers of sleep debt and sleepiness is also needed.

Other Diagnostic Technologies

In addition to the development of ambulatory strategies, efforts are also currently under way to utilize other techniques to diagnose individuals who suffer chronic sleep loss or sleep disorders. These strategies include the development of genetic and biochemical tests for narcolepsy, magnetic resonance imaging (MRI) to visualize the upper airway in children with OSA, and acoustic reflectometry (a noninvasive ultrasound technique) of the upper airway to quantify anatomic obstruction of the upper airway in children (Mignot et al., 2002; Arens et al., 2003; Monahan et al., 2002; Donnelly et al., 2004; Abbott et al., 2004). Tests such as the standardized immobilization test or biochemical/imaging measures of brain iron metabolism are being developed to assist in the diagnosis and quantification of severity in restless leg syndrome (Allen and Earley, 2001; Garcia-Borreguero et al., 2004; Trenkwalder et al., 2005). Actigraphy and other methods are also used to estimate leg movement frequency in outpatients (Kazenwadel et al., 1995; Sforza et al., 2005). Video technologies may also be of value, especially in the diagnosis of individuals with night terrors. Finally, there is a need to establish novel procedures to objectively identify abnormalities in insomnia beyond the changes generally observed using sleep questionnaires, logs, and polysomnography (Roth and Drake, 2004). These may involve the use of spectral analysis (Perlis et al., 2001), microstructural cyclic alternating patterns analysis (Parrino et al., 2004), and functional neuroimaging (Drummond et al., 2004; Nofzinger, 2005).

The development of polysomnograms that are performed in a local hospital and telemonitored by a central sleep laboratory could allow for a single technician to monitor multiple studies from a central location. However, the reliability of these procedures varies (Gagnadoux et al., 2002).

FUTURE DIRECTIONS

Given the cumbersome nature and cost of the diagnosis and treatment of sleep disorders and sleep loss, the resultant inequities with regard to access, and in order to ensure future quality care, greater investment in the development of new, and validation of existing, diagnostic and therapeutic technologies is required. Improvement in portable monitoring techniques will likely enhance access to sleep diagnostic services. With the inadequate availability of sleep centers and sleep technicians, not only in the United States but more so worldwide, access to portable diagnostic screening procedures and streamlining initiation of treatment would clearly be advantageous. In particular, portable monitoring at level III (limited channel polysomnogram of four or more cardiopulmonary bioparameters) or level IV (testing of only one or two cardiopulmonary bioparameters) would help lower health costs and shorten waiting lists. In selected patient populations, portable monitoring in conjunction with inpatient split-night polysomnography or unattended autotitration of nasal CPAP could prove to be the most cost-effective and rational approach to most patients with a clinical profile for moderate to severe sleep apnea syndrome. Research in the design and evaluation of existing and novel diagnostic technologies is also needed in the area of insomnia, hypersomnia, and restless legs syndrome and periodic limb movements.

However, the rational application of technology needs to be coupled with the following:

• A reexamination of the role of diagnostic testing in case identification and disease management, clarifying optimal use of objective physiological monitoring data (including data obtained from portable monitors) in clinical diagnostic and management algorithms.
• Recognition that the development of new physiological monitoring tools needs to be guided by research that clarifies the short- and long-term clinical predictive information of specific channels (including responses to clinical interventions), or combinations of data. This should include consideration of the extent to which data from new technologies complement those from other techniques.
• Standardization of diagnostic and treatment criteria, language, and technologies.
• Investigation of how information from laboratory and portable diagnosis may interface as complementary rather than competitive technologies.

• Investment by industry and the NIH in rigorous evaluation and outcome studies that are designed to test specific questions regarding technology applications in improving the efficiency of screening, case identification, and disease management.
• Assessment of technologies utilizing indexes to examine their cost-effectiveness.
• Development of technologies keeping in mind that treatment of sleep disorders requires a chronic care management scheme (see Chapter 9).
• Specific efforts to develop and modify technologies for children.

Recommendation 6.1: The National Institutes of Health and the Agency for Healthcare Research and Quality should support the validation and development of existing and new diagnostic and therapeutic technologies.

The National Center on Sleep Disorders Research—working with the Trans-NIH Sleep Research Coordinating Committee, the Agency for Health Care Policy and Research, other federal agencies, and private industry—should support the evaluation and validation of existing diagnostic and therapeutic technologies. Further, development of new technologies such as ambulatory monitoring, biological markers, and imaging techniques should be vigorously supported.

REFERENCES

AASM (American Academy of Sleep Medicine). 2005. *The International Classification of Sleep Disorders*. Westchester, IL: AASM.

Abbott MB, Donnelly LF, Dardzinski BJ, Poe SA, Chini BA, Amin RS. 2004. Obstructive sleep apnea: MR imaging volume segmentation analysis. *Radiology* 232(3):889–895.

Allen RP, Earley CJ. 2001. Restless legs syndrome: A review of clinical and pathophysiologic features. *Journal of Clinical Neurophysiology* 18(2):128–147.

Ancoli-Israel S, Clopton P, Klauber MR, Fell R, Mason W. 1997. Use of wrist activity for monitoring sleep/wake in demented nursing-home patients. *Sleep* 20(1):24–27.

Antle DW, Reid RA. 1988. Managing service capacity in an ambulatory care clinic. *Hospital and Health Services Administration* 33(2):201–211.

Arens R, McDonough JM, Corbin AM, Rubin NK, Carroll ME, Pack AI, Liu J, Udupa JK. 2003. Upper airway size analysis by magnetic resonance imaging of children with obstructive sleep apnea syndrome. *American Journal of Respiratory and Critical Care Medicine* 167(1):65–70.

Association of Polysomnographic Technologists. 1999. *The APT Demographic, Salary, and Educational Needs Survey*. Lenexa, KS: APT.

ATS (American Thoracic Society). 2004. Executive summary on the systematic review and practice parameters for portable monitoring in the investigation of suspected sleep apnea in adults. *American Journal of Respiratory and Critical Care Medicine* 169(10):1160–1163.

Ayas NT, Pittman S, Macdonald M, White DP. 2003. Assessment of a wrist-worn device in the detection of obstructive sleep apnea. *Sleep Medicine* 4(5):435–442.

Bader G, Gillberg C, Johnson M, Kadesjö B, Rasmussen P. 2003. Activity and sleep in children with ADHD. *Sleep* 26:A136.

Banno K, Kryger MH. 2004. Factors limiting access to services for sleep apnea patients. *Sleep Medicine Reviews* 8(4):253–255.

Barker SJ. 2002. "Motion-resistant" pulse oximetry: A comparison of new and old models. *Anesthesia and Analgesia* 95(4):967–972.

Benca RM. 2005. Diagnosis and treatment of chronic insomnia: A review. *Psychiatry Services* 56(3):332–343.

Callahan NM, Redmon WK. 1987. Effects of problem-based scheduling on patient waiting and staff utilization of time in a pediatric clinic. *Journal of Applied Behavioral Analysis* 20(2):193–199.

Christl HL. 1973. Some methods of operations research applied to patient scheduling problems. *Medical Progress Through Technology* 2(1):19–27.

Dauvilliers Y, Buguet A. 2005. Hypersomnia. *Dialogues in Clinical Neuroscience* 7(4):347–356.

Donnelly LF, Shott SR, LaRose CR, Chini BA, Amin RS. 2004. Causes of persistent obstructive sleep apnea despite previous tonsillectomy and adenoidectomy in children with Down syndrome as depicted on static and dynamic cine MRI. *American Journal of Roentgenology* 183(1):175–181.

Drummond SP, Smith MT, Orff HJ, Chengazi V, Perlis ML. 2004. Functional imaging of the sleeping brain: Review of findings and implications for the study of insomnia. *Sleep Medicine Reviews* 8(3):227–242.

Flemons WW, Littner MR. 2003. Measuring agreement between diagnostic devices. *Chest* 124(4):1535–1542.

Flemons WW, Littner MR, Rowley JA, Gay P, Anderson WM, Hudgel DW, McEvoy RD, Loube DI. 2003. Home diagnosis of sleep apnea: A systematic review of the literature. An evidence review cosponsored by the American Academy of Sleep Medicine, the American College of Chest Physicians, and the American Thoracic Society. *Chest* 124(4):1543–1579.

Flemons WW, Douglas NJ, Kuna ST, Rodenstein DO, Wheatley J. 2004. Access to diagnosis and treatment of patients with suspected sleep apnea. *American Journal of Respiratory and Critical Care Medicine* 169(6):668–672.

Fry JM, DiPhillipo MA, Curran K, Goldberg R, Baran AS. 1998. Full polysomnography in the home. *Sleep* 21(6):635–642.

Gagnadoux F, Pelletier-Fleury N, Philippe C, Rakotonanahary D, Fleury B. 2002. Home unattended vs hospital telemonitored polysomnography in suspected obstructive sleep apnea syndrome: A randomized crossover trial. *Chest* 121(3):753–758.

Garcia-Borreguero D, Larrosa O, de la Llave Y, Granizo JJ, Allen R. 2004. Correlation between rating scales and sleep laboratory measurements in restless legs syndrome. *Sleep Medicine* 5(6):561–565.

George CF. 2001. Reduction in motor vehicle collisions following treatment of sleep apnoea with nasal CPAP. *Thorax* 56(7):508–512.

Goodwin JL, Kaemingk KL, Fregosi RF, Rosen GM, Morgan WJ, Sherrill DL, Quan SF. 2003. Clinical outcomes associated with sleep-disordered breathing in Caucasian and Hispanic children—the Tucson Children's Assessment of Sleep Apnea Study (TuCASA). *Sleep* 26(5):587–591.

Iber C, Redline S, Kaplan Gilpin AM, Quan SF, Zhang L, Gottlieb DJ, Rapoport D, Resnick HE, Sanders M, Smith P. 2004. Polysomnography performed in the unattended home versus the attended laboratory setting—Sleep Heart Health Study methodology. *Sleep* 27(3):536–540.

Kapur V, Strohl KP, Redline S, Iber C, O'Connor G, Nieto J. 2002. Underdiagnosis of sleep apnea syndrome in U.S. communities. *Sleep and Breathing* 6(2):49–54.

Kazenwadel J, Pollmacher T, Trenkwalder C, Oertel WH, Kohnen R, Kunzel M, Kruger HP. 1995. New actigraphic assessment method for periodic leg movements (PLM). *Sleep* 18(8):689–697.

Kim H, Young T. 2005. Subjective daytime sleepiness: Dimensions and correlates in the general population. *Sleep* 28(5):625–634.

Krieger J, McNicholas WT, Levy P, De Backer W, Douglas N, Marrone O, Montserrat J, Peter JH, Rodenstein D, European Respiratory Society Task Force. 2002. Public health and medicolegal implications of sleep apnoea. *European Respiratory Journal* 20(6):1594–1609.

Lavie P, Schnall RP, Sheffy J, Shlitner A. 2000. Peripheral vasoconstriction during REM sleep detected by a new plethysmographic method. *Nature Medicine* 6(6):606.

Littner MR, Kushida C, Wise M, Davila DG, Morgenthaler T, Lee-Chiong T, Hirshkowitz M, Daniel LL, Bailey D, Berry RB, Kapen S, Kramer M. 2005. Practice parameters for clinical use of the multiple sleep latency test and the maintenance of wakefulness test. *Sleep* 28(1):113–121.

Mignot E, Lammers GJ, Ripley B, Okun M, Nevsimalova S, Overeem S, Vankova J, Black J, Harsh J, Bassetti C, Schrader H, Nishino S. 2002. The role of cerebrospinal fluid hypocretin measurement in the diagnosis of narcolepsy and other hypersomnias. *Archives of Neurology* 59(10):1553–1562.

Monahan KJ, Larkin EK, Rosen CL, Graham G, Redline S. 2002. Utility of noninvasive pharyngometry in epidemiologic studies of childhood sleep-disordered breathing. *American Journal of Respiratory and Critical Care Medicine* 165(11):1499–1503.

Mykytyn IJ, Sajkov D, Neill AM, McEvoy RD. 1999. Portable computerized polysomnography in attended and unattended settings. *Chest* 115(1):114–122.

Nieto FJ, Young TB, Lind BK, Shahar E, Samet JM, Redline S, D'Agostino RB, Newman AB, Lebowitz MD, Pickering TG. 2000. Association of sleep-disordered breathing, sleep apnea, and hypertension in a large community-based study. Sleep Heart Health Study. *Journal of the American Medical Association* 283(14):1829–1836.

Nofzinger EA. 2005. Functional neuroimaging of sleep. *Seminars in Neurology* 25(1):9–18.

Olivares VE. 1990. Scheduling strategies. *Radiology Management* 12(3):29–30.

Pack AI, Gurubhagavatula I. 1999. Economic implications of the diagnosis of obstructive sleep apnea. *Annals of Internal Medicine* 130(6):533–534.

Parrino L, Ferrillo F, Smerieri A, Spaggiari MC, Palomba V, Rossi M, Terzano MG. 2004. Is insomnia a neurophysiological disorder? The role of sleep EEG microstructure. *Brain Research Bulletin* 63(5):377–383.

Perlis ML, Smith MT, Andrews PJ, Orff H, Giles DE. 2001. Beta/Gamma EEG activity in patients with primary and secondary insomnia and good sleeper controls. *Sleep* 24(1):110–117.

Pittman SD, Ayas NT, MacDonald MM, Malhotra A, Fogel RB, White DP. 2004. Using a wrist-worn device based on peripheral arterial tonometry to diagnose obstructive sleep apnea: In-laboratory and ambulatory validation. *Sleep* 27(5):923–933.

Portier F, Portmann A, Czernichow P, Vascaut L, Devin E, Benhamou D, Cuvelier A, Muir JF. 2000. Evaluation of home versus laboratory polysomnography in the diagnosis of sleep apnea syndrome. *American Journal of Respiratory and Critical Care Medicine* 162(3 Pt 1):814–818.

Quan SF, Griswold ME, Iber C, Nieto FJ, Rapoport DM, Redline S, Sanders M, Young T. 2002. Short-term variability of respiration and sleep during unattended nonlaboratory polysomnography—the Sleep Heart Health Study. *Sleep* 25(8):843–849.

Redline S, Sanders M. 1999. A quagmire for clinicians: When technological advances exceed clinical knowledge. *Thorax* 54(6):474–475.

Redline S, Sanders MH, Lind BK, Quan SF, Iber C, Gottlieb DJ, Bonekat WH, Rapoport DM, Smith PL, Kiley JP. 1998. Methods for obtaining and analyzing unattended polysomnography data for a multicenter study. Sleep Heart Health Research Group. *Sleep* 21(7):759–767.

Rodsutti J, Hensley M, Thakkinstian A, D'Este C, Attia J. 2004. A clinical decision rule to prioritize polysomnography in patients with suspected sleep apnea. *Sleep* 27(4):694–699.

Ross SD, Sheinhait IA, Harrison KJ, Kvasz M, Connelly JE, Shea SA, Allen IE. 2000. Systematic review and meta-analysis of the literature regarding the diagnosis of sleep apnea. *Sleep* 23(4):519–532.

Roth T, Drake C. 2004. Evolution of insomnia: Current status and future direction. *Sleep Medicine* (suppl 1):S23–S30.

Ryan KL, Fedullo PF, Davis GB, Vasquez TE, Moser KM. 1988. Perfusion scan findings understate the severity of angiographic and hemodynamic compromise in chronic thromboembolic pulmonary hypertension. *Chest* 93(6):1180–1185.

Sforza E, Johannes M, Claudio B. 2005. The PAM-RL ambulatory device for detection of periodic leg movements: A validation study. *Sleep Medicine* 6(5):407–413.

Shahar E, Whitney CW, Redline S, Lee ET, Newman AB, Javier Nieto F, O'Connor GT, Boland LL, Schwartz JE, Samet JM. 2001. Sleep-disordered breathing and cardiovascular disease: Cross-sectional results of the Sleep Heart Health Study. *American Journal of Respiratory and Critical Care Medicine* 163(1):19–25.

Sharafkhaneh A, Richardson P, Hirshkowitz M. 2004. Sleep apnea in a high risk population: A study of Veterans Health Administration beneficiaries. *Sleep Medicine* 5(4):345–350.

Singh M, Drake C, Roehrs T, Koshorek G, Roth T. 2005. The prevalence of SOREMPs in the general population. *Sleep* 28(abstract suppl):A221.

Sulit L, Storfer-Isser A, Kirchner HL, Redline S. 2006. Differences in polysomnography predictors for hypertension and impaired glucose tolerance. *Sleep* 29(6):777–783.

Tachibana N, Ayas TA, White DP. 2005. A quantitative assessment of sleep laboratory activity in the United States. *Journal of Clinical Sleep Medicine* 1(1):23–26.

Tice JA. 2005. *Portable Devices for Home Testing for Obstructive Sleep Apnea.* San Francisco: California Technology Assessment Forum.

Trenkwalder C, Paulus W, Walters AS. 2005. The restless legs syndrome. *Lancet Neurology* 4(8):465–475.

Westbrook PR, Levendowski DJ, Cvetinovic M, Zavora T, Velimirovic V, Henninger D, Nicholson D. 2005. Description and validation of the apnea risk evaluation system: A novel method to diagnose sleep apnea-hypopnea in the home. *Chest* 128(4):2166–2175.

Whitney CW, Gottlieb DJ, Redline S, Norman RG, Dodge RR, Shahar E, Surovec S, Nieto FJ. 1998. Reliability of scoring respiratory disturbance indices and sleep staging. *Sleep* 21(7):749–757.

Zou D, Grote L, Peker Y, Lindblad U, Hedner J. 2006. Validation a portable monitoring device for sleep apnea diagnosis in a population based cohort using synchronized home polysomnography. *Sleep* 29(3):367–374.

7

Opportunities to Improve Career
Development in Somnology

CHAPTER SUMMARY   *The science and prevalence of sleep loss and sleep disorders necessitates a larger and more interdisciplinary workforce to advance the field's knowledge base and provide optimal clinical care. In 2004, there were only 253 principal investigators working on 319 sleep-related research projects (NIH R01). Of the 253 principal investigators, only 151 researchers are involved primarily in clinical sleep research, and 126 focus primarily on basic research projects. Further, only 54 doctorates were awarded with a focus on somnology or sleep medicine. This workforce is insufficient, given the burden of sleep loss and sleep disorders. The National Institutes of Health (NIH) and private foundations have not adequately invested in increasing the research workforce. Since 1997, there have been no new requests for application or program announcements for sleep-related fellowship, training or career development programs. Further, over the period encompassing 2000 to 2004 there was a decrease in the number of career development awards. Given all this, the field is ripe for expansion, but there are too few young and midcareer investigators. To improve the pipeline of individuals in the field, it is critical that the NIH commit to increasing the number of fellowship, training, and especially career development awards. Further, given the limited number of individuals clustered at a small number of institutes, the NIH should fully embrace flexible mentoring programs that are capable of meeting the challenges.*

The relative paucity of individuals trained and committed to careers in sleep and sleep disorders research has been recognized by the National Center on Sleep Disorders Research (NCSDR). It identified the need to train investigators as the highest priority among the 10 major sections of their 2003 research plan (NHLBI, 2003). Attracting, training, and supporting investigators in sleep-related research is critical for fueling the scientific efforts needed to make important discoveries into the etiology, pathogenesis, prevention, and treatment of chronic sleep loss and sleep disorders. Further, it is also important to train individuals whose major role will be master clinician, organizer and manager of care, and clinician-educator. In 2004, there were only 151 researchers who had a clinical sleep-related research project grant (R01) and only 126 investigators focused primarily on basic sleep-related research projects.[1] The small number of research project grants, 331 in 2004, can be substantially attributed to the limited number of individuals working in the field. It is, therefore, of critical importance that further investment be made to expand the number of well-trained investigators in the field.

Many of the strategies described in Chapter 5 to increase the awareness among health care professionals will also likely attract new investigators into the field. These strategies include targeting the career interests of high school and college students, as well as graduate students and students in allied health fields. Further, as will be described in detail in this chapter, increasing the number of investigators in the field will require the National Institutes of Health (NIH), professional societies, patient advocacy groups, and others to significantly increase their investment in career development programs. As a result of the current limited pool of senior investigators and concurrent clustering of senior people at a limited number of academic centers, it will be equally important to adopt flexible mentoring programs that are capable of meeting the challenges.

GROWTH OF THE SOMNOLOGY AND SLEEP MEDICINE FIELD

Somnology and sleep disorders research is a relatively young discipline that has grown significantly over the last 35 years. However, the current workforce is still not adequate, given the public health burden of the disorders (Chapters 3 and 4). Since the establishment of the first sleep center in 1970, clinical recognition of sleep disorders has grown but is still not widely

[1]Abstracts of all sleep-related R01s in the Computer Retrieval of Information on Scientific Projects (CRISP) database were analyzed under the following thesaurus terms: *insomnia, periodic limb movement disorder, restless legs syndrome, circadian rhythm, sudden infant death syndrome, sleep disorder, narcolepsy, sleep apnea, sleep, hibernation, and dream.* See Appendix A for further details.

acknowledged to be among the most common chronic health conditions (Chilcott and Shapiro, 1996; Young et al., 2002). Clinical advances have helped to attract and increase the number of clinicians and scientists to somnology and sleep medicine, as evidenced by the growth of membership in professional sleep societies. Since 1995, membership in the American Academy of Sleep Medicine (AASM) has more than doubled, while the Sleep Research Society (SRS) membership has almost tripled (Figure 7-1). However, the recent growth also emphasizes the need for a greater number of senior mentors and leaders in the field. The level of sleep-related research has grown, with over a 100 percent increase in the annual number of new NIH research project grants (R01) awarded in 1995 and 2004 (37 to 82). However, at the same time that the science and magnitude of the problem argues for greater investment, NIH funding of sleep-related activities has reached a plateau. Therefore, there are still substantial deficiencies in the workforce needed to address clinical somnopathy, and needs may be even greater relative to investment in research.

Growth in sleep-related research is limited by the paucity of funded investigators in the field. In 2004, only 253 investigators held active sleep-related NIH R01 grants. Although there has been an increase in the number of investigators since 1995, in comparison to other disorders, there are still too few sleep researchers. For instance, the absolute number of funded investigators with sleep-related projects is only around 80 percent of fields such as asthma,[2] which is a single disorder that affects 20 to 40 million. Further, funded investigators in sleep-related research tend to be older. The average age of all NIH investigators when awarded their first R01 has steadily risen and now is between 42 and 44 years of age (NIH, 2006b). However, in 2004, the average age of recipients at the time of their first R01 sleep-related grant was 51 (personal communication, M. Snyder, NIH Office of Scientific Affairs, November 8, 2005), which suggests an emergent need to replenish the pipeline with new investigators who can sustain the field and make it grow.

The limited number of researchers is clustered at a limited number of institutions. Of the 253 funded primary investigators in 2004, 33 percent of all investigators were at the top 10 academic sleep programs (ranking by the total number of somnology and/or sleep disorders grants), and 60 percent of all investigators were at the top 25 institutes (Appendix J). Likewise, 34 percent of all sleep-related R01 grants are awarded to the top 10 sleep

---

[2]314 individuals with asthma grants were identified by analyzing all 2004 R01 grants. Asthma grants were identified by all R01 grants that contained the word *asthma* as a thesaurus term. It is important to note that because only one search term was used, this search was not as thorough as the search performed for somnology and somnopathy R01 grants. Therefore, it may represent a significant under representation of the asthma field.

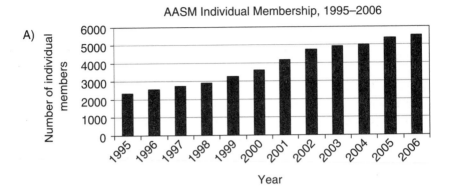

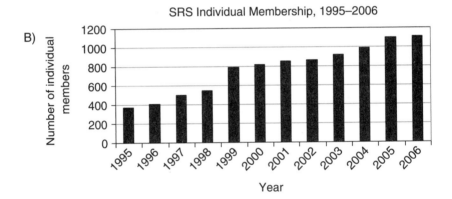

FIGURE 7-1 Individual membership in the AASM (A) and the SRS (B) has continued to grow over their history.
SOURCE: Personal communication, J. Barrett, AASM and SRS, (January, 2006).

academic programs, and 59 percent of all R01 grants are clustered in 25 institutions. In 2004, Harvard University, the University of Pennsylvania, and the University of Pittsburgh received 46 percent of sleep-related career development awards. Further, although many sleep disorders disproportionately affect minorities (Rosen et al., 2003), the number of minority investigators in the field is poorly representative (Spilsbury et al., 2004). In 2004, only 15 percent of all investigators with an R01 identified themselves as belonging to a minority ethnicity (Asian, African American, Hispanic, Pacific Islander, or other) (personal communication, M. Snyder, NIH Office of Scientific Affairs, November 8, 2005). As minority clinicians and investigators are more likely to work in underserved areas (Urbina et al., 1994), a dearth of minority investigators may limit clinical research that requires access to minority populations and ultimately limit the translation of research advances to these important populations.

Barriers to Sleep Research Career Development

Barriers to attracting, training, and sustaining a critical mass of sleep investigators include the poor awareness among the general public and health care professionals and the availability of appropriate mentors to provide scientific and career guidance to new investigators.

Exciting basic science research and the dissemination of this excitement to a broad group of potential trainees are necessary and potentially rate-limiting steps in attracting new investigators from a limited pool of individuals committed to academic careers. In 2005, there were 204 student members of the SRS; only 54 individuals received a doctorate in sleep-related research, as compared to 158 in pain and 630 in cancer.[3] Given the total number of principal investigators in the field, it appears that the majority of individuals with sleep-related doctorates do not remain in the field. Therefore, although there have been some remarkable successes in scientific investigation aimed at elucidating fundamental sleep physiology and biology (e.g., discovery of a mammalian *Clock* gene (Antoch et al., 1997; King et al., 1997; Tei et al., 1997) and the cause of narcolepsy (Lin et al., 1999; Chemelli et al., 1999; Mignot et al., 1999; Thannickal et al., 2000; Peyron et al., 2000), the future pace of scientific discovery is limited by the small numbers of active researchers pursuing basic investigation. Fundamental scientific discoveries play critical roles in galvanizing interest in any scientific discipline. Recruiting and retaining trainees in somnology and sleep medicine competes with other more established fields, many of which have made highly publicized advances, enjoy widespread respect across medical centers, and are more established as an academic discipline.

Investigators, particularly new ones who commit to interdisciplinary sleep-related research, are challenged to prove their value in academic medical centers that are accustomed to recognizing and rewarding individuals with "departmentally" defined research foci. Resource allocation needed to support new investigators may require complex negotiations among academic departments, which may deter new investigators or otherwise limit their access to needed support. In addition, identification of optimal mentoring relationships, critical for career development, will likely require sustained relationships among individuals with competing institutional commitments.

---

[3]Data were collected through a keyword search, using either *sleep, pain,* or *cancer,* of the Dissertation Abstracts database through DIALOG.

As for all scientific fields, new investigators require protected time and support as they transition to independent funding. Increasing fiscal pressures and, for physicians, demands to spend more time on clinical services, are threats to protected time critical for career development. New investigators are also often burdened with substantial debt from school loans, providing disincentives to participate in prolonged postdoctorate training.

NIH TRAINING AND CAREER DEVELOPMENT PROGRAMS

A variety of NIH-funded career development and academic training awards have been sponsored over the past decade (see Appendix H). In particular, there has been growth in the recognition and investment by the NIH in a broad variety of individual and institution-based career training programs, with a recent emphasis on clinical, translational, and interdisciplinary research training. Programs have been developed with the aims of attracting new trainees and developing the research and academic skills, and supporting their transition to independent and externally funded investigators (K01, K02, K08, K23, and K25). Other awards support midcareer development and mentorship skills (K24, K26). National Research Service Award Institutional Training Grants (T32) provide institutions with funds to support the training of individual postdoctoral candidates. The K30 and K12 series of NIH institutional training awards provide institutional support to develop new or expanded training programs and curriculum development.

NIH Support of Sleep-Related Training Activities

To determine the current investment in the field and how the grant portfolio has changed over the last 10 years, this committee performed a detailed review and analysis of the portfolio of NIH sleep-related awards in career training (K), fellowship (F), and training (T). Abstracts of all K, F, and T awards in the Computer Retrieval of Information on Scientific Projects (CRISP) database were analyzed. This database collects information on the number of federally funded biomedical research projects. Data from the CRISP database were used to assess the number of awards that were classified under the following thesaurus terms: *insomnia, periodic limb movement disorder, restless legs syndrome, circadian rhythm, sudden infant death syndrome, sleep disorder, narcolepsy, sleep apnea, sleep, hibernation,* and *dream.* To limit the number of grants that were not relevant to somnology or sleep disorders, the committee included only grants in which the key words appeared in both the thesaurus terms and the abstract and not the abstract alone. Temporal trends and distributions of awards across NIH institutes and to academic institutions were examined (see Appendixes H and J for compiled findings). The committee did not have access to the applications that were submitted and not funded; therefore, it is not pos-sible to conclusively determine if changes in investment are the result of NIH policy, the number and/or quality of submissions in each area, compo-sition of grant review committees, or combination of these factors.

Temporal Analysis of Sleep Training Awards

Although there is a statistically significant increase in the total num-ber of K awards from 1996 to 1998 (Appendix H), there was a relative leveling of total awards from 1998 to 2004—despite the establishment by the NIH of three new career development programs and significant in-creases in extramural funding. Further, since 1997, the NIH has not in-vested in a single sleep-related request for application (RFA) or program announcement (PA) career development program (Appendix F). Analysis of the number of sleep-related T and F awards shows an increase between 2000 and 2004 (Figure 7-2). However, the number of K awards decreased over the same time period and a larger proportion went to a smaller group of academic institutions. Three institutions, Harvard University, Univer-sity of Pennsylvania, and University of Pittsburgh, accounted for 27 per-cent of all sleep-related T, K, and F grants received in 2000, 35 percent in 2004. This concentration is even greater if only K award distribution is analyzed. The same three institutions received 29 percent of all K awards in 2000, and 46 percent in 2004. This may reflect the extensive develop-ment of these programs and concentration of senior investigators.

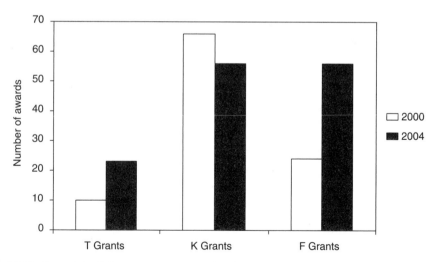

FIGURE 7-2 Total sleep training, career development, and fellowship grants in 2000 and 2004.

Support of training grants may also diminish. The NIH reported that in response to rising tuitions and steady budgets that if the current formula used to determine the number of awards is not altered there would be an overall loss of 4,000 training grant slots by 2015 (Bhattacharjee, 2005a).

Institute-Specific Funding of Career Development Awards

Career development awards in sleep are sponsored by numerous NIH institutes (see Appendix H). In general, for any given award category, with few exceptions no more than one new career development award was granted in any given year between 2000 and 2004. Since 2000, investment in career development awards for clinical scientists, K08 and K23, has varied. The National Institute of Mental Health (NIMH) and the National Heart, Lung, and Blood Institute (NHLBI) awarded the greatest number of grants. In 2003 and 2004 there was only one new K08 award. Although there has been greater investment in the K23 series, it is still minimal with five new awards in 2003 by four different institutes. K24 awards for mid-career development have also been minimal in 2003 and 2004, with no new awards in 2003 and only three in 2004—two of which were by the NHLBI.

There has also been very limited investment in the K07 academic career awards, designed to improve curricula and emphasize development of scientist leadership skills. Apart from the Sleep Academic Award program, there has been very little investment through the K07 mechanism, no new awards were granted in 2003, and only three in 2004. Further, no institute apart from the NHLBI has supported this mechanism for sleep-related awards.

Over the 5-year period between 2000 and 2004, there has been even less investment in career development awards for mentored research (K01), independent scientists (K02), and senior scientists (K05). All three of these mechanisms historically have been used to support basic research. NIMH was the first institute that supported these three mechanisms for sleep-related activities, but in recent years there has been a marked decrease. For example, in 2002, the NIMH supported six sleep-related K01 awards, seven K02 awards, and two K05 awards. In 2004, these numbers have decreased to two K01 awards, two K02 awards, and one K05 award. These latter statistics underscore the relatively small amount of investment of any given institute in sleep research training, with no evidence that any institute or the Trans-NIH Sleep Research Coordinating Committee has assumed leadership in this area. Although the decrease in career development awards is dramatic, it is important to note that over the same period, there has been an increase in fellowship awards (Appendix I).

Of the 314 career development awards that were funded during the five years between 2000 and 2004, NHLBI sponsored 94 (29 percent), and the NIMH sponsored 162 (52 percent). One third (32 of the 94) of sleep-related

NHLBI-sponsored training grants were K07 awards devoted to the Sleep Academic Award program, which were designed to support the development of curricula and educational leadership, not research training. The vast majority of the Trans-NIH Sleep Research Coordinating Committee member institutes—many of whom have a large portion of the sleep-related research project grant portfolio (Appendix G)—have minimally supported career development. The underlying reasons may be multiple, including poor or low numbers of applications, insufficient sleep-related research expertise on study sections (which is also partially affected by a limited number of senior members of the field), and lack of awareness of the extent of the problem. Further, K awards are expensive; consequently, institutes are often reluctant to invest heavily in the K awards, especially in periods of budget constraints.

One potential strategy to offset the lack of investment would be to leverage the combined resources from multiple member institutes of the Trans-NIH Sleep Research Coordinating Committee to develop a larger pool of money for training programs. In 2003, the NIH supported 845 K23 career development awards at a total cost of over $114 million, or an average annual cost of $135,000 per award. If four institutes were to cosponsor a K23 program in somnology or sleep medicine, this would cost each institute approximately $34,000 annually per award, a 75 percent decrease in expense. The committee strongly recommends joint investment in training programs; it does so recognizing that there are potentially increased overhead costs associated with tracking and implementing an annual transfer of funds between institutes. Further, mechanisms need to be developed to enable all institutes contributing to a joint effort to be acknowledged in congressional goals for new grants.

NIH Roadmap Initiatives

As part of the NIH director's research agenda, a series of roadmap initiatives was identified to foster the development of interdisciplinary training for investigators at all levels of their careers. These initiatives emphasize translational research, behavioral/social sciences, and quantitative sciences. Between 2004 and 2005, $8 million was invested in the establishment of seven K12 Multidisciplinary Clinical Research Training Programs (NIH, 2006a). Because sleep-related research is particularly well suited to interdisciplinary and translational strategies, it could serve as one of several key programs for these new initiatives

New NIH Career Award Support

Recognizing the difficulty of becoming an independent researcher and in response to the Institute of Medicine's and National Academies' report,

Facilitating Interdisciplinary Research, on fostering independence among young biomedical researchers, the NIH recently announced the creation of three new initiatives (Bhattacharjee, 2005b). Each initiative is designed to facilitate postdoctoral fellows into independent faculty positions. The first—the NIH Pathway to Independence Award program—is a 5-year award composed of two phases (NIH, 2006b). The initial phase (K99) is a 1- to 2-year mentored period designed to allow investigators to complete their supervised research work, publish results, and search for an independent faculty position. The second, independent phase (R00) would comprise the remaining 3 years of the award and is structured to provide financial support to awardees who secure an assistant professorship while they establish their own research program and successfully apply for an NIH investigator-initiated (R01) grant. The second mechanism is an independent research grant program, which does not require preliminary data. The final initiative is to speed up the R01 grant application turnaround time for new researchers who fail to receive an award on their first attempt.

Summary of NIH Support of Career Development Programs

In summary, analysis shows that no single NIH institute has made substantive investments into sleep-related research career development or training awards. There are alarming downward temporal trends in level of support for research training and career development, suggested by the recent drop in funded K awards, with further clustering of funding to fewer institutions. Institutes that support large levels of sleep research funding should also be encouraged to make a significant investment in career development initiatives. Funding trends also suggest that there are very few individuals with training support to develop careers in basic sleep science. There are many existing training grants or large research programs in disciplines related to somnology or sleep medicine (e.g., internal medicine, neurology, psychiatry, psychology, otolaryngology, nursing, epidemiology, neuroscience, and health services research). Given the interdisciplinary nature of the field, these programs provide an additional mechanism for increasing the number of somnology and sleep medicine trainees. Although there is an exciting national movement toward supporting interdisciplinary and translational research highlighted in roadmap initiatives, existing programs largely have not recognized the potential of the somnology and sleep medicine field as a prototype for these initiatives. This represents a great opportunity to both foster development of sleep research and to forge new interdisciplinary approaches.

Professional Organization and Foundation Support
of Career Development

Professional societies have played important roles in sponsoring career development across a wide variety of disciplines. Well-established career training awards are available from professional organizations with interest in somnology and sleep disorders, such as the American Heart Association, American Diabetes Association, American College of Chest Physicians, American Lung Association, and the American Thoracic Society, among others. Table 7-1 shows the number of career development awards several organizations made in 2004. Since sleep-related research is relevant to several of these organizations, the number of sleep-related training grants is also provided. It is worth noting that investment in sleep-related research is low for all professional organizations profiled below; for example, despite the significant association of sleep disorders and cardiovascular disease, only 2 of the 845 awards given by the American Heart Association's career training program portfolio supported sleep-related research. One impediment leading to the limited support from these organizations is that they might not recognize the important role they have in fostering interdisciplinary research, as they are focused on more traditional organ-based research.

There are two primarily sleep-focused organizations that have training awards: the National Sleep Foundation (NSF)'s Pickwick Club Award, and the American Sleep Medicine Foundation (ASMF)'s Faculty Career Advancement Award.

The ASMF, affiliated with the American Academy of Sleep Medicine, annually sponsors between four and six fellowship awards, each as much as 2 years in duration and for a maximum annual funding level of $60,000. From 2003 to 2005 the program received on average 18 applications (personal communication, R. Money, AASM, November 9, 2005). In 2005, the

TABLE 7-1 Career Training Awards by Professional
Organizations with Secondary Interests in Sleep (2004)

	Total Awards	Sleep Awards
American Heart Association	845	2
American Diabetes Association	9	0
American College of Chest Physicians	11	1
American Lung Association	115	2
American Thoracic Society	6	0

NOTE: The information contained in this table was obtained from personal communication with appropriate staff members at each organization.

ASMF also developed the AASM/Pfizer Scholars Grant Program in Sleep Medicine to provide support for career development of junior faculty in somnology and sleep medicine.

The Pickwick Club Fellowship of the NSF, an independent public health advocacy organization, awards two to four fellowships of 1 to 2 years in duration for postdoctorate trainees in sleep-related research. Support is primarily for annual salary support ($35,568 to $45,048). In 2004, investment in research training by the NSF is estimated at approximately $180,000.

Foundations, such as the Francis Family Foundation, have made notable contributions to training pulmonary scientists through the Parker B. Francis Fellowship Program. Over the last 30 years, this foundation has contributed nearly $40 million in support of more than 600 fellows, some of whom have worked in the somnology and sleep medicine field. Each award is for 3 years, and provides stipends, fringe benefits, and travel expenses to postdoctoral fellows or newly appointed assistant professors to enable their research development related to pulmonary disease and lung biology. A survey of former fellows demonstrated that greater than 90 percent of respondents are currently employed in academic settings and spend a significant portion of their time on research.

Summary of Foundation Support of Career Development Programs

Given the overall paucity of support, further investment is required by private foundations for career development. Foundations, such as the Parker B. Francis Foundation and the Cystic Fibrosis Foundation (Box 7-1) are excellent models of sustained foundation support for research career development. Although professional organizations cannot directly support research fellowships, through associated foundations they have made moderate to large investments in research career development, including funding for some trainees with a primary somnology and somnopathy focus. Funds for these programs have been derived from endowments and well-organized, targeted fund-raising efforts. This analysis identifies the potential availability of funding for sleep training from multi- and interdisciplinary initiatives available through professional organizations with secondary interests related to sleep loss and/or sleep disorders, in addition to the need for organizations with primary sleep-related agendas to invest more heavily in developing the next generations of investigators. Similar to the committee's call for multiple institutes of the Trans-NIH Sleep Research Coordinating Committee to combine resources to support career development programs, private foundations should also explore mechanisms to coordinate their efforts. This will ensure that the maximal effect from these efforts is realized.

BOX 7-1
Model Investment by a Foundation into
Career Development: The Cystic Fibrosis Foundation

An example of a scientific community that has rallied to support the career development of research trainees is in cystic fibrosis. Despite the relative rarity of this condition in the population (30,000 children and adults), and the relatively small pool of researchers available to recruit from, foundation support has succeeded in developing a cadre of productive researchers, who largely have a strong history of sustained academic contributions. Three key programs have been developed through the Cystic Fibrosis Foundation: the Clinical Fellowship Program, the LeRoy Mathews Program, and the Harry Shwachman Fellowship. Together, these programs provide support for the full spectrum of trainees: combined clinical/research fellowship training, early research career development (enrolling fellows within the first 4 years of training), and junior faculty development. Support for these programs is derived from well-organized fund-raising and philanthropy. The combined support for these training programs represents approximately 2 percent of the annual Cystic Fibrosis Foundation budget.

The Clinical Fellowship Programs expose fellows early in their training to working in a multidisciplinary team environment. Annually, approximately 23 fellows are supported, at a total cost of $1.2 million. It supports first and second years for the clinic, and during the third and fourth year supports time for basic, translational, or clinical research. Fellows receive an annual base salary of $52,000 with an additional $10,000 for research supplies. Most junior and many senior faculty members who staff the 115 accredited Cystic Fibrosis Foundation centers have derived some support through this program.

The LeRoy Mathews program is a smaller program, with an annual cost of approximately $345,000. It targets the development of fellows and their transition to a junior faculty role. Each awardee is supported for 6 years. Two fellows are supported at any given time. Fellows may be accepted into the program up to their fourth year of specialty training.

The Harry Shwachman fellowships are 3-year programs that target junior faculty with the goal of supporting their development as independent investigators. These awards are considered to be equivalent to NIH K08 awards in the scope of support for protected time and in the requirement for mentored research.

The Cystic Fibrosis Foundation also utilizes these programs to create a "community" of scholars through sponsorship of fellows to attend special sessions at national meetings.

The Role of Mentoring and Availability of Sleep Mentors

Numerous studies have documented the pivotal role of mentoring in career development (Chilcott and Shapiro, 1996; Palepu et al., 1998; Young et al., 2002; Lieff et al., 2003). The Council of Graduate Schools promoted the concept that: "Mentors are advisors, people with career experience willing to share their knowledge; supporters, people who give emotional and moral encouragement; tutors, people who give specific feedback on one's performance; masters, in the sense of employers to whom one is apprenticed; sponsors, sources of information about and aid in obtaining opportunities; models of the kind of person one should be to be an academic" (Zelditch, 1995). The cornerstone of most training programs, including NIH and foundation-funded programs, is evidence of a strong mentor-mentee relationship. Multiple mentors are required for multidisciplinary research training. Many advocate for formal oversight committees for trainees and junior faculty. Successful peer-reviewed training awards include clearly articulated roles for mentors as the responsible agents for overseeing the entire scope of the trainee's career development program.

The availability of appropriate mentors to provide scientific and career guidance to new investigators (as well as to serve as a catalyst to attract such individuals to the field) is limited, with some variation across institutions. There is currently a concentration of investigators and grants at a limited number of academic institutions. Even highly established sleep academic centers have a paucity of senior mentors. This often requires senior mentors to be responsible for several mentees, potentially reducing the effectiveness of the mentorship relationship. The availability of mentors is also limited by the fiscal constraints of academic medical systems and structures, which normally do not always recognize the contribution of mentoring to the institute's mission. Increasing fiscal pressures at academic centers require faculty to be increasingly accountable for justifying their effort in relationship to compensation. Mentoring is, in general, not a compensated activity. Thus, there are growing disincentives for potential mentors to assume new mentorship relationships.

The limited availability of appropriate mentors has far-reaching consequences to the growth of the field. Trainees may make decisions to enter certain fields because of the reputation of accessible mentors. Securing protected time and research support from external sources requires commitment by at least one strong mentor. Young investigators benefit enormously by relationships with a mentor who can help negotiate complex academic settings, prioritize goals and work, critically examine research methods and data interpretation, refine presentation and scientific and grant-writing skills, and develop high levels of professionalism.

OPPORTUNITIES TO ACCELERATE SOMNOLOGY AND SLEEP MEDICINE CAREER DEVELOPMENT

Each challenge also presents opportunities to develop novel strategies for career development, to enhance the recognition of somnology and sleep disorders research as an interdisciplinary field and more effectively interface with other related disciplines, and to build upon existing NIH and private foundation initiatives. In addition to strategies described in Chapter 5, additional strategies include the following:

• Training in somnology and sleep medicine can be structured to complement those of other programs and vice versa, by interactively engaging trainees in other programs. The interdisciplinary organization of the field creates a foundation for trainees from multiple fields to participate and apply their methods or expand their initial foci to questions relevant to somnology and somnopathy. The NIH can foster this by adopting trans-institutional training programs.

• The NIH Roadmap explicitly emphasizes the importance of interdisciplinary research, especially aimed at achieving translational research objectives. As academic institutions vie for support from NIH Roadmap programs, incorporation of somnology and sleep disorders research as a translational research focus may provide a competitive edge.

• The innovation of the new NIH K12 training programs—which provide support to an educational institution for career development experiences for clinicians leading to research independence—and their sensitivity to respond to the scientific needs of the community make these programs desirable avenues for providing support for both mentors and mentees interested in somnology and sleep disorders. Modern communication technologies make long-distance mentoring feasible and effective.

• Recent loan repayment policies have been initiated at the NIH, which may substantially reduce the burden of loan repayment in return for evidence of scientific activity and further investment in academic training. Targeting sleep-related research trainees and junior faculty for NIH loan repayment is suggested as a potentially important recruitment tool. Availability of NIH and foundation training programs are a crucial source of support to ensure protected time and resource investment in new investigators.

• The growing strength of several private organizations (e.g., foundations, professional societies, industry) committed to promoting sleep health and somnology and sleep disorders professionals is a largely untapped resource for support for trainees.

Potential Mechanisms to Improve Training

A particular challenge for development of investigators in sleep research is that currently few institutions have the critical mass of established investigators in this area to provide mentorship and training. This suggests that mechanisms need to be sought to leverage the intellectual resources at these few institutions.

Remote Mentoring Programs

Successful career development awards require the identification of a strong mentor. However, if such mentors may only be located at the candidate's home institution, there would be little growth of somnology and/or sleep disorders research expertise in institutions other than the few large academic programs. Further, educating grant reviewers of career development applications allows more flexibility in the range of mentorship relationships—a flexibility needed to allow the field to grow.

There are several NIH mechanisms to support midcareer development and mentorship skills (K24, K25). In 2004, however, only three individuals were awarded a new K24 grant in somnology and/or sleep medicine (no new grants were awarded in 2003), and there were no new K25 awards in somnology and/or sleep medicine for the same year. The new K12 Translational Research Institutional Training program also provides salary support for mentees. However, no K12 scholars identified a sleep-related focus in their research application. These data indicate the need for greater NIH investment in developing and supporting the effort of mid- to senior-level investigators as mentors and to provide support for mentoring time.

Specialized NIH programs have also been developed to facilitate the creation of national networks of mentors and mentees. However, due to budgetary constraints, some NIH institutes are no longer funding undergraduate programs. Two programs were very successful in developing mentoring skills of mentors, creating new mentor-mentee relationships, and exposing trainees to intensive research experiences—Brown University's Summer Sleep and Chronobiology Research Apprenticeship (see Chapter 5) and the Summer Research Institute in Geriatric Psychiatry (Box 7-2) (Halpain et al., 2001).

Another approach to efficiently "matching" mentors and mentees across institutions is through networks supported by professional societies. The American Thoracic Society established a mentoring program in 1999 and serves as a clearinghouse for mentors and mentees with complementary issues (and sometimes concordant gender). The American Thoracic Society provided venues for matched mentors and mentees to meet with the goal of facilitating the mentoring relationship.

**BOX 7-2
Summer Research Institute:
A Model Program for Mentor-Mentee Networks**

The Summer Research Institute is a 10-year-old program that has created a national network of mentors in a relatively small field (geriatric psychiatry). The Summer Research Institute provides a useful model for attracting new investigators to a defined field and for bridging and shortening the transition period from fellowship to first research funding. The program offers a 1-week "boot camp" in research career survival skills for postdoctorates and junior faculty. At the end of each program, a workshop facilitates interactions and sharing of research among all trainees. The program's success is evidenced by the career trajectories of trainees. Of the approximately 300 program alumni (postdocs, junior faculty), 80 percent now hold full-time academic positions, and 50 percent or so have competed successfully for extramural research from the NIH and foundations.

In 2005, the SRS and the AASM also initiated a long-distance mentor-mentee program. This program is still under development; too few data are available to evaluate its effectiveness or level of participation.

In summary, the pivotal role of mentorship in attracting trainees to sleep medicine and facilitating their academic success is clear. Given the relatively small numbers of available mentors, additional efforts are needed to encourage NIH, professional societies, and foundations to provide support for developing mentors. In addition, creative use of national networks of mentors and mentees needs to be encouraged. Funding agencies need to recognize the role of long-distance mentorship plans, if those plans adequately address important issues in successful mentor-mentee relationships.

Given all this, the field is ripe for expansion, but there are too few young and midcareer investigators.

*Integration of Somnology and Sleep Medicine with
Other Training Programs*

Another strategy to be considered is providing additional training positions to already established training grants in relevant disciplines, such as neuroscience and clinical epidemiology. This, when combined with the remote mentorship model, would have considerable benefit. It would not only provide a new mechanism to provide training to trainees, but also the mentor with expertise in the primary discipline, such as neuroscience or clinical epidemiology, at the host institution might also become interested in sleep research.

The development of midcareer mentoring awards for 1 to 2 years would allow midcareer investigators in institutions with little sleep expertise but relevant skills (e.g., neuroscience or clinical epidemiology) to get retrained in sleep research. They would do so in collaboration with one of the comprehensive sleep centers described elsewhere in this report. Such mentoring could be a combination of time spent at the comprehensive sleep center and remote mentorship while at their own institution. The home institution would need to indicate its commitment to developing a sleep research program for this to be a viable, productive strategy.

Somnology—the branch of science devoted to the study of sleep and wakefulness—requires a larger interdisciplinary research workforce. This can be accomplished by both attracting individuals from other related fields and by establishing a new cohort of researchers who work specifically on sleep-related topics. As presented in this chapter, the current status of the sleep research field requires new mechanisms to be considered to seed institutions that currently lack the intellectual resources.

Recommendation 7.1: The National Institutes of Health and private foundations should increase investment in interdisciplinary somnology and sleep medicine research training and mentoring activities.

The National Institutes of Health, foundations, and professional societies should utilize and develop further funding mechanisms to attract young investigators into the field of somnology and sleep medicine. As a reflection of the interdisciplinary nature of somnology and sleep medicine, members of the Trans-NIH Sleep Research Coordinating Committee should be encouraged to combine resources to sponsor grants for disciplinary and cross-disciplinary training and mentoring activities (T, F, and K funding mechanisms) of medical students, graduate students, postdoctoral fellows, clinical fellows, and junior faculty.

To implement this recommendation the following should be considered:
- The Trans-NIH Sleep Research Coordinating Committee should establish a somnology and sleep medicine career development program. This program should support trainees for a significant number of years, spanning research training in fellowship and research career development as a faculty member. It should also

facilitate mid-career training opportunities (e.g., K21, K24), the Academic Career Award for Education and Curriculum Development program (K07), and research education grants (R25).
- Existing training grants or large research programs in disciplines related to somnology or sleep medicine (e.g., internal medicine, neurology, psychiatry, psychology, otolaryngology, nursing, epidemiology, neuroscience, health services research) should allow for the addition of a sleep medicine trainee. Where pertinent expertise is not available on-site, remote mentoring at other institutions should be encouraged.

REFERENCES

Antoch MP, Song EJ, Chang AM, Vitaterna MH, Zhao Y, Wilsbacher LD, Sangoram AM, King DP, Pinto LH, Takahashi JS. 1997. Functional identification of the mouse circadian *Clock* gene by transgenic BAC rescue. *Cell* 89(4):655–667.

Bhattacharjee Y. 2005a. NIH career awards. Universities may have to pay more in support of graduate training. *Science* 310(5754):1601.

Bhattacharjee Y. 2005b. NIH career awards. Young scientists get a helping hand. *Science* 310(5754):1601.

Chemelli RM, Willie JT, Sinton CM, Elmquist JK, Scammell T, Lee C, Richardson JA, Williams SC, Xiong Y, Kisanuki Y, Fitch TE, Nakazato M, Hammer RE, Saper CB, Yanagisawa M. 1999. Narcolepsy in orexin knockout mice: Molecular genetics of sleep regulation. *Cell* 98(4):437–451.

Chilcott LA, Shapiro CM. 1996. The socioeconomic impact of insomnia. An overview. *Pharmacoeconomics* 10(suppl 1):1–14.

Halpain MC, Jeste DV, Katz IR, Reynolds CF. 2001. Summer Research Institute: Enhancing research career development in geriatric psychiatry. *Academy of Psychiatry* 25:48–56.

King DP, Zhao Y, Sangoram AM, Wilsbacher LD, Tanaka M, Antoch MP, Steeves TD, Vitaterna MH, Kornhauser JM, Lowrey PL, Turek FW, Takahashi JS. 1997. Positional cloning of the mouse circadian *Clock* gene. *Cell* 89(4):641–653.

Lieff SJ, Tolomiczenko GS, Dunn LB. 2003. Effect of training and other influences on the development of career interest in geriatric psychiatry. *American Journal of Geriatric Psychiatry* 11(3):300–308.

Lin L, Faraco J, Li R, Kadotani H, Rogers W, Lin X, Qiu X, de Jong PJ, Nishino S, Mignot E. 1999. The sleep disorder canine narcolepsy is caused by a mutation in the hypocretin (orexin) receptor 2 gene. *Cell* 98(3):365–376.

Mignot E, Young T, Lin L, Finn L. 1999. Nocturnal sleep and daytime sleepiness in normal subjects with HLA-DQB1*0602. *Sleep* 22(3):347–352.

NHLBI (National Heart, Lung, and Blood Institute). 2003. *National Sleep Disorders Research Plan, 2003.* Bethesda, MD: National Institutes of Health.

NIH (National Institutes of Health). 2006a. *Roadmap Initiative to Provide Training for Future Leaders of Clinical Research.* [Online]. Available: http://nihroadmap.nih.gov/clinicalresearch/clinicaltraining/futureleaders.asp [accessed January 25, 2006].

NIH. 2006b. *Resources for New Investigators.* [Online]. Available: http://grants2.nih.gov/grants/new_investigators/ [accessed January 25, 2006].

Palepu A, Friedman RH, Barnett RC, Carr PL, Ash AS, Szalacha L, Moskowitz MA. 1998. Junior faculty members' mentoring relationships and their professional development in U.S. medical schools. *Academy of Medicine* 73(3):318–323.

Peyron C, Faraco J, Rogers W, Ripley B, Overeem S. 2000. A mutation in a case of early onset narcolepsy and a generalized absence of hypocretin peptides in human narcoleptic brains. *Nature Medicine* 6(9):991–997.

Rosen CL, Larkin EK, Kirchner HL, Emancipator JL, Bivins SF, Surovec SA, Martin RJ, Redline S. 2003. Prevalence and risk factors for sleep-disordered breathing in 8- to 11-year-old children: Association with race and prematurity. *Journal of Pediatrics* 142(4): 383–389.

Spilsbury JC, Storfer-Isser A, Drotar D, Rosen CL, Kirchner LH, Benham H, Redline S. 2004. Sleep behavior in an urban U.S. sample of school-aged children. *Archives of Pediatrics and Adolescent Medicine* 158(10):988–994.

Tei H, Okamura H, Shigeyoshi Y, Fukuhara C, Ozawa R, Hirose M, Sakaki Y. 1997. Circadian oscillation of a mammalian homologue of the Drosophila period gene. *Nature* 389(6650):512–516.

Thannickal TC, Moore RY, Nienhuis R, Ramanathan L, Gulyani S, Aldrich M, Cornford M, Siegel JM. 2000. Reduced number of hypocretin neurons in human narcolepsy. *Neuron* 27(3):469–474.

Urbina C, Hickey M, McHarney-Brown C, Duban S, Kaufman A. 1994. Innovative generalist programs: Academic health care centers respond to the shortage of generalist physicians. *Journal of General Internal Medicine* 9(4 suppl 1):S81–S89.

Young T, Peppard PE, Gottlieb DJ. 2002. Epidemiology of obstructive sleep apnea: A population health perspective. *American Journal of Respiratory and Critical Care Medicine* 165(9):1217–1239.

Zelditch M. 1995. *A Conversation About Mentoring: Trends and Models*. Washington, DC: Council of Graduate Medical Schools.

8

Bolstering Somnology and Sleep Disorders Research Programs

CHAPTER SUMMARY *The National Center on Sleep Disorders Research (NCSDR) and the Trans-NIH Sleep Research Coordinating Committee were established to coordinate the sleep-related research, training, and education activities at the National Institutes of Health (NIH). At the same time that the science and magnitude of the public health and economic burden requires greater investment, the output from the NCSDR and Trans-NIH Sleep Research Coordinating Committee has not kept pace. As a consequence, NIH funding for sleep-related activities has reached a plateau, and the future outlook for somnology and sleep medicine is unclear. A detailed examination of the past and current investment in sleep-related research demonstrates that there are only 331 funded research projects and 253 independent investigators, far below the requirements of the field. Further, of the 253 principal investigators only 151 researchers are primarily involved in clinical sleep research and 126 primarily focus on basic research projects. The challenge for the field is to develop a collaborative and focused approach with a strong research infrastructure. To bolster clinical and basic research efforts, catalyze collaborative research efforts, and attract the breadth of talented researchers who will be able to move somnology and sleep disorders research and clinical care forward to achieve optimal outcomes requires a coordinated and integrated strategy. The NCSDR, its advisory board, and the Trans-NIH Sleep Research Coordinating Committee need to take a proactive role in providing continued leadership. Further, a research network is of particular importance in the*

254

SLEEP DISORDERS AND SLEEP DEPRIVATION

field because of the need for a coordinated interdisciplinary research approach to basic and clinical research, clinical care, public education, and training. Therefore, the NIH should establish Somnology and Sleep Medicine Centers of Excellence within a National Somnology and Sleep Medicine Research and Clinical Network.

The field of somnology and sleep medicine is poised to take great strides in elucidating and addressing the etiology, pathogenesis, and public health burden of chronic sleep loss and sleep disorders. This strong position is the result of the National Institutes of Health (NIH) establishing the Trans-NIH Sleep Research Coordinating Committee and the National Center on Sleep Disorders Research (NCSDR). However, at the same time that the science and magnitude of the problem requires greater investment, NIH funding to sleep-related activities has reached a plateau. Consequently, the future outlook for somnology and sleep medicine is unclear. The next significant advances necessitate leveraging these resources to their utmost potential in conducting research and refining diagnosis and treatment interventions for sleep loss and sleep disorders.

This chapter provides an overview of the current coordination of sleep-related activities at the NIH, including an evaluation of the NCSDR. Included in the evaluation is a detailed a summary of sleep-related research activities sponsored by the NIH between 1995 and 2004. The chapter culminates with a discussion on the next steps required to accelerate progress, including the establishment of a National Somnology and Sleep Medicine Research and Clinical Network.

NIH COORDINATION OF SLEEP-RELATED ACTIVITIES

To a greater extent than many medical and research disciplines, the field of somnology and sleep medicine cuts across many disciplines, including but not limited to cardiology, dentistry, endocrinology, epidemiology, geriatrics, molecular biology, neurology, neurosciences, nursing, nutrition, otolaryngology, pediatrics, pharmacology, psychiatry, and pulmonology. In 2004, there were 331 sleep-related research project grants sponsored by 17 institutes at the NIH (Table 8-1, Appendix G). The NIH has two mechanisms to coordinate its sleep-related activities, the Trans-NIH Sleep Research Coordinating Committee and the NCSDR.

TABLE 8-1 NIH Institute Support of Somnology and Sleep Disorders Research Project Grants (R01) in 2004

Institute	Number of Grants
National Heart, Lung, and Blood Institute	102
National Institute of Mental Health	88
National Institute of Neurological Disorders and Stroke	49
National Institute on Aging	31
National Institute of General Medical Sciences	22
National Institute of Nursing Research	19
National Eye Institute	15
National Institute on Drug Abuse	13
National Institute on Alcohol Abuse and Alcoholism	12
National Institute of Diabetes and Digestive and Kidney Diseases	11
National Institute of Child Health and Human Development	10
National Cancer Institute	7
National Institute of Arthritis and Musculoskeletal and Skin Diseases	5
National Institute on Deafness and Other Communication Disorders	4
National Center for Complementary and Alternative Medicine	3
National Institute of Allergy and Infectious Diseases	1
Fogarty International Center	1

NOTE: Institutes and centers in bold are not members of the Trans-NIH Sleep Research Coordinating Committee.

Trans-NIH Sleep Research Coordinating Committee

In 1986, the Director of the NIH established the Trans-NIH Sleep Research Coordinating Committee to facilitate an interchange of information about somnology and sleep disorders research. This coordinating committee meets every 2 to 3 months to discuss current sleep-related activities within the NIH and develop new programs. Currently 13 NIH institutes and offices are members of the Trans-NIH Sleep Research Coordinating Committee. The director of the NCSDR chairs the Coordinating Committee, and its members are program staff from the various NIH institutes with an interest in somnology and sleep disorders. Although most institutes that support sleep-related research are members of the coordinating committee, a few are not (Table 8-1), including the National Institute of General Medical Sciences and the National Eye Institute. In 2004 these two institutes each supported more sleep-related grants than 8 of the 13 current members—close to 10 percent of all sleep-related research project grants.

The Trans-NIH Sleep Research Coordinating Committee offers the somnology and sleep medicine field an exceptional resource for increasing and coordinating NIH support of interdisciplinary sleep-related research and career development programs. Over the last 10 years, through requests for applications (RFAs) and program announcements (PAs), members of the coordinating committee have cosponsored 16 out of the 18 research project grant initiatives (Appendix F). This has the advantage of spreading out the costs of an initiative over multiple institutes, thus being able to support greater investment. However, as will be discussed in greater detail later in this chapter, recently the coordinating committee has not taken a proactive role in developing new research programs.

National Center on Sleep Disorders Research

In direct response to the 1993 report of the National Commission on Sleep Disorders Research, *Wake Up America: A National Sleep Alert*, a provision of the NIH Revitalization Act instructed the Director of the NIH and the National Heart, Lung, and Blood Institute (NHLBI) to establish the NCSDR. As described in the congressional language, the mission of the NCSDR is to "conduct and support of biomedical and related research and research training, the dissemination of health information, and the conduct of other programs with respect to various sleep disorders, the basic under-standing of sleep, biological and circadian rhythm research, chronobiology and other sleep related research" (U.S. Congress, Senate, 1993). As man-dated by Congress the NCSDR has the authority:

- for the conduct and support of research, training, health informa-tion dissemination, and other activities with respect to sleep disorders, in-cluding biological and circadian rhythm research, basic understanding of sleep, chronobiological and other sleep-related research; and
- to coordinate the activities of the NCSDR with similar activities of other federal agencies, including the other agencies of the NIH, and similar activities of other public entities and nonprofit entities. (See Appendix D for complete congressional language.)

The NCSDR establishment within the NHLBI allowed it to call upon the existing successful programs at the NHLBI in sleep-disordered breath-ing as well as the NHLBI's expertise in public education programs. It was realized at the inception of the NCSDR that there was a major need to educate both public and health care professionals about sleep and sleep disorders. Because many NIH institutes have a strong interest in somnology and sleep disorders research and fund portfolios of grants in this area, it was not envisioned that all funding for sleep-related programs would be done through the NCSDR. Rather, the NCSDR would facilitate develop-ment of research and training programs in areas of identified need. In addi-tion, it would be a center that facilitated and coordinated research across the many institutes of the NIH with an interest in sleep-related research, as well as across the many federal agencies that have an interest in sleep deprivation and sleep disorders. These agencies include: the Centers for Disease Control and Prevention (CDC) (prevalence and impact of sleep disorders, inadequate sleep); the Department of Defense (impact of sleep deprivation and nighttime activity on human performance); the Department of Transportation (crashes occurring from falling asleep at the wheel); the Occupational Safety and Health Administration (impact of sleep deprivation and sleep disorders on industrial accidents and shift work sleep disorder); and the Department of Veterans Affairs (VA) (impact of sleep disorders on health of veterans, posttraumatic stress disorder). It is of note that although one out of every five Americans perform shift work, the Department of Labor withdrew its membership from the NCSDR advisory board in 2003. Following the departure of the department's representative the Department of Labor chose not to appoint a replacement member. The committee hopes that the Department of Labor will reconsider this, as it can make an important contribution to the national effort to decrease the burden of sleep loss and sleep disorders.

Several federal agencies have research and public education programs including the Department of Defense, the Department of Transportation, and the CDC. However, the NCSDR has not made clear or demonstrated far-reaching coordination of these activities, with potential missed opportunities for integrating sleep-related programs among federal agencies and departments. The original mandate to the NCSDR, as envisioned in the authorizing legislation, saw the CDC playing a major role in public education and surveillance. As described in Chapter 5, the CDC is involved in many public education campaigns and national surveys. Apart from the recent addition of sleep-related questions in the National Health and Nutrition Examination Survey (NHANES), this has not occurred. There are insufficient data about the sleep patterns of Americans, and the CDC's expertise should be sought in conducting surveillance, monitoring sleep disorders and sleep habits, and developing public health campaigns about sleep loss and sleep disorders.

The NCSDR budget is a line item on the NHLBI administrative budget and includes the director, a public health analyst, an executive assistant, and an office assistant. From a separate NHLBI budget source, the NCSDR receives an allocation each year to support the activities of the Sleep Disorders Research Advisory Board and other programmatic activities, including workshops. Thus, the budget available to the director of the NCSDR is limited. The member institutes in the Trans-NIH Sleep Research Coordinating Committee provide support for their representative to the Committee, and NCSDR provides administrative support as needed for the Trans-NIH Sleep Research Coordinating Committee from its fiscal resources already described. The Office of Prevention, Education, and Control support other NHLBI personnel who work on educational programs and two such individuals (personal communication, M. Twery, NIH, January 24, 2006).

The Advisory Board of the National Center on Sleep Disorders Research

The original NCSDR authorizing legislation established an advisory board to the NCSDR, composed of 12 members of the public—8 scientific members and 4 public members who either are advocates for or have a particular sleep disorder. Included in the advisory board are 10 ex officio members who represent relevant federal agencies (Table 8-2). The advisory board meets biannually. As directed in the authorizing congressional language "The advisory board shall advise, assist, consult with, and make recommendations to the Director of the National Institutes of Health and the Director of the Center concerning matters relating to the scientific activities carried out by and through the Center and the policies respecting such activities, including recommendations with respect to the [research] plan" (U.S. Congress, Senate, 1993). As will be discussed in further detail below, throughout the 12 years since its establishment the advisory board has had varying levels of activity in these responsibilities.

Since its inception, the advisory board has had 29 members. It is NIH policy that the appointed members of advisory councils or other mandated boards cannot serve for terms of more than 4 years and that reappointment is not permitted. This presents a strain on a small field such as somnology and sleep medicine, as those most knowledgeable about the field are frequently selected. It is important that the composition of the advisory board consists of members who are credible and who have the respect of the somnology and sleep medicine community, as well as an understanding of large research and educational enterprises, background as a practicing

---

TABLE 8-2 Ex Officio Members of the NCSDR Advisory Board

Director of the National Institutes of Health (NIH)
Director of the National Center on Sleep Disorders Research (NCSDR)
Director of the National Heart, Lung, and Blood Institute (NHLBI)
Director of the National Institute of Mental Health
Director of the National Institute on Aging
Director of the National Institute of Child Health and Human Development
Director of the National Institute of Neurological Disorders and Stroke
Assistant Secretary for Health
Assistant Secretary of Defense (Health Affairs)
Chief Medical Director of the Veterans Affairs (VA)

researcher, and awareness of a wide variety of public policy issues. Individuals who have been involved in the advisory board are provided in Appendix E, together with, where appropriate, their academic honors and area of expertise. As a result of the small numbers of senior members in the field, the tradition of academic leadership has been difficult to maintain on the advisory board. The board would benefit from advice made by senior investigators who have credibility and a sound understanding of both scientific and clinical advances, as well as an appreciation for policy issues. It is the opinion of this committee that after an appropriate interval senior members of the somnology and sleep medicine fields should be permitted to be reappointed to serve an additional term on the advisory board, along with the most promising juniors member of the field. This should be permitted until the field has a large enough cadre of experienced leaders.

NATIONAL SLEEP DISORDERS RESEARCH PLAN

One of the requirements of the advisory board is to periodically develop a comprehensive research plan. The first research plan was published in 1996. Its recommendations were based on analyses of the needs of the field and the investment in sleep-related programs by the federal government. The recommendations reflected the need to support three areas of research: (1) basic research using state-of-the-art approaches to elucidate the functions of sleep and the fundamental molecular and cellular processes underlying sleep; (2) patient-oriented research to understand the cause, evaluate the scope, and improve the prevention, diagnosis, and treatment of sleep disorders; and (3) applied research to evaluate the scope and consequences of sleepiness and to develop new approaches to prevent impaired performance during waking hours (NHLBI, 1996). Sixteen specific recommendations were crafted in such a way that the outcomes of the effort were easily measurable (see grant analysis below).

The second research plan, published in 2003, provided a brief overview of each topic area and an update of the research progress made since the 1996 report. The report contained over 191 individual recommendations. It has yet to be established, but the large number of recommendations may decrease the effectiveness of the document. The report did provide relative weight to some recommendations, but this may limit the implementation of the remaining recommendations. Based on the recommendations the advisory board identified a limited number of research priorities:

- Understand the neurobiology and function of sleep.
- Assess the impact of reduced sleep across age.
- Find the causes of various sleep disorders.
- Establish normative standards for sleep need and sleep variables.

- Discover/improve treatments for sleep disorders.
- Study if sleep disorders are associated with, and how they affect, the progression of other diseases.
- Educate health care professionals and the public about healthy sleep habits and sleep disorders.
- Apply novel technologies to the study of sleep.
- Develop data and examine prevention, intervention, treatment, and other sleep-related programs specific to women and minorities.

In the research plan, training was considered the highest priority and a separate category was created to underline its importance.

Although the 2003 plan is more comprehensive than the 1996 plan, it lacks specificity in each recommendation, and no strategy was established to advance the research agenda. The large number of recommendations and the broad focus make it difficult to establish measures to evaluate the research plan's effectiveness. The 2003 research plan laid out an ambitious set of priorities but did not provide a strategy to implement the recommendations.

Scientific Advances Since the 2003 Sleep Disorders Research Plan

Below is a brief update of the state of science since 2003. However, as only 2 years have passed since the publication of the 2003 plan, this review is not meant to serve as an in-depth evaluation of the plan or an in-depth review of the current state of the field. Rather, its purpose is to demonstrate the potential the field has to continue to make great scientific strides. The outline for this update uses the organization originally used in the executive summary of the 2003 National Sleep Disorders Research Plan. As the following sections will demonstrate, although there has been scientific progress leading to an even greater number of unanswered questions, over the last few years the field has not grown but has reached a plateau.

Circadian Neurobiology

Research in this area is expanding because of advances in basic research. The major molecular and anatomical components associated with the generation of circadian rhythms have been known for about a decade. Genetic variants associated with delayed and advanced sleep phase are increasingly reported in a small minority of patients with familial occurrence (Xu et al., 2005). However, the clinical implications of altered circadian rhythms are yet to be explored. Some examples include the need to better define the causes and consequences of delayed phase in adolescence and to understand advanced phase in the elderly (Carskadon et al., 2004; Monk, 2005).

The importance of circadian rhythms extends beyond the brain. It is now recognized that the circadian clock does not solely operate within the suprachiasmatic nucleus but also at multiple levels in peripheral and central organs (Yamazaki et al., 2000; Yoo et al., 2004). Researchers have continued to elucidate with increasing detail the molecular mechanisms regulating these multiple molecular clocks. For example, peripheral clock markers can now be generated and studied in human fibroblasts (Brown et al., 2005). In addition, the genetic disruption of molecular mechanisms regulating circadian rhythms is recognized as deleterious at multiple levels within the organism. For example, the *Clock*-mutated mouse was found to suffer from metabolic abnormalities and to be prone to obesity (Turek et al., 2005). It is also increasingly likely that *Clock* genes have effects on the sleep process itself. This research may explain, for example, why shift workers are prone to certain diseases (Harrington, 1994; Boggild and Knutsson, 1999).

Sleep Neurobiology and Basic Sleep Research

The importance of the hypothalamus in sleep regulation, beyond the generation of circadian rhythms and their genesis within the suprachiasmatic nuclei, is increasingly clear (Saper et al., 2005). The recognition of the ventrolateral preoptic area as a sleep generator, together with the identification of the hypocretin (orexin) system as a wake promoting system, has fueled intense research in this area. How these two systems interact neuroanatomically, and how they affect other classical neurobiological systems, such as the monoamine and cholinergic systems, is being elucidated (Saper et al., 2005). Projection sites and novel sleep regulatory nuclei are being identified. The impact of this research is being felt beyond the field; for example, the role of the hypocretin system in regulating dopaminergic systems and addiction potential for drugs of abuse is the subject of intense investigation (Harris et al., 2005).

The function of sleep is also increasingly explored through phylogenetic approaches—the study of sleep in various animal species (Rattenborg et al., 2004; Lyamin et al., 2005). Sleep is a vital behavior conserved across evolution, suggesting it serves one or more critical functions. One important function may be the development of the neonatal brain, as many animals sleep a lot just after birth. The necessity of sleep may also be seen in animals that are in constant motion (e.g., swimming aquatic mammals or migrating birds) as they have developed unihemispheric sleep to allow for the generation of sleep under these difficult ecological circumstances. Interestingly, several reports are now suggesting that in specific instances, sleep can be suppressed completely for very long periods (up to months), such as during long-range migration in certain birds (Rattenborg et al., 2004) or even more surprisingly just after birth in some cetaceans (Lyamin et al.,

2005). These recent results suggest it may be possible to sustain life without sleep in special circumstances, which challenges existing dogma and suggests an area ripe for further advances.

This field of research is also benefiting from genetic studies in animal models. Knockout mice models (mice that are bred so that they lack certain genes) are now systematically being evaluated for sleep abnormalities. Gene variants, including a number of variants that affect sleep, have been isolated in various mouse strains that have specific electroencephalogram patterns (Tafti et al., 2003). These and other genetic mechanisms should be explored in future studies (Maret et al., 2005).

Sleep Disorders in Neurology

The discovery in 1999 and 2000 that hypocretin/orexin is involved in the pathophysiology of most narcolepsy-cataplexy cases is now being translated into clinical practice. Measuring cerebral spinal fluid (CSF) hypocretin-1 (orexin-A) is used in some cases to diagnose narcolepsy and is listed as a diagnostic tool in the revised *International Classification of Sleep Disorders* (AASM, 2005; Bader et al., 2003; Mignot et al., 2003). This diagnostic procedure may be especially important considering the recent report of high prevalence of sleep onset during rapid eye movement (REM) sleep instead of during nonrapid eye movement (NREM) sleep in the general population, a finding that may suggest a large number of false positives for this test and/ or a high prevalence of narcolepsy without cataplexy (Singh et al., 2005).

Sleep disturbances are recognized as a major issue in Parkinson's and Lewy body disease (Rye, 2004), also suggesting a role for dopamine in sleep regulation. Not only can Parkinson's disease patients have a narcolepsy-like daytime sleepiness, but REM behavior disorder is now recognized as an important component of these disorders, often preceding Parkinson's disease by several decades. Investigators are also increasingly interested in other disorders where hypocretin abnormalities might explain sleep disturbances (Nishino and Kanbayashi, 2005), most notably Huntington's chorea, a disorder where mice models show a preferential hypocretin cell loss (Petersen et al., 2005). Similar sleep studies are also occurring with Alzheimer's dementia and stroke patients, where central and obstructive sleep apnea (OSA) may play an important role in both causing and exacerbating the condition.

Finally, rapid progress is occurring in our understanding of restless legs syndrome (Trenkwalder et al., 2005). Pathophysiology and treatment may be closely linked to the dopaminergic system and iron metabolism. Genetic studies suggest the existence of at least three potential loci, located on chromosomes 12, 14, and 9, and investigators are narrowing down on possible candidate genes. It is likely that those actually causing diseases will soon be identified (Manconi et al., 2004).

Sleep-Disordered Breathing

Genetic epidemiological studies conducted over the prior decade have clearly established that sleep-disordered breathing, although a complex trait, has a strong genetic basis with evidence of oligogenic inheritance (Buxbaum et al., 2002). Areas of linkage for the apnea-hypopnea index (AHI) appear to differ by ethnicity (Palmer et al., 2003, 2004). Association and fine mapping studies have quantified the potential role of several candidate genes in the pathogenesis of sleep apnea (Gottlieb et al., 2004b; Larkin et al., 2005a), with results implicating a gene near the *APOe4* locus (Larkin et al., 2005a). There is also evidence that sleep-disordered breathing and obesity, a major public health problem, are partly linked by pleiotropic genetic mechanisms (Palmer et al., 2003, 2004). Thus, future studies of the genetics of sleep-disordered breathing also likely will illuminate the genetic basis of obesity. Applying advances in genome association methods to population studies of sleep apnea will be important in discovering genes for this and related diseases.

Large scale epidemiological studies in the 1990s quantified the prevalence of OSA in middle aged and elderly populations (Ancoli-Israel et al., 1991, 1995; Young et al., 1993). More recently, population-based studies also identified sleep-disordered breathing to be common in American school-aged children, with an especially high prevalence in African American children (Rosen et al., 2003). Other studies have identified the predilection of other groups to sleep apnea. These include commercial drivers (Howard et al., 2004), whose occupations place them at particular risk for sleepiness-associated injuries (Gurubhagavatula et al., 2004). Further work is needed to develop and apply screening approaches for identifying individuals at high risk for sleep apnea (see technology section). However, in the case of commercial drivers, a two-stage screening strategy using questionnaires and simplified tests was shown to be effective (Gurubhagavatula et al., 2004). Given that commercial drivers with sleep apnea are likely to be at an increased risk for crashes, occupational screening of this group may provide an important opportunity to test the model for occupational screening for sleep disorders.

There is developing evidence that sleep apnea leads to oxidative stress (Lavie, 2003). This likely results from the cyclical doxygenation-reoxygenation, akin to ischemia reperfusion, that occurs with apneic events, causing free radial production and increased levels of inflammatory molecules. C-reactive protein, a biomarker for cardiovascular disease, may be elevated in OSA. C-reactive protein declines with treatment with continuous positive airway pressure (CPAP) (Yokoe et al., 2003). Increasing oxidative stress is not only relevant to the cardiovascular risk of sleep apnea but also to its effects on neurocognition. Cyclical intermittent hypoxia leads to oxidative damage of various groups of neurons: hippocampal neurons with resulting learning deficits (Row et al., 2003); hypoglossal motoneurons, a mechanism that may accelerate disease progression (Veasey et al., 2004b), as well as wake active neurons (Veasey et al., 2004a). The latter may be the mechanism by which residual sleepiness occurs in patients with OSA even when they are well treated with nasal CPAP.

There is ongoing evidence from prospective studies that OSA is a risk factor for cardiovascular events and mortality, and this evidence is becoming more compelling based on large prospective cohort studies. Such studies show that patients with sleep apnea, in particular severe sleep apnea (i.e., AHI greater than 30 episodes per hour), have increased rates of cardiovascular events, strokes, mortality independent of other risk factors, and hypertension (Yaggi et al., 2005; Marin et al., 2005). Patients with severe sleep apnea who were not treated have an increased rate of cardiovascular events and deaths compared to controls with similar degrees of obesity who do not have sleep apnea (Marin et al., 2005). When patients with severe sleep apnea are treated with CPAP, both the rate of cardiovascular events and cardiac deaths drop to control rates (Marin et al., 2005). Although this provides strong support for a role of OSA in atherogenesis, the critical proof for a causal association, and further defining a need for early treatment, requires randomized trials designed to assess the impact of OSA on cardiovascular events.

The Sleep Heart Health Study has added further support for sleep apnea being a risk factor for insulin resistance independent of the effects of obesity (Punjabi et al., 2004). In this large study the presence of sleep apnea (i.e., AHI greater than 15 events per hour) was independently associated with insulin resistance even after controlling for body mass index and waist-to-hip ratio, a measure of visceral obesity (Punjabi et al., 2004). Moreover, data suggest that treating patients with OSA by nasal CPAP significantly increases insulin sensitivity as measured by the euglycemic clamp method (Harsch et al., 2004). This effect was, however, most evident in relatively nonobese subjects, with questions regarding the extent to which sleep apnea treatment improves glucose tolerance in obese individuals with sleep apnea and may help prevent diabetes. A small study suggests that this is so; improvement is particularly found in those with high levels of a specific type of hemoglobin that is a marker for poor glucose control (Babu et al., 2005).

Although much of the focus of research continues to be on OSA, progress is also being made in other aspects of sleep-disordered breathing. Obesity-hypoventilation syndrome, a condition in which individuals hypoventilate during sleep (due to an increased respiratory load from the increased weight) and have elevated daytime arterial P_{CO_2} levels, has been shown to be common yet frequently unrecognized in obese hospitalized patients. Obese patients with this problem have poorer medical outcomes (Nowbar et al., 2004).

Thus, this research in sleep and sleep disorders is vibrant and has great potential to improve public health problems related to sleep-disordered breathing.

Insomnia

A turning point in this area may have been the recent NIH-sponsored State-of-the Science Conference on chronic insomnia (Dolan-Sewell et al., 2005). In this conference, a decision was made to abandon the concept of secondary insomnia. The rationale for this change was that it is difficult in most cases to distinguish causes and consequences for insomnia. The possibility that insomnia is associated with abnormalities of sleep microarchitecture and brain metabolism, as measured by imaging studies, is also increasingly recognized. This, together with the concept of hyperarousal in patients with insomnia (Nofzinger et al., 2004), is leading to the discovery of objective markers and a pathophysiological model for insomnia. It was also recognized that insomnia is not only frequently associated with depression but may be an independent predictor of it (Roth and Roehrs, 2003).

Treatment modalities for insomnia are changing. Prescribed hypnotic use is reported in children and adolescents, a pattern that raises concern as there are limited data in this area (Owens et al., 2003). An increasing number of well-designed studies are showing efficacy and safety for cognitive-behavioral therapies (Morin, 2004). This, together with the introduction and development of a large number of new hypnotics of various modes of action, is changing clinical practice in insomnia.

Pediatric Sleep Sciences

There have been several advances in the field of pediatric sleep medicine in the last two years: the discovery of the gene for congenital central hypoventilation syndrome, improved understanding of the pathogenesis and epidemiology of sleep apnea, and better understanding of the complications associating OSA in children. However, pediatric sleep remains relatively understudied, and there are still many gaps in the knowledge base. For example, although the Back to Sleep Campaign has been very successful there is still very little information concerning the etiology of sudden infant death syndrome (SIDS).

In 2003, Amiel and colleagues described a mutation of the *PHOX2B* gene in 62 percent of their patients with congenital central hypoventilation syndrome (Amiel et al., 2003). Following refinement of the technique, 97 percent of patients have been shown to have a mutation of the gene (Weese-Mayer et al., 2003), which is dominant and usually a de novo mutation. This finding has already become useful in clinical practice, with clinical testing and amniocentesis now available.

There has been increasing research in the area of pediatric sleep-disordered breathing. Several studies have provided a better understanding of the pathophysiology of OSA in children, including the role of upper airway reflexes in this disease (Gozal and Burnside, 2004; Marcus et al., 2005). Major advances have been made in understanding the complications of childhood OSA. In particular, work from a number of different labs has shown that very mild obstructive apnea, and perhaps even primary snoring, is associated with changes in neurocognitive and behavioral function in children (Fregosi et al., 2003; Rosen et al., 2004; Gottlieb et al., 2004a). Other studies have shown that childhood OSA is associated with cardiac hypertrophy (Amin et al., 2005), inflammation (Tauman et al., 2004; Larkin et al., 2005b), and the metabolic syndrome (de la Eva et al., 2002), potentially putting children at risk for cardiovascular complications later in life. Of great interest is the observation of adverse outcomes in individuals with a very mild sleep apnea (including habitual snoring without appreciable levels of overnight hypoxemia). Given that almost all of the work to date has been descriptive, it is imperative that interventional studies assess whether early diagnosis and treatment would modify short- or long-term health outcomes. In this regard, there is also a need to identify the efficacy of sleep apnea treatment in children, including tonsillectomy and adenoidectomy, for which there has not yet been a single randomized controlled study of treatment for sleep apnea.

Sleep Deprivation

The impact of sleep deprivation and shift work on driving and industrial accidents has been known for more than a decade. Unfortunately, change, especially in the area of commercial driving, has been difficult to implement. Modafinil, a wake-promoting agent, may be effective for the treatment of shift work disorder and prove to be useful in this setting (Czeisler et al., 2005). Sleep deprivation is also increasingly recognized as being associated with poor school performance, especially when school re-starts after an extended number of days off. This may be mediated by delayed sleep phase, early school start time, and increased sleep need during adolescence (Carskadon et al., 2004).

Recent studies have shown that sleep deprivation causes medical errors among physicians (Lockley et al., 2004; Landrigan et al., 2004; Barger et al., 2005). Attentional lapses and errors can be improved by reducing work hours and increasing sleep (Lockley et al., 2004; Landrigan et al., 2004).

These findings are leading to rapid changes in the on-call requirements for physicians in training (Cavallo et al., 2004).

The impact of chronic sleep restriction on human health and endocrinological status is also increasingly recognized. Associations among short sleep, obesity, diabetes, and mortality have been reported (Alvarez and Ayas, 2004; Gottlieb et al., 2005). A large number of studies have shown cross-sectional association between short sleep and obesity (Cizza et al., 2005). A trend for a longitudinal association between shortening sleep and gaining weight is also typically found. The biological mediation of these changes may be through alterations in leptin and ghrelin, two major appetite regulatory hormones (Taheri et al., 2004; Spiegel et al., 2004). The levels of these hormones are altered in health subjects if sleep is restricted for a few nights.

Sleep Education and Training

Although a top priority of the 2003 research plan, the NIH has not established any new large-scale programs in training or career development. In fact, as has been described in Chapter 7, there has been a decrease in the number of career development grants pertaining to sleep. Further, although a few private foundations and professional societies have invested some in professional development, as discussed in Chapter 5, increased efforts are required to fully embrace the need to increase education and training programs. Thus, progress in this critical area has been quite limited.

ANALYSIS OF NIH-SPONSORED RESEARCH PROJECT GRANTS

Currently, assessment of the success of the sleep research effort at NIH seems to be based largely on the total dollars being committed by various institutes to the field (for more information see the 2001 to 2004 annual reports of the Trans-NIH Sleep Research Coordinating Committee). NIH funding for somnology research has increased by more than 150 percent since the NCSDR became fully operational in 1996, reaching a total of $196.2 million (0.07 percent of the NIH budget) in fiscal year 2004 (NHLBI, 2003). However, this growth occurred during the same period that the overall budget to the NIH doubled.

At the same time that the science and magnitude of the problem requires greater investment, over the last few years NIH funding to sleep-related activities has plateaued. This has partially overlapped the period when the overall NIH budget has plateaued. Consequently, the future outlook for somnology and sleep medicine is unclear. In 2004, for the first time since the NCSDR was established, there was a decrease of $846,000 in annual expenditures for sleep-related projects. This decrease raises even greater concern because it occurred in the same year that the NCSDR included the expenditures of three additional institutes not included in previous fiscal reports. A comparison of research funding for the institutes in 2003 fiscal year analysis reveals a decrease of $1.142 million. Further, between 2003 and 2004 there were fewer research project grants funded, and this trend may continue as the number of new research project grants funded in 2004 also decreased (Appendix G). There must be incremental growth in this field to meet the public health and economic burden caused by sleep loss and sleep disorders.

It is difficult to accurately track the commitment of different NIH institutes to somnology and sleep disorders, in part because there is no uniform accounting system. Some NIH institutes count only a proportion of a grant when only a component of the grant is related to sleep research, but others count the entire grant, even though sleep-related research is only a minor part of the grant. This is particularly problematic for large program project or center grants. More important, however, these financial data do not allow the advisory board or leadership of the NCSDR to track the type of research being conducted and hence help identify areas of need. Originally the NCSDR Advisory Board took an active role in assessing the then current portfolio of sleep research grants, such as the analysis that was published in the journal *Sleep* in 1999 (Gillette et al., 1999). The committee presents its analysis below and urges the advisory board to continue to take an active role in this and perform a similar analysis on an annual basis.

Somnology and Sleep Disorders RFAs and PAs

The 1996 research plan was based on analyses of currently funded grants and led to a number of specific RFAs and PAs. Recently, there has been a marked reduction in the number of sleep-related RFAs that provide an important mechanism to develop research programs in specific areas of need. They identify a narrowly defined area for which one or more NIH institutes have set aside funds for awarding grants. This is different from PAs, which identify areas of increased priority or emphasis but typically do not have specific funds set aside (except for PAS announcements).

Over the last 3 years, the NCSDR has only sponsored two programs, one PA and one RFA—Research on Sleep and Sleep Disorders: PA-05-046 (in 2004) (NIH, 2004) and Mechanisms Linking Short Sleep Duration and Risk of Obesity or Overweight: RFA-HL-06-003 (in 2005) (NIH, 2005). The marked reduction over recent years in efforts identifying and developing RFAs and PAs is seen by examining the list of RFAs and PAs in sleep disorders research since the inception of the NCSDR (Appendix F).

The recent efforts of the NCSDR can be compared to those of the National Center for Medical Rehabilitation Research (NCMRR), which is a similarly structured center in the National Institute of Child Health and

Human Development. The NCMRR supports research on enhancing the functioning of people with disabilities in daily life. Compared to the 1 RFA established by the NCSDR in fiscal year 2004, the NCMRR established 6 RFAs and 4 PAs. Further, between 2001 and 2004 the NCMRR established 20 RFAs, while the NCSDR established only 4 RFAs. It is unclear why there is such a dramatic difference in the activity of these two centers.

Protocol for Research Project Grant Analysis

This committee performed a detailed analysis of the 1995 and 2004 portfolios of NIH somnology and sleep disorders research project grants (R01) to determine the current investment in the field and to examine how the grant portfolio has changed over the last 10 years. To do so, abstracts of all sleep-related R01s in the Computer Retrieval of Information on Scientific Projects (CRISP) database were analyzed. This database collects information on the number of federally funded biomedical research projects. Sleep-related R01s were collected by searching the CRISP database for all abstracts that were classified under the following thesaurus terms: *insomnia, periodic limb movement disorder, restless legs syndrome, circadian rhythm, SIDS, sleep disorder, narcolepsy, sleep apnea, sleep, hibernation,* and *dream.* To limit the number of grants that were not relevant to somnology or sleep disorders, the committee only included grants in which the key words appeared in both the thesaurus terms and abstract and not the abstract alone. It should be noted that the following conclusions are based on the number of grants awarded in each area. The committee did not have access to the applications that were submitted and not funded; therefore, it is not possible to conclusively determine if changes in investment are the result of NIH policy, the number and/or quality of submissions in each area, composition of grant review committees, or a combination of these factors.

General Findings

The CRISP search identified 156 sleep-related grants for 1995 and 397 for 2004. Upon review of their abstracts a number of these were determined to be unrelated to sleep. This resulted in 116 total sleep-related grants in 1995 and 331 sleep-related grants in 2004, a 2.85 fold increase (Table 8-3). The number of the grants deemed not relevant to sleep-related research— 34 out of 156 in 1995, and 59 out of 397 in 2004—represents a relatively constant percentage (i.e., 21 percent and 15 percent, respectively; supplemental grants and grants with no abstract were also not classified). Thus, use of this methodology to track temporal trends in number of grants seems appropriate. Of the relevant sleep R01 grants there were 253 principal

TABLE 8-3 Analysis of Somnology and Sleep Disorders Research Project Grants (R01): 1995 and 2004

	1995		2004		Number in 2004 / Number in 1995
	Number of Sleep Grants	Percentage of Sleep Grants	Number of Sleep Grants	Percentage of Sleep Grants	
Grants Analyzed					
Number of grants analyzed	156		397		2.54
Number of grants relevant to sleep	116		331		2.85
Number of principal investigators	100		253		2.53
Clinical or Basic Research					
Clinical research projects	71	61	179	54	2.52
Basic research projects (not circadian rhythm)	28	24	61	18	2.18
Circadian rhythm projects	19	16	97	29	5.11
Type of Sleep Disorder					
Restless legs syndrome and periodic limb movements	0	0	5	2	N/A
Insomnia	10	9	22	7	2.20
Narcolepsy/hypersomnia	5	4	6	2	1.20
Circadian rhythm	7	6	22	7	3.14
Parasomnia	1	1	0	0	N/A
Sleep deprivation	3	3	18	5	6.00
Sleep apnea	19	16	65	20	3.42
Sleep neurological, other	3	3	6	2	2.00
Drug abuse	2	2	11	3	5.50
Sleep medical, other	15	13	23	7	1.53
Sleep psychiatric disorder	13	11	10	3	-0.23

Research Strategy					
Systems neuroscience	32	28	62	19	1.94
Electrophysiology	26	22	70	21	2.69
Pharmacology	13	11	36	11	2.77
Cell biology	27	23	57	17	2.11
Molecular	10	9	70	21	7.00
Genetic	5	4	53	16	10.60
Observational study	36	31	84	25	2.33
Intervention study	22	19	54	16	2.45
Epidemiology	10	9	24	7	2.40
Hormone/biomarker	13	11	71	22	5.46
Clinical trial	12	10	27	8	2.25
Assessment of devices	4	3	5	2	1.25
Species					
Human, no age specified	26	22	68	21	2.62
Human, child and adolescent	12	10	23	7	1.92
Human, adult	18	16	51	15	2.83
Human, elderly	17	15	30	9	1.76
Rat	21	18	77	23	3.67
Mouse	2	2	32	10	16.00
Drosophila	2	2	15	5	7.50
Other or not specified	32	28	60	18	1.88

NOTE: Percentages were rounded. N/A = Not applicable.

investigators in 2004, a 2.53 fold increase from 1995 (100 principal investigators). Given that an estimated 50 to 70 million Americans have sleep-related health challenges, the current investment of 0.07 percent of the NIH budget and presumably a lesser proportion across other agencies, we believe, is not sufficient.

Clinical, Basic, and Circadian Rhythm Research Projects

Each grant was categorized to determine if the research was primarily basic or clinical in nature. Fifty-four percent of the grants in 2004 focused on clinical sleep disorders. Seventeen percent of 2004 grants were focused on basic sleep research projects, and 29 percent were devoted to the study of circadian rhythms. The total percentage of nonclinical research projects devoted to circadian rhythms rose from 40 percent of nonclinical research projects in 1995 to 61 percent in 2004. There has been over the last 10 years a disparate growth in these areas. Investment in circadian rhythms research projects increased by 5.11-fold; however, basic research unrelated to circadian rhythms only increased by 2.53-fold, well below the need. Not surprisingly, this largely reflects where much scientific advance has occurred.

Sleep Disorders

Since 1995, there has also been growth in the number of grants focused on sleep disorders. The current analysis suggests that research funding is disproportional to the public health burden and the known prevalence and consequences of the disorders. In a few cases, research has actually decreased or barely grown. These areas include parasomnia research (from one grant in 1995 to none in 2004), sleep in psychiatric disorders (0.23-fold decrease), and narcolepsy (1.20-fold increase). The lack of research regarding parasomnias is troublesome, considering the prevalence of these conditions. Similarly, the decrease in research grants in the area of sleep disturbances in psychiatric diseases is disturbing, considering the growing recognition that insomnia is a major risk factor for depression (see the Scientific Advances Since the 2003 Sleep Disorders Research Plan). This last observation should be mitigated by the relatively hefty increase in insomnia research.

Research in the area of narcolepsy and hypersomnia sleep disorder research also stayed flat. This last finding was disappointing, considering the recent discovery of hypocretin deficiency as the main cause of narcolepsy with cataplexy and the growing recognition that a large number of patients have milder forms of centrally mediated hypersomnolence, narcolepsy without cataplexy, and idiopathic hypersomnia. Research in this area may be uniquely poised to make progress, but funding has not increased. Not a single grant was identified on the study of idiopathic hypersomnia or Kleine-Levin syndrome. The latter is admittedly a rare condition.

Over the 10-year span between 1995 and 2004 there has been no growth in research examining the etiology and pathophysiology of SIDS. In 1995 seven R01s were identified as focusing, at least partially, on SIDS, but in 2004 there were only six grants. Although the prevalence of SIDS has decreased since the Back to Sleep public education campaign began, this is still an area of research that warrants attention.

Selected areas grew more rapidly. There has been increasing interest in restless legs syndrome/periodic leg movements research; but the current investment is still low. There were no grants with a primary focus in these areas in 1995 and six in 2004. Given the high prevalence of restless legs syndrome and its negative impact (Chapter 3), the small number of grants is, however, still surprising. Further, although the number of insomnia research project grants has also grown from 10 grants in 1995 to 22 grants in 2004 (2.20-fold growth), this growth is modest given the high prevalence of insomnia. Clinical research project grants focused on the elucidation of sleep apnea demonstrated an increase in support that is reflected in the increased appreciation of its public health burden that occurred over the same period—19 grants in 1995 (15 percent of total grants) and 65 in 2004 (22 percent of total grants), a growth of 3.42-fold.

Assessment of Devices

The committee also noted that research assessing new devices barely grew from 1995 to 2004 (1.25-fold increase). This was also a troubling trend, as the study group identified the need to validate and increase the use of ambulatory monitoring devices in the diagnosis and assessment of sleep disorders, most notably sleep-disordered breathing (see Chapter 6).

Research Strategy

The committee also examined the primary research strategy proposed in each project. The striking trends in this area have been the dramatic growth in studies employing molecular (7.00-fold growth) and genetic (10.60-fold growth) strategies. Although this partially reflects the trends in modern biomedical research, the NHLBI, the National Institute of Mental Health, and the National Institute of Child Health and Human Development sponsored an RFA in 1996 to advance the understanding of the molecular and genetic basis of sleep and sleep disorders (RFA-HL-96-015). This RFA provided researchers funding for research projects that had molecular and genetic strategies.

Species

In this area there are also key trends. The growth in studies using mice is staggering, 16-fold from 1995 to 2004. There were only two grants using mice in 1995 and 32 in 2004. This is likely to be in direct response to the NHLBI, the National Institute of Mental Health, the National Institute on Aging, and the National Institute of Neurological Disorders and Stroke sponsoring an RFA in 1998 to develop improved molecular, cellular, and systems approaches to investigate sleep and circadian phenotypes in mice (RFA-HL-99-001).

There has also been a major increase in studies utilizing *Drosophila* as a model organism (7.50 fold increase). The use of *Drosophila* to study sleep was originally recommended at a workshop held by the NCSDR in 1995 and was included in the previously mentioned 1996 RFA to advance the understanding of the molecular and genetic basis of sleep and sleep disorders (RFA-HL-96-015). There are also a large number of grants that are in the "Other" category for species.

There are, as expected, a large number of studies on humans. The total number of grants in humans in 1995 was 73, but in 2004 it was 172, a 3.35-fold increase. It is concerning, however, that there are still only 23 grants studying sleep and its disorders in children and adolescents. This represents only 13 percent of total grants in humans, and the increase in pediatric sleep grants (1.92-fold) is lower than that for all grants (2.35-fold) and for all grants in humans (3.35-fold increase). The number of grants studying sleep and its disorders in the elderly, a population with a particularly high prevalence of sleep disorders, is also only 30. The growth in this area (1.77-fold) is also less than in other categories. Finally, although there has been growth in human subjects research, there has been a limited number of long-term clinical outcomes intervention studies that have examined strategies to improve the scientific base and treatments.

Composition of Grant Review Panels

An analysis of relevant NIH review panel expertise was also performed. To do so, the composition of review panels that received applications with sleep was analyzed. A total of 24 review panels, including special emphasis panels and standing integrated review groups (IRG), were included. Reviewers were subjected to Medline searches with the keywords *sleep* and *circadian*. Names were also visually inspected by multiple members of the committee who had expertise in various aspects of somnology and sleep medicine. Membership to sleep or circadian rhythms societies was noted, together with area of expertise. Only reviewers with a major sleep or circadian research focus, as judged by their publication record or professional society, were considered.

Twenty-eight reviewers with knowledge in sleep or circadian biology were identified in the 24 review panels. It is important to note that although some review panels may not have experts in the field, often the Center of Scientific Review will appoint ad hoc reviewers when specific expertise is absent on the review panel. One third of the reviewers (12 out of 36 reviewers) were concentrated in a single study section, the Biological Rhythms and Sleep Study Section. Another third (9 reviewers) were in NHLBI special emphasis panels. Eleven of the total 28 (39 percent) reviewers were primarily interested in circadian rhythm research, rather than basic sleep research or clinical sleep disorders. Four other NHLBI review panels had more than 2 reviewers with sleep and circadian expertise; these included the mentored patient-oriented carrier development (K23) grant review panel (2 reviewers); a NHLBI special emphasis panel on T32 grants (2 reviewers); a small business activities special emphasis panel (4 reviewers) and the Respiratory Integrative Biology and Translational Research panel (2 reviewers). It was notable that two study sections with *sleep* in their title (and mandate) had one or no reviewers with a sleep expertise: the Neural Basis of Psychopathology panel, addictions and sleep disorders (1 reviewer); and the cardiovascular and sleep epidemiology study section (no reviewers with sleep expertise).

As expected, there was an association between reviewer expertise and types of grants funded. A notable finding was the low percentage of reviewers with clinical research expertise (36 percent) covering all of the different sleep disorders outlined in earlier chapters. This finding may be one potential reason why clinical research was the area with the least growth. However, because the committee was unable to examine and categorize all the grants that were submitted and not funded, it is difficult to interpret this finding. Further, the limited number of sleep reviewers, as well as the small number of funded grants, may also be a direct reflection of the limited number of scientists (especially senior investigators) in specific areas of this field.

Value of Grant Analysis Protocol

Categorizing each research project grant offers researchers and policy makers the opportunity to examine the current investment in particular areas, identify areas in need of greater investment, and provide a quantifiable metric to examine the success of specific RFA and PA programs. This committee strongly encourages the NCSDR Advisory Board to perform a similar annual analysis of all somnology and sleep disorders grants, including research (R), training (T), fellowship (F), career development (K), program (P), and cooperative (U) activities sponsored by the NIH, the CDC, and Department of Defense, Department of Transportation, Department of Labor, and other relevant federal agencies. This committee also believes that the Center for Scientific Review should gather basic keyword information on submitted grants and reviewers to address adequacy of review expertise on review panels. This information would be helpful to the NIH at large and to the NCSDR as it develops a more proactive research plan.

Although the success of an RFA is dependent on the number and quality of grant applications, this analysis demonstrates the value an RFA may have in expanding interest and awareness in specific areas of a field. Therefore, this committee recommends that the NCSDR Advisory Board use their annual analysis to identify priority research and training areas and annually recommend an RFA to appropriate advisory councils of the Trans-NIH Sleep Coordinating Committee and other federal agencies including the CDC.

NEXT STEPS IN ACCELERATING PROGRESS

Given the multiple and varied sources of federal and private funding and support for the field and the numerous disciplines involved in research and clinical care, the challenge for the field of sleep medicine is to develop a collaborative and focused approach with a strong research infrastructure. To bolster clinical and basic research efforts, catalyze collaborative research efforts, and attract the breadth of talented researchers who will be able to move somnology and sleep disorders research and clinical care forward to achieve the therapeutic solutions requires a coordinated and integrated strategy.

Strengthen the NCSDR and Its Advisory Board

It is an opportune time for coordination of sleep-related activities throughout the federal government. The NCSDR and its advisory board should take the lead in reinvigorating a coordinated strategy. To assist in this coordination, annually the directors of the NCSDR and the NCSDR Advisory Board should meet with all institute directors who are members of the Trans-NIH Sleep Coordinating Committee and directors of other relevant federal agencies. Further, institutes at the NIH that manage a large sleep-related portfolio should be encouraged to appoint appropriate representatives of the field of Somnology and Sleep Medicine to their advisory councils and program project review committees.

Recommendation 8.1: The National Center on Sleep Disorders Research and its advisory board should play a more proactive role in stimulating and coordinating the field.

The National Center on Sleep Disorders and Research (NCSDR) should have adequate staff and resources to ensure its ability to fulfill its mission of coordinating and stimulating training, research, and health information dissemination relevant to somnology and sleep disorders. All relevant institutes with significant sleep portfolios should become members of the Trans-NIH Sleep Research Coordinating Committee. Further, the NCSDR Advisory Board should take a more proactive role in advising the director of the NCSDR. On an annual basis, the NCSDR and its advisory board should:

- Identify specific objectives that address each of the three NCSDR missions and evaluate specific actions taken to accomplish each objective. This assessment should be reported in an annual meeting to the Trans-NIH Sleep Coordinating Committee, the institute directors of its members, and to the director of the NIH.
- Directors of the other federal agencies that fund significant sleep-related activities, such as Department of Defense, Department of Commerce, Department of Education, Department of Labor, and Department of Transportation should report annually on their activities to the NCSDR Advisory Board.
- The NCSDR Advisory Board should annually review the current NIH portfolio of sleep-related grants, as well as requests for applications, and program announcements, assess them for responsiveness to the program plan and identify gaps in research and training.
- The NCSDR Advisory Board should annually recommend new, or modify existing, requests for applications that can be presented to appropriate NIH institutes and other federal agencies including the Centers for Disease Control and Prevention and Department of Defense. Multiple members of the Trans-NIH Sleep Coordinating Committee are encouraged to continue to cosponsor sleep-related grants.

Enhance Research Collaborations

Clinical advances in treatments for chronic sleep loss and sleep disorders depends on the quality and integration of fundamental knowledge from multiple laboratory and clinical disciplines; including but not limited to: cardiology, dentistry, endocrinology, epidemiology, molecular biology, neurology, neurosciences, nursing, nutrition, otolaryngology, pediatrics, pharmacology, psychiatry, and pulmonology. Historically the field has been clinically focused and has not integrated the efforts of its clinical and basic research scientists. For the field to make its next set of advances it will require a strengthened research infrastructure that will feature the development of combined clinical and research centers of excellence focused on somnology and sleep medicine and a structured network to facilitate and ensure collaborative interdisciplinary approaches.

Centers of excellence are required to establish and enhance somnology and sleep disorders research. A critical feature of these centers will be their ability to foster collaborations among the many research and clinical disciplines through a coordinated and integrated effort. They should promote interdisciplinary research, which is needed to explore the interrelationship between sleep and an individual's health (e.g., common medical illnesses). The proposed research network described below will integrate the efforts of the broad array of researchers (both investigators at centers of excellence and from other institutions) who study or are involved in somnology and sleep medicine and other relevant avenues of therapeutic intervention for chronic sleep loss and sleep disorders.

Establish Centers of Excellence

The committee urges a strong continued commitment by the NIH to designate and support Somnology and Sleep Medicine Centers of Excellence. These centers would provide the interdisciplinary environment that is essential to accelerate the development of future advances in treating chronic sleep loss and sleep disorders. They would facilitate interactions between laboratory, clinical, and population scientists. Further, the centers would create an environment to support cross-cutting research that requires collaboration among scientists who work in different intellectual contexts. These would not only be "research centers," but they would be sites for collaborations focused on the close association between research, clinical care, education, and dissemination of information.

Modeled after the National Cancer Institute's Cancer Center Program (NCI, 2004), these comprehensive centers of excellence would offer expanded laboratory facilities; focused interactions among preclinical researchers, clinical researchers, and patients; and central sites for clinical trial design. They would serve as the centerpiece of the nation's effort to reduce morbidity and mortality from chronic sleep loss and sleep disorders. This investment would likely draw new senior-level researchers into the somnology and sleep medicine field and would heighten the interest of young investigators in devoting their research interests to chronic sleep loss and sleep disorders treatment. Further, structuring these centers to include strong integrated and coordinated clinical and basic research programs will help facilitate translational research. The centers would deliver medical advances to patients, educate health care professionals and the public, and reach out to underserved populations.

As described in detail in Chapters 5 and 7, enhancing career opportunities for researchers at all points in their careers is vital to accelerating progress in somnology and sleep medicine research. The committee believes that strengthening the research infrastructure through the development of new comprehensive centers will be the impetus needed to attract and retain early career, mid-career, and senior researchers. At these centers they will have the opportunity to fully engage in their own research initiatives, in addition to having the resources to develop and nurture trainees and sustain a full research effort.

These centers should be supported with the infrastructure needed to promote and enhance the institutional development of somnology and sleep medicine and treatment capabilities. This includes core research laboratory equipment, tools, and facilities; an emphasis on training programs; strong basic and clinical research components; and a structured plan for research priorities. However, the committee does not call on any specific organizational model, recognizing the diversity of academic settings that include well organized, freestanding centers; a center matrix within an academic institution; or a formal consortium under centralized leadership. The centers should also have the capacity to facilitate clinical trials; develop best practices and clinical guidelines; educate the community; screen and counsel individuals with chronic sleep loss and sleep disorders; and educate health professionals about state-of-the-art diagnostic, preventive, and treatment techniques. These centers of excellence should serve as the cornerstone of a National Somnology and Sleep Medicine Research and Clinical Network designed to coordinate and support somnology and sleep medicine research efforts.

Similar to the organization of the cancer centers, this committee envisions both Somnology and Sleep Medicine Centers and Comprehensive Somnology and Sleep Medicine Centers (NCI, 2004). Somnology and Sleep Medicine Centers should have a scientific agenda primarily focused on basic, population science, or clinical research, or any two of these three components. Similar to comprehensive cancer centers with a clinical component, the centers with clinical components are expected to conduct early phase clinical trials (NCI, 2004). A comprehensive somnology and sleep medicine center is expected to have reasonable depths and breadths of research in each of these areas. As with the National Cancer Institute designated comprehensive centers, Comprehensive Somnology and Sleep Medicine Centers are expected to disseminate information to the public and health care professionals about medical advances developed within the center. They should also establish formal programs for teaching, screening, therapy, and/or preventative interventions.

As identified by the National Cancer Institute, there are six essential characteristics of a designated cancer center: facilities, organizational capabilities, interdisciplinary and transdisciplinary collaboration and coordination, cancer focus, institutional commitment, and center director (Box 8-1). Each of these attributes—substituting somnology and sleep medicine focus for cancer—is also likely to be critical for establishing and sustaining efficient and productive somnology and sleep medicine centers of excellence.

BOX 8-1
The Six Essential Characteristics of a National Cancer Institute-Designated Cancer Center

Facilities: Dedicated resources to the conduct of cancer-focused research and to the center's shared resources, administration, and research dissemination should be appropriate and adequate to the task.

Organizational capabilities: Adequate capacity for the conduct of research and the evaluation and planning of center activities should take maximum advantage of the parent institution's capabilities in cancer research.

Interdisciplinary and transdisciplinary collaboration and coordination: Substantial coordination, interaction, and collaboration among center members from a variety of disciplines should enhance and add value to the productivity and quality of research in the center.

Cancer focus: A defined scientific focus on cancer research should be clear from the center members' grants and contracts, and from the structure and objectives of its programs.

Institutional commitment: The center should be recognized as a formal organizational component with sufficient space, positions, and resources to ensure organizational stability and fulfill the center's objectives.

Center director: The director should be a highly qualified scientist and administrator with the leadership experience and institutional authority appropriate to manage the center.

SOURCE: National Cancer Institute (2004).

Develop Comprehensive Somnology and Sleep Medicine Centers of Excellence

The establishment of Somnology and Sleep Medicine Centers of Excellence requires large programs that can support and foster excellence in research, clinical care, and population science. This committee recognizes that there are few academic programs that currently have this capacity. However, to facilitate other academic centers achieving this goal, the NIH Exploratory Center award (P20) may be used for this endeavor. These awards are intended to facilitate the development of collaborative research teams of established investigators by providing support for collaborative research projects and core services for investigating leading-edge research questions not currently being addressed in optimal ways (NIMH, 2006). Further, the mechanism supports planning for new programs, expansion or modification of existing resources, and feasibility studies to explore various approaches to the development of interdisciplinary programs that offer potential solutions to problems of special significance (NIH, 2006a). Support is typically limited to 5 years and is not renewable.

The Silvio O. Conte Centers to Develop Collaborative Neuroscience Research provide a good example. These centers, supported through a P20 mechanism, support early-stage development of collaborative teams of high-caliber investigators from diverse disciplines to study basic and/or clinical neuroscience issues. They are characterized by the following:

- the capacity to bring together a team of collaborative investigators with different scientific perspectives.
- an organization that supports innovative creativity, and potentially high-risk/high-import research questions that require collaborative research.
- interactive research projects and core facilities to support projects.
- a program director with a demonstrated ability to organize, administer, and direct the center.
- opportunities for young investigators and close coordination between the center and relevant predoctoral and/or postdoctoral research training programs.
- outreach that makes the public aware of the importance and implications of the center's research.

A developing center must have a clearly articulated plan to develop a set of scientific core functions that will enhance and expand the capacity to move somnology and/or sleep disorders research and treatment into community settings.

NIH Institutional Clinical and Translational Science Award

The NIH has established the Institutional Clinical and Translational Science Award, which has the purpose of developing programs to overcome the growing barriers between clinical and basic research, facilitate the sharing of knowledge to the clinic and back again to the basic research laboratory, and aid academic institutes in developing efficient capabilities to perform clinical and translational science. Through these programs, the NIH aims to: (1) attract and develop a cadre of well-trained multi- and interdisciplinary investigators and research teams; (2) develop programs that spawn innovative research tools and information technologies; and (3) synergize multi- and interdisciplinary clinical and translational research and researchers to catalyze the application of new knowledge and techniques to clinical practice at the front lines of patient care (NIH, 2006b). As supported by all the same arguments already presented throughout this report, somnology and sleep medicine programs are ideal recipients.

As the NIH highlights, to ensure the successful establishment and long-term sustenance of these groundbreaking programs, it is important that the developed program accrue significant institutional support, be granted status as a major administrative entity within the applicant institution, and that the program director have authority, perhaps shared with other high-level institutional officials, over requisite space, resources, faculty appointments, protected time, and promotion (NIH, 2006b).

National Somnology and Sleep Medicine Research Network

A research network is of particular importance in the field because of the need for a coordinated interdisciplinary research approach to basic and clinical research, clinical care, public education, and training. The proposed National Somnology and Sleep Medicine Research Network would improve the efficiency and capacity to research on rare sleep disorders. The Somnology and Sleep Medicine Centers of Excellence discussed above would spearhead this dedicated focus on basic, clinical, and translational research and would promote collaborations among all sites conducting research relevant to somnology and sleep medicine. Similar to cancer centers, the Somnology and Sleep Medicine Centers of Excellence would act as local, regional, and national resources for the scientific community and the community at large. This will require coordination among all participating centers. Although online technologies greatly enhance the nearly instantaneous sharing of ideas across the nation and globally, the research network envisioned by the committee would involve not only a strong virtual component but also a structured plan for periodic and regular meetings and workshops to set priorities and strengthen interactions.

The committee strongly believes that the somnology and sleep medicine field is now sufficiently mature for the development of a National Somnology and Sleep Medicine Research Network and could successfully compete for network funding from the NHLBI and other members of the Trans-NIH Sleep Research Coordinating Committee that have substantial commitments to somnology and sleep disorders research. Individual Somnology and Sleep Medicine Centers of Excellence could compose the cornerstone of this network, and institutions that do not have sufficient scope and size to successfully compete for a Somnology and Sleep Medicine Center of Excellence would be active affiliate members of this network. The committee envisions a sustained network for somnology and sleep medicine in the United States that would facilitate public education, career development opportunities, translational research, and implementation of multi-center clinical trials.

The process of developing components of the National Somnology and Sleep Medicine Research Network can draw on the experiences of several such networks that already exist, but with more focused objectives, such as the aforementioned National Cancer Institute centers. The NHLBI currently sponsors 12 networks. The National Institute of Child Health and Human Development sponsors the National Center for Medical Rehabilitation Research regional research networks. Each network is coordinated and administered out of one academic institution, which coordinates the efforts of institutions that are affiliated with the network. The leading coordinating institutions are structured to facilitate major collaborations among affiliated institutions, with the potential to connect with researchers from other facilities within the region. They support multidisciplinary research cores, information transfer, and pilot projects with the goal of facilitating ongoing projects and stimulating the development of future research activities in medical rehabilitation (NCMRR, 2005).

Another example of a regional network is the Muscular Dystrophy Cooperative Research Centers. Cosponsored by the National Institute of Arthritis and Musculoskeletal and Skin Diseases, the National Institute of Neurological Disorders and Stroke, the National Institute of Child Health and Human Development, as well as the Muscular Dystrophy Association, these centers work collaboratively on both basic and clinical research projects. Each center has one or more core facility to support them and must also make core resources or services available to the national muscular dystrophy research community.

The National Somnology and Sleep Medicine Research Network envisioned by the committee would be structured to facilitate and require active involvement of the participants and substantive interactions between basic and clinical researchers. As will be described in detail in Chapter 9, the committee calls on new and existing academic programs in somnology and sleep medicine to be organized to meet the criteria of three types of interdisciplinary sleep programs—Type I, Type II, or Type III. A Type I clinical interdisciplinary sleep program is designed to provide optimal interdisciplinary clinical care for individuals who suffer sleep loss or sleep disorders. Although not consisting of large research components, a Type I program should have a data collection and management system that provides clinical data to a coordinating center within the network. A Type II training and research interdisciplinary sleep program includes the characteristics of a Type I program, but in addition is designed to provide optimal education, training, and research in somnology and sleep medicine. A Type III regional interdisciplinary sleep program coordinator includes the characteristics of Type I and II programs; however, a Type III program is designed to serve as a regional comprehensive center and coordinator for education, training, basic research, and clinical research in somnology and sleep medicine within the National Somnology and Sleep Medicine Research Network. The Committee also envisions that all Type I and II programs would be affiliate members of the National Somnology and Sleep Medicine Network.

Although there are only a limited number of academic institutions that currently have the capacity to be a Type III regional interdisciplinary sleep program, this should not delay the establishment of the research network. Initially the network could consist of a limited number of programs. The network would benefit greatly from cultural, ethnic, and environmental diversity. Therefore, a long-range goal should be to have 8 to 10 geographically distributed regional coordinating centers.

In summary, the National Somnology and Sleep Medicine Research Network should do the following:

- Coordinate and support the current cadre of basic and clinical researchers.
- Train new investigators and fellows through local and remote mentoring programs.
- Provide core facilities for basic research.
- Support multisite clinical research in children, adolescents, adults, and elderly people.
- Create and support virtual networking centers to facilitate the sharing of data and resources online and enhance collaborations with researchers not working in research centers.
- Create a data coordinating center that includes an Internet-based clearing house for the publication of all data produced in cooperation with the research and clinical network.
- Work with the CDC to integrate and support surveillance and population-based research.
- Create and coordinate public health education campaigns.

Efforts to develop a National Somnology and Sleep Medicine Research and Clinical Network are consistent with many of the goals of the NIH Roadmap (NIH, 2006b), including an emphasis on translational research that results in clinically useful therapies and a need for multidisciplinary efforts to be used to address this complex medical condition.

Recommendation 8.2: The National Institutes of Health should establish a National Somnology and Sleep Medicine Research Network.

The National Center on Sleep Disorders Research, in collaboration with the Trans-NIH Sleep Research Coordination Committee, should establish a National Somnology and Sleep Medicine Research Network. Type III regional interdisciplinary sleep programs designated by the National Institutes of Health would act as regional centers working with basic research laboratories and sleep cores at NIH-designated clinical translational research centers. It is envisioned that the networks would do the following:

- Coordinate and support the current and future cadre of basic and clinical researchers.
- Train new investigators and fellows.
- Provide core capabilities for basic, clinical, and translational research.
- Support multisite clinical research in children, adolescents, adults, and elderly.
- Create and support virtual networking centers to facilitate the standardization and sharing of data and resources online and enhance collaborations with researchers not working in research centers.
- Create a data coordinating center that includes an Internet-based clearing house for the publication of all data produced in cooperation with the research and clinical network.
- Together with the Agency for Healthcare Research and Quality develop standards for research, outcomes, and clinical practice.
- Work with the Centers for Disease Control and Prevention to integrate and support surveillance and population-based research.

Establish Sleep Laboratories in the NIH Clinical Research Program

As described in the 2003 research plan, "[t]he role of sleep disturbances and sleep disorders in the morbidity of most chronic conditions is understudied . . . [and] poorly understood"(NHLBI, 2003). The report further went on to call for greater study of the "bidirectional relationship between sleep processes and disease development, progression, and morbidity." Given these priorities, it is of note that the intramural clinical research program at the NIH does not have a sleep laboratory. Consequently, many experimental sleep therapies and the relationship between sleep processes and disease development are not being examined. If there is adequate investment in extramural sleep-related programs, the field can continue to make great strides; therefore, the committee does not support use of limited resources to invest in an intramural somnology and sleep disorders research program. However, because appropriate sleep patterns constitute one of the basic tenets of health, the committee strongly urges the NIH intramural clinical research program to ascertain the need for potentially establishing a sleep study laboratory so that evaluation of sleep may be integrated into ongoing relevant clinical research protocols at NIH.

Recommendation 8.3: The National Institutes of Health should ascertain the need for a transdisciplinary sleep laboratory that would serve as a core resource in its intramural clinical research program.

The director of the National Institutes of Health Intramural Research Program should ascertain the need for a transdisciplinary sleep laboratory within the intramural clinical research program that would serve as a core resource for the community of intramural clinical investigators across all institutes.

REFERENCES

AASM (American Academy of Sleep Medicine). 2005. *The International Classification of Sleep Disorders*. Westchester, IL: AASM.

Alvarez GG, Ayas NT. 2004. The impact of daily sleep duration on health: A review of the literature. *Progress in Cardiovascular Nursing* 19(2):56–59.

Amiel J, Laudier B, Attie-Bitach T, Trang H, de Pontual L, Gener B, Trochet D, Etchevers H, Ray P, Simonneau M, Vekemans M, Munnich A, Gaultier C, Lyonnet S. 2003. Polyalanine expansion and frameshift mutations of the paired-like homeobox gene *PHOX2B* in congenital central hypoventilation syndrome. *Nature Genetics* 33(4):459–461.

Amin RS, Kimball TR, Kalra M, Jeffries JL, Carroll JL, Bean JA, Witt SA, Glascock BJ, Daniels SR. 2005. Left ventricular function in children with sleep-disordered breathing. *American Journal of Cardiology* 95(6):801–804.

Ancoli-Israel S, Kripke DF, Klauber MR, Mason WJ, Fell R, Kaplan O. 1991. Sleep-disordered breathing in community-dwelling elderly. *Sleep* 14(6):486–495.

Ancoli-Israel S, Klauber MR, Stepnowsky C, Estline E, Chinn A, Fell R. 1995. Sleep-disordered breathing in African-American elderly. *American Journal of Respiratory and Critical Care Medicine* 152(6 Pt 1):1946–1949.

Babu AR, Herdegen J, Fogelfeld L, Shott S, Mazzone T. 2005. Type 2 diabetes, glycemic control, and continuous positive airway pressure in obstructive sleep apnea. *Archives of Internal Medicine* 165(4):447–452.

Bader G, Gillberg C, Johnson M, Kadesjö B, Rasmussen P. 2003. Activity and sleep in children with ADHD. *Sleep* 26:A136.

Barger LK, Cade BE, Ayas NT, Cronin JW, Rosner B, Speizer FE, Czeisler CA, Harvard Work Hours HaS Group. 2005. Extended work shifts and the risk of motor vehicle crashes among interns. *New England Journal of Medicine* 352(2):125–134.

Boggild H, Knutsson A. 1999. Shift work, risk factors and cardiovascular disease. *Scandinavian Journal of Work Environment Health* 25(2):85–99.

Brown SA, Fleury-Olela F, Nagoshi E, Hauser C, Juge C, Meier CA, Chicheportiche R, Dayer JM, Albrecht U, Schibler U. 2005. The period length of fibroblast circadian gene expression varies widely among human individuals. *PLoS Biology* 3(10):e338.

Buxbaum SG, Elston RC, Tishler PV, Redline S. 2002. Genetics of the apnea hypopnea index in Caucasians and African Americans: I. Segregation analysis. *Genetic Epidemiology* 22(3):243–253.

Carskadon MA, Acebo C, Jenni OG. 2004. Regulation of adolescent sleep: Implications for behavior. *Annals of the New York Academy of Science* 1021:276–291.

Cavallo A, Mallory ML, Association of Medical School Pediatric Department Chairs Inc. 2004. Sleep deprivation, residency training, and ACGME rules: Practical guidelines. *Journal of Pediatrics* 145(6):717–718.

Cizza G, Skarulis M, Mignot E. 2005. A link between short sleep and obesity: Building the evidence for causation. *Sleep* 28(10):1217–1220.

Czeisler CA, Walsh JK, Roth T, Hughes RJ, Wright KP, Kingsbury L, Arora S, Schwartz JR, Niebler GE, Dinges DF. 2005. Modafinil for excessive sleepiness associated with shift-work sleep disorder. *New England Journal of Medicine* 353(5):476–486.

de la Eva RC, Baur LA, Donaghue KC, Waters KA. 2002. Metabolic correlates with obstructive sleep apnea in obese subjects. *Journal of Pediatrics* 140(6):654–659.

Dolan-Sewell RT, Riley WT, Hunt CE. 2005. NIH State-of-the-Science Conference on Chronic Insomnia. *Journal of Clinical Sleep Medicine* 1(4):335–336.

Fregosi RF, Quan SF, Kaemingk KL, Morgan WJ, Goodwin JL, Cabrera R, Gmitro A. 2003. Sleep-disordered breathing, pharyngeal size and soft tissue anatomy in children. *Journal of Applied Physiology* 95(5):2030–2038.

Gillette MU, Roth T, Kiley JP. 1999. NIH funding of sleep research: A prospective and retrospective view. *Sleep* 22(7):956–958.

Gottlieb DJ, Chase C, Vezina RM, Heeren TC, Corwin MJ, Auerbach SH, Weese-Mayer DE, Lesko SM. 2004a. Sleep-disordered breathing symptoms are associated with poorer cognitive function in 5-year-old children. *Journal of Pediatrics* 145(4):458–464.

Gottlieb DJ, DeStefano AL, Foley DJ, Mignot E, Redline S, Givelber RJ, Young T. 2004b. APOE ε4 is associated with obstructive sleep apnea/hypopnea: The Sleep Heart Health Study. *Neurology* 63(4):664–668.

Gottlieb DJ, Punjabi NM, Newman AB, Resnick HE, Redline S, Baldwin CM, Nieto FJ. 2005. Association of sleep time with diabetes mellitus and impaired glucose tolerance. *Archives of Internal Medicine* 165(8):863–867.

Gozal D, Burnside MM. 2004. Increased upper airway collapsibility in children with obstructive sleep apnea during wakefulness. *American Journal of Respiratory and Critical Care Medicine* 169(2):163–167.

Gurubhagavatula I, Maislin G, Nkwuo JE, Pack AI. 2004. Occupational screening for obstructive sleep apnea in commercial drivers. *American Journal of Respiratory and Critical Care Medicine* 170(4):371–376.

Harrington JM. 1994. Shift work and health—A critical review of the literature on working hours. *Annals of the Academy of Medicine, Singapore* 23(5):699–705.

Harris GC, Wimmer M, Aston-Jones G. 2005. A role for lateral hypothalamic orexin neurons in reward seeking. *Nature* 437(7058):556–559.

Harsch IA, Schahin SP, Radespiel-Troger M, Weintz O, Jahreiss H, Fuchs FS, Wiest GH, Hahn EG, Lohmann T, Konturek PC, Ficker JH. 2004. Continuous positive airway pressure treatment rapidly improves insulin sensitivity in patients with obstructive sleep apnea syndrome. *American Journal of Respiratory and Critical Care Medicine* 169(2):156–162.

Howard ME, Desai AV, Grunstein RR, Hukins C, Armstrong JG, Joffe D, Swann P, Campbell DA, Pierce RJ. 2004. Sleepiness, sleep-disordered breathing, and accident risk factors in commercial vehicle drivers. *American Journal of Respiratory and Critical Care Medicine* 170(9):1014–1021.

Landrigan CP, Rothschild JM, Cronin JW, Kaushal R, Burdick E, Katz JT, Lilly CM, Stone PH, Lockley SW, Bates DW, Czeisler CA. 2004. Effect of reducing interns' work hours on serious medical errors in intensive care units. *New England Journal of Medicine* 351(18):1838–1848.

Larkin EK, Patel SR, Redline S, Mignot E, Elston RC, Hallmayer J. 2005a. Apolipoprotein E and obstructive sleep apnea: Evaluating whether a candidate gene explains a linkage peak. *Genetic Epidemiology* 30(2):101–110.

Larkin EK, Rosen CL, Kirchner HL, Storfer-Isser A, Emancipator JL, Johnson NL, Zambito AM, Tracy RP, Jenny NS, Redline S. 2005b. Variation of C-reactive protein levels in adolescents: Association with sleep-disordered breathing and sleep duration. *Circulation* 111(15):1978–1984.

Lavie L. 2003. Obstructive sleep apnoea syndrome—An oxidative stress disorder. *Sleep Medicine Reviews* 7(1):35–51.

Lockley SW, Cronin JW, Evans EE, Cade BE, Lee CJ, Landrigan CP, Rothschild JM, Katz JT, Lilly CM, Stone PH, Aeschbach D, Czeisler CA, Harvard Work Hours HaS Group. 2004. Effect of reducing interns' weekly work hours on sleep and attentional failures. *New England Journal of Medicine* 351(18):1829–1837.

Lyamin O, Pryaslova J, Lance V, Siegel J. 2005. Animal behaviour: Continuous activity in cetaceans after birth. *Nature* 435(7046):1177.

Manconi M, Govoni V, De Vito A, Economou NT, Cesnik E, Casetta I, Mollica G, Ferini-Strambi L, Granieri E. 2004. Restless legs syndrome and pregnancy. *Neurology* 63(6):1065–1069.

Marcus CL, Katz ES, Lutz J, Black CA, Galster P, Carson KA. 2005. Upper airway dynamic responses in children with the obstructive sleep apnea syndrome. *Pediatric Research* 57(1):99–107.

Maret S, Franken P, Dauvilliers Y, Ghyselinck NB, Chambon P, Tafti M. 2005. Retinoic acid signaling affects cortical synchrony during sleep. *Science* 310(5745):111–113.

Marin JM, Carrizo SJ, Vicente E, Agusti AG. 2005. Long-term cardiovascular outcomes in men with obstructive sleep apnoea-hypopnoea with or without treatment with continuous positive airway pressure: An observational study. *Lancet* 365(9464):1046–1053.

Mignot E, Chen W, Black J. 2003. On the value of measuring CSF hypocretin-1 in diagnosing narcolepsy. *Sleep* 26(6):646–649.

Monk TH. 2005. Aging human circadian rhythms: Conventional wisdom may not always be right. *Journal of Biological Rhythms* 20(4):366–374.

Morin CM. 2004. Cognitive-behavioral approaches to the treatment of insomnia. *Journal of Clinical Psychiatry* 65(suppl 16):33–40.

NCI (National Cancer Institute). 2004. *The Cancer Centers Branch of the National Cancer Institute: Policies and Guidelines Relating to the Cancer Center Support Grant.* [Online]. Available: http://www3.cancer.gov/cancercenters/CCSG_Guide12_04.pdf [accessed December 19, 2005].

NCMRR (National Center for Medical Rehabilitation Research). 2005. *NCMRR Research Networks.* [Online]. Available: http://www.nichd.nih.gov/about/ncmrr/networks.htm [accessed December 19, 2005].

NHLBI (National Heart, Lung, and Blood Institute). 1996. *National Sleep Disorders Research Plan, 1996.* Bethesda, MD: National Institutes of Health.

NHLBI. 2003. *National Sleep Disorders Research Plan, 2003.* Bethesda, MD: National Institutes of Health.

NIH (National Institutes of Health). 2004. *Program Announcement: PA-05-046.* [Online]. Available: http://grants.nih.gov/grants/guide/pa-files/pa-05-046.html [accessed March 6, 2006].

NIH. 2005. *Request For Applications: RFA-HL-06-003.* [Online]. Available: http://grants.nih.gov/grants/guide/rfa-files/RFA-HL-06-003.html [accessed March 6, 2006].

NIH 2006a. *Program Announcement PAR-05-144: Developing Centers for Innovation in Services and Intervention Research (DCISIR).* [Online]. Available: http://grants.nih.gov/grants/guide/pa-files/PAR-05-144.html [accessed January 27, 2006].

NIH. 2006b. *Request For Applications: RFA-RM-06-002.* [Online]. Available: http://grants.nih.gov/grants/guide/rfa-files/RFA-RM-06-002.html [accessed February 6, 2006].

NIMH (National Institute of Mental Health). 2006. *Program Announcement: PAR-02-123.* [Online]. Available: http://grants.nih.gov/grants/guide/pa-files/PAR-02-123.html [accessed January 27, 2006].

Nishino S, Kanbayashi T. 2005. Symptomatic narcolepsy, cataplexy and hypersomnia, and their implications in the hypothalamic hypocretin/orexin system. *Sleep Medicine Reviews* 9(4):269–310.

Nofzinger EA, Buysse DJ, Germain A, Price JC, Miewald JM, Kupfer DJ. 2004. Functional neuroimaging evidence for hyperarousal in insomnia. *American Journal of Psychiatry* 161(11):2126–2128.

Nowbar S, Burkart KM, Gonzales R, Fedorowicz A, Gozansky WS, Gaudio JC, Taylor MR, Zwillich CW. 2004. Obesity-associated hypoventilation in hospitalized patients: Prevalence, effects, and outcome. *American Journal of Medicine* 116(1):1–7.

Owens JA, Rosen CL, Mindell JA. 2003. Medication use in the treatment of pediatric insomnia: Results of a survey of community-based pediatricians. *Pediatrics* 111(5 Pt 1):e628–e635.

Palmer LJ, Buxbaum SG, Larkin E, Patel SR, Elston RC, Tishler PV, Redline S. 2003. A whole-genome scan for obstructive sleep apnea and obesity. *American Journal of Human Genetics* 72(2):340–350.

Palmer LJ, Buxbaum SG, Larkin EK, Patel SR, Elston RC, Tishler PV, Redline S. 2004. Whole genome scan for obstructive sleep apnea and obesity in African-American families. *American Journal of Respiratory and Critical Care Medicine* 169(12):1314–1321.

Petersen A, Gil J, Maat-Schieman ML, Bjorkqvist M, Tanila H, Araujo IM, Smith R, Popovic N, Wierup N, Norlen P, Li JY, Roos RA, Sundler F, Mulder H, Brundin P. 2005. Orexin loss in Huntington's disease. *Human Molecular Genetics* 14(1):39–47.

Punjabi NM, Shahar E, Redline S, Gottlieb DJ, Givelber R, Resnick HE, Sleep Heart Health Study Investigators. 2004. Sleep-disordered breathing, glucose intolerance, and insulin resistance: The Sleep Heart Health Study. *American Journal of Epidemiology* 160(6):521–530.

Rattenborg NC, Mandt BH, Obermeyer WH, Winsauer PJ, Huber R, Wikelski M, Benca RM. 2004. Migratory sleeplessness in the white-crowned sparrow (*Zonotrichia leucophrys gambelii*). *PLoS Biology* 2(7):E212.

Rosen CL, Larkin EK, Kirchner HL, Emancipator JL, Bivins SF, Surovec SA, Martin RJ, Redline S. 2003. Prevalence and risk factors for sleep-disordered breathing in 8- to 11-year-old children: Association with race and prematurity. *Journal of Pediatrics* 142(4): 383–389.

Rosen CL, Storfer-Isser A, Taylor HG, Kirchner HL, Emancipator JL, Redline S. 2004. Increased behavioral morbidity in school-aged children with sleep-disordered breathing. *Pediatrics* 114(6):1640–1648.

Roth T, Roehrs T. 2003. Insomnia: Epidemiology, characteristics, and consequences. *Clinical Cornerstone* 5(3):5–15.

Row BW, Liu R, Xu W, Kheirandish L, Gozal D. 2003. Intermittent hypoxia is associated with oxidative stress and spatial learning deficits in the rat. *American Journal of Respiratory and Critical Care Medicine* 167(11):1548–1553.

Rye DB. 2004. The two faces of Eve: Dopamine's modulation of wakefulness and sleep. *Neurology* 63(8 Suppl 3):S2–S7.

Saper CB, Scammell TE, Lu J. 2005. Hypothalamic regulation of sleep and circadian rhythms. *Nature* 437(7063):1257–1263.

Singh M, Drake C, Roehrs T, Koshorek G, Roth T. 2005. The prevalence of SOREMPs in the general population. *Sleep* 28(Abstract Suppl):A221.

Spiegel K, Tasali E, Penev P, Van Cauter E. 2004. Brief communication: Sleep curtailment in healthy young men is associated with decreased leptin levels, elevated ghrelin levels, and increased hunger and appetite. *Annals of Internal Medicine* 141(11):846–850.

Tafti M, Petit B, Chollet D, Neidhart E, de Bilbao F, Kiss JZ, Wood PA, Franken P. 2003. Deficiency in short-chain fatty acid beta-oxidation affects theta oscillations during sleep. *Nature Genetics* 34(3):320–325.

Taheri S, Lin L, Austin D, Young T, Mignot E. 2004. Short sleep duration is associated with reduced leptin, elevated ghrelin, and increased body mass index. *PLoS Medicine* 1(3):210–217.

Tauman R, Ivanenko A, O'Brien LM, Gozal D. 2004. Plasma C-reactive protein levels among children with sleep-disordered breathing. *Pediatrics* 113(6):e564–e569.

Trenkwalder C, Paulus W, Walters AS. 2005. The restless legs syndrome. *Lancet Neurology* 4(8):465–475.

Turek FW, Joshu C, Kohsaka A, Lin E, Ivanova G, McDearmon E, Laposky A, Losee-Olson S, Easton A, Jensen DR, Eckel RH, Takahashi JS, Bass J. 2005. Obesity and metabolic syndrome in circadian *Clock* mutant mice. *Science* 308(5724):1043–1045.

U.S. Congress, Senate. 1993. *National Institutes of Health Revitalization Act of 1993; bill to establish a National Center on Sleep Disorders Research within the National Heart, Lung, and Blood Institute.* 103rd Cong., S.104:285b–287.

Veasey SC, Davis CW, Fenik P, Zhan G, Hsu YJ, Pratico D, Gow A. 2004a. Long-term intermittent hypoxia in mice: Protracted hypersomnolence with oxidative injury to sleep-wake brain regions. *Sleep* 27(2):194–201.

Veasey SC, Zhan G, Fenik P, Pratico D. 2004b. Long-term intermittent hypoxia: Reduced excitatory hypoglossal nerve output. *American Journal of Respiratory and Critical Care Medicine* 170(6):665–672.

Weese-Mayer DE, Berry-Kravis EM, Zhou L, Maher BS, Silvestri JM, Curran ME, Marazita ML. 2003. Idiopathic congenital central hypoventilation syndrome: Analysis of genes pertinent to early autonomic nervous system embryologic development and identification of mutations in *PHOX2b*. *American Journal of Medical Genetics: Part A* 123(3):267–278.

Xu Y, Padiath QS, Shapiro RE, Jones CR, Wu SC, Saigoh N, Saigoh K, Ptacek LJ, Fu YH. 2005. Functional consequences of a *CKIdelta* mutation causing familial advanced sleep phase syndrome. *Nature* 434(7033):640–644.

Yaggi HK, Concato J, Kernan WN, Lichtman JH, Brass LM, Mohsenin V. 2005. Obstructive sleep apnea as a risk factor for stroke and death. *New England Journal of Medicine* 353(19):2034–2041.

Yamazaki S, Numano R, Abe M, Hida A, Takahashi R, Ueda M, Block GD, Sakaki Y, Menaker M, Tei H. 2000. Resetting central and peripheral circadian oscillators in transgenic rats. *Science* 288(5466):682–685.

Yokoe T, Minoguchi K, Matsuo H, Oda N, Minoguchi H, Yoshino G, Hirano T, Adachi M. 2003. Elevated levels of C-reactive protein and interleukin-6 in patients with obstructive sleep apnea syndrome are decreased by nasal continuous positive airway pressure. *Circulation* 107(8):1129–1134.

Yoo SH, Yamazaki S, Lowrey PL, Shimomura K, Ko CH, Buhr ED, Siepka SM, Hong HK, Oh WJ, Yoo OJ, Menaker M, Takahashi JS. 2004. PERIOD2::LUCIFERASE real-time reporting of circadian dynamics reveals persistent circadian oscillations in mouse peripheral tissues. *Proceedings of the National Academy of Sciences of the United States of America* 101(15):5339–5346.

Young T, Palta M, Dempsey J, Skatrud J, Weber S, Badr S. 1993. The occurrence of sleep-disordered breathing among middle-aged adults. *New England Journal of Medicine* 328(17):1230–1235.

9

Building Sleep Programs in Academic Health Centers

CHAPTER SUMMARY *New organizational structures for interdisciplinary sleep programs in academic health centers are necessary. This chapter makes the case for why interdisciplinary sleep programs are needed nationwide. It then offers a framework for establishing academic somnology and sleep medicine programs. Without being prescriptive, the chapter discusses operating principles gleaned from interdisciplinary somnology and sleep medicine programs that have flourished, as well as from others that have struggled. Finally, the chapter unveils the committee's recommendation for a three-tier structure that ensures all academic health centers provide adequate interdisciplinary clinical care, with subsequent tiers also emphasizing training and research components. If these components and guiding principles are followed, interdisciplinary sleep programs can thrive, whether as a freestanding department or as a program within an existing department or division. Although not a trivial undertaking, it is necessary that all academic health centers strive to develop or transform their current sleep activities into interdisciplinary sleep programs. Some academic health centers are close to, or already have, achieved strong clinical programs. Once a sleep program is established, whether multidimensional or not, it can generate higher revenues than costs, according to a fiscal analysis presented in this chapter. To ensure improved care and scientific advances, the committee recommends clinical accreditation standards be updated to address patient care needs.*

Building sleep programs at academic health centers is not a matter of bricks and mortar. It is a matter of crumbling the organizational walls that separate a variety of traditional scientific and medical disciplines to function more appropriately to meet patient care needs and to facilitate research and training. In this chapter, the committee lays out a vision for each of the nation's 125 academic health centers to formally establish an interdisciplinary somnology and sleep medicine program. Building sleep programs nationwide will strengthen Somnology and Sleep Medicine as a recognized medical specialty. There is too much at stake—a large patient population, high levels of underdiagnosis, and high public health toll—for inaction.

RATIONALE FOR SLEEP PROGRAMS IN ACADEMIC HEALTH CENTERS

The rationale for sleep programs has been presented throughout this report. This section of the chapter recapitulates those arguments concerning the magnitude of the public health problem and the lack of appropriate education at every level of academic instruction. It also answers the specific question—why is a sleep program optimally interdisciplinary?

Public Health Burden Is High

Chronic sleep loss and sleep disorders are serious and common problems, affecting an estimated 50 to 70 million Americans (NHLBI, 2003). These conditions have a bearing upon nearly every facet of public health—morbidity, mortality, productivity, accidents and injuries, quality of life, family well-being, and health care utilization. Earlier chapters of this report documented the prevalence of sleep problems and their health consequences. Sleep loss and sleep-disordered breathing, for example, are associated with obesity, diabetes, hypertension, cardiovascular disease, and stroke (Chapter 3).

Nearly all types of sleep problems affect personal as well as public health (Chapter 4). The foremost symptom of sleep loss and most sleep disorders—daytime sleepiness—affects performance and cognition. When these functions are perturbed, whether at work, in school, or in the community, serious consequences can ensue. One of the most serious comes in the form of motor vehicle injuries. More broadly, the annual direct and indirect costs of sleep problems reach well beyond $100 billion (Chapter 4).

Most Patients Remain Undiagnosed and Untreated

Most individuals with sleep disorders remain undiagnosed and thus untreated. Two large epidemiological studies, each with thousands of subjects, found that the vast majority, up to 90 percent, of individuals with sleep-disordered breathing had not been diagnosed (Young et al., 1997; Kapur et al., 2002). Narcolepsy and insomnia are also infrequently detected (Benca, 2005; Singh et al., 2005). All of the findings reported above are consistent with surveys indicating that primary care physicians infrequently ask questions about sleep problems (Chung et al., 2001; Reuveni et al., 2004).

Patients with Sleep Loss and Sleep Disorders Require Long-Term Care and Chronic Disease Management

Sleep disorders are chronic conditions with complex treatments. They are frequently comorbid with other sleep disorders, as well as other complex conditions (e.g., cardiovascular disease, depression, and diabetes) (Chapter 3). Sleep disorders also are dynamic, meaning that the underlying condition or its treatment changes with age and onset of new comorbidities.

Despite the importance of early recognition and treatment, the primary focus of most existing sleep centers is on diagnosis rather than on comprehensive management of sleep loss and sleep disorders as chronic conditions. The narrow focus of sleep centers may largely be the unintended result of accreditation criteria, which emphasize diagnostic standards, as explained later, as well as a result of reimbursement, which is for diagnostic testing.

There are numerous reasons for a paradigm shift to chronic disease management. Proper treatment for most sleep disorders—as for other chronic diseases such as congestive heart failure, diabetes, asthma, and depression—requires a period of time for fine-tuning, extended follow-up, and lifestyle changes. Sleep disorders cannot be adequately treated in a single visit.

The need for chronic care management is even more pressing for the many patients (probably up to 30 percent) with combined sleep pathologies. These patients are difficult to manage without multiple clinicians being involved. For example, 20 to 50 percent of narcoleptics have obstructive sleep apnea (OSA); 40 percent of narcoleptics have insomnia; 40 percent of narcoleptics have periodic leg movements disorder (Baker et al., 1986; Cherniack, 2005; Chung, 2005). Residual daytime sleepiness is common in patients with sleep apnea adequately treated with continuous positive airway pressure (CPAP); it may require additional pharmacotherapy. Similarly, a large portion of patients with sleep apnea have insomnia and vice versa. Insomnia plus sleep apnea is a difficult combination, as it makes it more challenging for patients to tolerate CPAP and thus increases the likelihood of failure if the combination is not addressed.

Sleep disorders are also common in patients with various medical and psychiatric conditions. For example, increased sleep apnea is found in obese subjects with or without the metabolic syndrome and in patients with stroke or various neurodegenerative disorders. Restless legs syndrome can occur in the context of iron deficiency, renal failure, and pregnancy. Rapid-eye-movement (REM) behavior disorder is often an antecedent of Parkinson's disease and Lewy body disease. Hypersomnia is a common symptom in Parkinson's disease, depression, and various neurological conditions. Similarly, insomnia can occur in the context of various medical and psychiatric conditions and is associated with depression. These patients often require coordinated care across disciplines. As will be described below, interdisciplinary sleep programs provide the best structure to facilitate this type of care.

Inadequate Numbers of Training and Research Programs

Training of health professionals seldom deals with sleep hygiene, sleep loss, and sleep disorders (Chapters 5 and 7). Although there have been some improvements, challenges lie ahead for training of medical, nursing, and pharmacy students. Research opportunities for medical residents, subspecialty residents, and doctoral and postdoctoral researchers are also limited. Most sleep researchers are clustered in a handful of institutions, according to the grants analysis presented in Chapter 7. Because mentoring is critical to success in clinical or basic research, the concentration of mentors at so few institutions leaves students elsewhere with few opportunities to successfully enter the field, thereby constricting the pipeline of new clinicians and researchers.

Large Body of Knowledge

Given the limited number of sleep experts nationwide and their clustering in a handful of institutions, is there a sufficient knowledge base and need to justify creation of an interdisciplinary somnology and sleep medicine program at each of the nation's academic health centers? The simple answer is yes. Over the last 25 years, the field has grown to the point that a large base of knowledge now exists regarding diagnosis and treatment. Several recent milestones for the field attest to the achievement of a critical mass of knowledge. Sleep medicine is a medical subspecialty now recognized by the American Board of Medical Specialties. The Accreditation Council for Graduate Medical Education (ACGME) now accredits fellowship training programs. Numerous educational resources, including curriculum, are available from the American Academy of Sleep Medicine. The standard 1,500-page textbook, *Principles and Practice of Sleep Medicine*, is in its fourth edition. There is also a vibrant body of research, described in previous chapters, on the basic science of sleep and sleep disorders. The number of recipients of National Institutes of Health (NIH) R01 grants in sleep has risen from 100 to 253 over the last 10 years (Chapter 8).

Why Is Somnology and Sleep Medicine Program Optimally Interdisciplinary?

Medicine has historically drawn strength from compartmentalizing into distinct specialties and subspecialties. But sleep medicine is not an ordinary subspecialty; its purview spans multiple organ systems. Consequently, complications that arise as a result of sleep loss and sleep disorders require attention from health care professionals in many disciplines. Further, sleep cycles and perturbations exert physiological effects. The major circadian rhythm that originates in the brain influences body temperature, heart rate, muscle tone, and the secretion of hormones. There are also circadian clocks in the heart and other organs. Beyond maintaining proper health and normal cognitive and motor function, sleep is required for survival (Rechtschaffen et al., 1989). Disturbance of sleep or loss of sleep has widespread metabolic implications (Chapter 2). Finally, the scientific study of sleep loss and sleep disorders integrates the efforts of many disciplines, including but not limited to neuroscience, epidemiology, molecular and cellular biology, and genetics.

Thus, by its very nature, the field is at the interface of many medical and scientific disciplines. Therefore, it is not surprising that board certification in sleep medicine is under the auspices of four different medical boards—the American Boards of Internal Medicine, Pediatrics, Otolaryngology, and Psychiatry and Neurology.

To harness the needed specialties, sleep programs must be multidisciplinary. But being multidisciplinary is not sufficient. A true interdisciplinary program is an orientation, approach, or philosophy that seeks to go beyond the sum of the parts to build a new enterprise (Figure 9-1). It is not necessary for sleep medicine to be housed in a stand-alone department or division. Many interdisciplinary sleep programs thrive in a department (see below). However, sleep programs that are restricted to a single department that does not allow for interdisciplinary treatment and care tend to struggle. This is partly because they fail to provide a sense of identity; they lack a career path for faculty, which in turn, makes it difficult to recruit students and additional faculty—the very ingredients needed to establish and rejuvenate a field. Further, fragmented programs lack the collaborative spirit necessary for excellence in clinical care, training, and research.

The field of somnology and sleep medicine is an excellent example of an interdisciplinary field because it strives to integrate ideas, tools, and perspectives from several disciplines in order to advance understanding beyond the scope of a single discipline or field of research practice. The field is being forged from existing fields of cardiology, dentistry, endocrinology, geriatrics, neurology, neuropsychopharmacology, neuroscience, nursing, otolaryngology, pediatrics, psychiatry, psychology, and pulmonology (Box 9-1). Although

A) Interdisciplinary

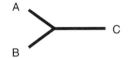

A
B
C

Joined together to work on a common question or problem. Interaction may forge a new research field or discipline.

B) Multidisciplinary

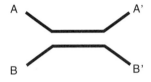

A   A'
B   B'

Disciplines joined together to work on a common question or problem, split apart when work is complete, having likely gained new knowledge, insight, strategies from other disciplines.

FIGURE 9-1 Interdisciplinary and multidisciplinary research.
SOURCE: NAS (2004).

not all of these disciplines are essential for starting a sleep program, each enriches the sleep field in transcendent ways. Two of the most advanced and successful sleep programs, at Harvard University and the University of Pennsylvania, attest to the productivity and vibrancy of an interdisciplinary approach. The success of the program at the University of Pennsylvania also demonstrates that the success of an interdisciplinary sleep program is not dependent on it being its own stand-alone department.

Many types of health professionals are needed to guide the chronic management of sleep disorders. Individuals with sleep loss and sleep disorders have a multitude of health-related problems that require attention from a number of medical disciplines. However, given the limited number of certified health care professionals in sleep medicine and depending on the size and structure of an interdisciplinary sleep program, an individual often may need to be referred to a specialist in another department who may not be certified in sleep medicine. These physicians come from a variety of medical specialties, including internal medicine, pediatrics, otolaryngology, pulmonology, neurology, and psychiatry. Psychologists are essential in behavioral management of sleep disorders.

Nurses and nurse practitioners also play an important role in patient support, patient teaching (especially in sleep hygiene and use of CPAP), follow-up, and promoting adherence to prescribed medical therapies (Epstein and Bootzin, 2002; Lee et al., 2004b). For example, in one of the

---

BOX 9-1
Examples of Interdisciplinary Approaches
to Somnology and Sleep Medicine

Several major accomplishments of somnology and sleep medicine have critically depended on the insights and perspectives of disparate disciplines:

Cardiology
Contributions of cardiology and large cohorts such as the Framingham study led to the Sleep Heart Health Study. This large cohort study has shown that sleep apnea is a risk factor for hypertension, cardiovascular disease, and insulin resistance (Nieto et al., 2000; Shahar et al., 2001; Punjabi et al., 2004).

Endocrinology
Cumulative sleep loss led to reduced leptin and increased ghrelin and hence increased appetite (Spiegel et al., 2004; Taheri et al., 2004). This led to the hypothesis that a hormonally mediated increase in appetite may help to explain why short sleep is a risk factor for obesity.

Pulmonary
Pulmonologists, with their knowledge of pulmonary physiology and ventilators, led the development of nasal CPAP, the most efficacious and common treatment for OSA (Sullivan et al., 1981).

Neurobiology and Genetics
Contributions of neurobiologists led to the demonstration that the rest period in the fruit fly (*Drosophila*) is analogous to mammalian sleep (Shaw et al., 2000; Hendricks et al., 2000).This provides a powerful new genetic model to study sleep mechanisms.

Nursing
Nursing's focus on quality of life led to development of the Functional Outcomes of Sleepiness Questionnaire (Weaver et al., 1997). This instrument, which measures functional capacity in relation to sleep, is now used in clinical trials.

---

few studies of its kind, group education sessions with a pulmonary nurse practitioner were found to enhance CPAP compliance over a 2-year period (Likar et al., 1997). Other nursing interventions, such as appropriately timed exercise, relaxation, and meditation, have also been shown to have beneficial effects on sleep in patients with chronic illnesses such as cancer and those in the acute care setting (Davidson et al., 2001; Mock et al., 2001; Richards et al., 2003; Allison et al., 2004). The role that poor sleep plays in enhancing other symptoms such as depression, fatigue, and pain is also receiving increased attention by nurse clinicians and researchers in an attempt to improve overall symptom management (Miaskowski and Lee, 1999; Lee et al., 2004a; Miaskowski, 2004; Parker et al., 2005).

Despite its promise, the field, like any enterprise that strives to cut across traditional disciplines, is fragile—even in the most supportive environments (NAS, 2004). Sleep clinicians or researchers often face daunting obstacles and disincentives, most of which arise from the customs and practices of individual academic departments. Those obstacles are discussed later in this chapter.

CONSTRAINTS FACING INTERDISCIPLINARY SLEEP PROGRAMS

Many of the most promising new lines of academic pursuit fall outside of traditional disciplines (Ehrenberg and Epifantseva, 2001). Yet interdisciplinary programs, even under the best of circumstances, face barriers and impediments within the confines of academic or research institutions (Ehrenberg et al., 2003; Lach and Schankerman, 2003). A recent National Academies report focusing on ways to facilitate interdisciplinary research was unambiguous about the difficulties confronting these programs, despite their promise. The report observed that, "Researchers interested in pursuing [interdisciplinary research] often face daunting obstacles and disincentives." Some of these obstacles take the form of personal communication or culture barriers; others are related to the tradition in academic institutions of organizing research and teaching activities by discipline-based departments—a tradition that is commonly mirrored in funding organizations, professional societies, and journals (NAS, 2004). This is a generic problem, regardless of whether the interdisciplinary research program deals with nanotechnology or the perception of pain.

The problem of departmental silos permeates interdisciplinary programs within any setting: academic health centers, universities, national laboratories, or industry. The following section presents a series of constraints that together limit the achievement of interdisciplinary programs. These constraints were identified on the basis of an analysis of six sleep programs using methods from operations research that the committee commissioned (see below). Several of the other constraints described in the following sections stem from organizational structures that were established prior to the advent of interdisciplinary research: interdisciplinary programs challenge institutional reward systems; interdisciplinary requirements impose obstacles, different administrative jurisdictions, and lack of appropriately trained staff for sleep studies; and service demand outstrips service supply.

Different Administrative Jurisdictions

As a corollary of the interdisciplinary nature of sleep programs, another constraint is that the services offered by a sleep program often occur at different locations under different administrative jurisdictions. Coordinating all the different types of personnel, lines of authority, policy and procedures, and quality control measures across organizational boundaries is challenging. Who bears the costs and their alignment with benefits and the various revenue streams is neither obvious nor consistent.

Interdisciplinary Programs Challenge the Institutional Reward System

Most institutional reward systems are organized within traditional disciplines or academic departments. These are the units that control what most professionals covet: hiring capacity, tenure and promotion decisions, and space allocation. Interdisciplinary programs challenge this discipline-based reward system, as well as the culture accompanying each discipline (i.e., the customs and shared values that create group cohesion).

The National Academies report on interdisciplinary research conducted three surveys of different groups either working within or overseeing interdisciplinary programs: individual professionals, provosts, and attendees of a conference on interdisciplinary research. In all, some 500 people responded to the surveys (NAS, 2004). The report acknowledges that the samples were not random. But since these are the only surveys of their kind, it is worth noting that the overwhelming majority of respondents (70.7 percent) reported that there were impediments at their institution. The leading barriers identified by individual professionals and provosts: promotion criteria, budget control, control on use of indirect costs, compatibility with university's strategic plans, and space allocation (Figure 9-2).

Interdisciplinary Requirements Impose Obstacles

Interdisciplinary sleep programs, at a minimum, require multidisciplinary participation. As explained earlier, an interdisciplinary program moves beyond being multidisciplinary and is one in which multiple disciplines collaborate in a way that forges a new discipline or endeavor. Provision of clinical services in sleep medicine call upon professionals from internal medicine and its relevant subspecialties (e.g., pulmonology, cardiology, neurology, psychiatry, otolaryngology, pediatrics, and geriatrics) and other disciplines such as nursing, dentistry, and psychology. Research includes genetics, endocrinology, neuroscience, statistics, pharmacology, and epide-

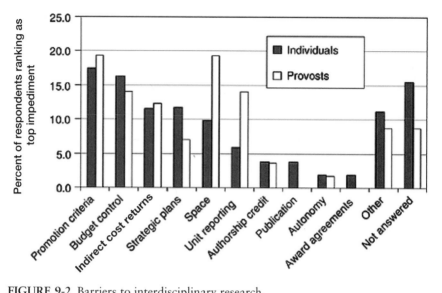

FIGURE 9-2 Barriers to interdisciplinary research.
SOURCE: NAS (2004).

miology. Similar issues exist in teaching undergraduate, graduate, and physicians in their residencies, fellowships, and postdoctoral work.

The unintended consequence is to produce barriers to interdisciplinary patient care, training, and research. Barriers include the length and depth of training in a single field necessary to develop scientists successful at competing for funds, the difficulty in forging a successful career path outside the single disciplinary structure, impediments to obtaining research funding for interdisciplinary research, and the perceived lack of outlets for the publication and dissemination of interdisciplinary research results.

Lack of Appropriately Trained Staff for Sleep Studies

By nearly universal consensus, one sleep technician can monitor at one time two uncomplicated diagnostic studies or one complicated study. Yet, the number of certified technicians nationally is inadequate to meet this need. As with any market in which the supply is less than demand, costs of certified technicians is rising faster than the average rate of inflation or the average rate of medical costs. This has two likely consequences: sleep programs are forced to provide on-the-job training for their technicians; and private-sector organizations are able to adjust their payment structures more readily than academic health centers. Thus, academic centers often provide training, but higher salaries in the private sector lure the experienced technologists. The net consequence is that the lack of trained technicians can act as a serious structural impediment to developing interdisciplinary sleep programs.

Demand Outstrips Supply

Estimates suggest that 50 to 70 million Americans suffer from a chronic disorder of sleep and wakefulness (NHLBI, 2003). As discussed in detail in Chapter 6, the predicted number of individuals with sleep disorders greatly outstrips the ability to provide services using trained personnel (Tachibana et al., 2005). Although there are over 3,250 American Board of Sleep Medicine (ABSM) diplomats, inadequate staffing results in long wait time until next appointment. Analysis commissioned on behalf of the committee indicated that wait times could range by as much as 4 weeks to 4 months.

KEY COMPONENTS AND GUIDING PRINCIPLES FOR BUILDING SLEEP PROGRAMS

In this section, the committee offers guidance to academic health centers about the missions and roles of sleep programs. There is no single way to create or expand an interdisciplinary sleep program. The committee recognizes that every institution has established—often over many decades—its own policies, procedures, institutional organization, and lines of authority. The committee offers principles that can guide development of somnology and sleep medicine programs. For each of these key components and guiding principles, the committee draws on its experience with programs that have been successful, as well as those that have struggled. It also draws on the formidable barriers identified in the previous section. If these components and guiding principles are followed, interdisciplinary sleep programs can thrive, whether as a freestanding department or as a program within an existing department or division.

Key Components of Interdisciplinary Sleep Programs

Strong Linkages from Diagnostic Testing Centers to Comprehensive Care

Diagnostic sleep centers need to establish strong linkages with treatment providers. The emphasis of sleep centers may be too narrowly focused on diagnosis. The committee heard testimony and anecdotal reports that many patients, once tested, are lost to follow-up. Once diagnosed, severe sleep apnea, for instance, optimally should be followed up by a physician certified in sleep medicine. Less severe forms of apnea may warrant watching or referral to a dentist for preparation of dental devices, if a dental problem is etiologically related.

A Chronic Disease Management Model

Responding to the well-documented problem that most Americans with chronic diseases receive suboptimal care (IOM, 2000; 2001), Wagner and colleagues have developed and tested a model for improved management of chronic illness in the primary care setting. Components of the model have been demonstrated to lower health care costs or lower use of health care services (Bodenheimer et al., 2002). The model's six components are:

- community resources (e.g., exercise programs, senior centers, and self-help groups)
- health care organization (a provider organization and its relationships with purchasers, insurers, and other providers)
- self-management support (ways to help families acquire the skills and confidence to manage their chronic illnesses)
- delivery system design (structuring medical practice to create teams, including nonphysician personnel, for patient support and follow-up)
- decision support (access to specialists that does not necessarily require a specialty referral)
- clinical information systems (e.g., reminder systems, feedback to physicians, registries for planning patient care)

Education and Training

Few health professionals receive adequate training in somnology and sleep medicine, as summarized earlier in this chapter and considered in depth in Chapters 5 and 7. At a minimum, medical students need basic training in sleep disorders, as do pharmacy, public health, dentistry, and nursing students. This training should cover the public health burden of sleep loss and sleep disorders and the importance of diagnosis and treatment throughout the life span. Sleep disorders and sleep medicine should be covered in greater depth in residency and fellowship training programs in all primary care specialties, as well as specialties related to sleep (e.g., otolaryngology), but without formal ACGME-accredited sleep fellowship programs. Research training—for clinical fellows, as well as for graduate and postgraduate researchers—is a key component for more specialized sleep programs (Type II and III; see below).

Clinical, Basic, and Translational Research

The field, as an interdisciplinary enterprise, garners momentum from the many clinical and basic disciplines at its core. The translational opportunities inherent in the field were among the motivations behind the formation by the NIH, in 1986, of the Trans-NIH Sleep Research Coordinating Committee (Chapter 8). The coordination and integration of many scientific fields will maximize these efforts.

Participation in Proposed Research Network

The committee recommended in Chapter 8 the creation of a National Somnology and Sleep Medicine Research and Clinical Network. The purpose of the proposed network is to advance the field by providing a means to connect individual investigators, research programs, and research centers. The network would provide a resource for education, training, collaborations, core facilities, data coordination, and access to multisite clinical research trials. Most sleep programs could benefit greatly from participation in the proposed network. For the network to be successful, all participating programs should be required to submit research and clinical data to whatever joint projects the network undertakes. This concept parallels the structure of many existing networks supported by NIH, as noted in Chapter 8.

Guiding Principles of Interdisciplinary Sleep Programs

Leadership

Leadership, so easily recognizable but elusive to define, is the single greatest success factor in forming a new program. The most successful programs developed over the past two decades are largely traceable to the conviction, determination, and persistence of committed leaders. These programs have served as beacons to others, facilitating their establishment. In a survey of 186 principal investigators, the IOM and National Academies committee on interdisciplinary research asked, "If you could recommend one action that principal investigators could take that would best facilitate interdisciplinary research, what would that be?" The leading recommendation from this survey was to increase leadership support of team-forming activities (NAS, 2004).

Revenue Generation and Fiscal Independence

Established sleep programs can generate higher revenues than costs, according to the analysis that the committee commissioned. This has resulted in individual departments taking "ownership" of the sleep program, thereby limiting reinvestment potential. But this is a shortsighted strategy. As emphasized throughout this report, there is enormous opportunity both in terms of clinical service and research. Academic centers, which adopt budgeting strategies that offer individual incentives to work together, should be better positioned to promote interdisciplinary research. Moreover, deans can facilitate interdisciplinary research by specifically giving chairpersons incentives for this type of activity. Such strategies give deans a very specific role in development of and support of somnology and sleep medicine as an interdisciplinary discipline.

Transparent Policies and Procedures

Sleep programs that are administered as divisions within individual departments may be at a disadvantage. They are not represented at the level of the school of medicine and hence may not be directly involved in strategic planning initiatives of the academic medical center. Further, the program competes for faculty positions in a structure that is not focused on development of interdisciplinary programs. On the other hand, entities that have medical-school-wide structures that support the interdisciplinary nature of sleep medicine have the converse—they are involved in strategic planning, there is financial transparency with budget authority, and they have the ability to advocate for faculty positions.

ORGANIZATIONAL AND FISCAL STRUCTURES FOR SUSTAINING OR EXPANDING A SLEEP PROGRAM

How can programs in somnology and sleep medicine be organized to sustain themselves and grow? This was the driving question behind an analysis the committee commissioned. The analysis focused on organization and fiscal structure of five interdisciplinary sleep programs—each with clinical, teaching, and research capacity. By studying programs with distinct organizational structures, the analysis sought to determine which were most conducive to sustaining or expanding their sleep program.

The analysis was undertaken using methods from operations research, a field that examines the impact of organizational structure on a program's capacity to achieve its mission. Operations research has shown that a program's success not only depends on leadership and quality of faculty and students, but also on its organization. It has identified organizational structure as being associated with success in producing doctorates (Ehrenberg and Epifantseva, 2001), acquiring grants (Ehrenberg et al., 2003), and developing patented technology (Luszki, 1958; Lach and Schankerman, 2001; 2003). This section of the chapter summarizes the specific questions, methods, and major findings of the commissioned paper. It is important to point out that the choice of programs was meant neither to be representative of all sleep programs, nor to cover the question of how to start a program de novo. Consequently, although the general findings are consistent, any conclusions drawn from the analysis may be limited and may not transcend every medical center.

Specific Questions and Methodology

The analysis addresses three specific questions: (1) Can sleep programs generate revenue in excess of their costs? (2) Which revenue streams produce the largest net revenue available for program development? (3) What organizational structure maximizes control over resources for program development? Parametric analysis applying the principles of operations research was used to examine these three questions. Semistructured interviews were conducted at five academic sleep programs with varying organizational structures: Emory University, George Washington University, Stanford University, University Hospital of Cleveland, and University of Pennsylvania. The interviews dealt with the topics in Box 9-2. Financial data were obtained from each program, and direct observations were performed, including the provision of clinical services and the effect of teaching on patient throughput. Major priorities of the analysis were to develop an operational framework to categorize organizational structures, to delineate specific constraints affecting sleep programs, to identify major cost structures and major funding streams, and to develop a "business plan" for each major organizational variant most likely to sustain or expand its program.

Direct Costs

The analysis identified three major direct costs: clinical services, teaching, and research. Clinical services consist of obtaining a reliable clinical history from a patient, determining what studies to conduct and, based on findings, establishing a diagnosis and developing a treatment plan. Diagnostic sleep studies are constrained by the fact that a sleep technician simultaneously can run, at best, two studies. "Reading" of studies requires frequent technician and clinician "calibration" for quality assurance purposes. Most programs are able to generate approximately 30 readings a week per full-time equivalent. Incorrect staffing ratios (e.g., medical assistant to provider ratios lower than 2 to 1) often produce longer patient wait times, which negatively affect patient throughput. No-show rates typically increase beyond a 2-week "next appointment" wait time. The direct costs of performing a sleep study are rising rapidly, primarily as a result of personnel costs. The changes in direct service costs between 1994, 2000, and 2005 are depicted in Figure 9-3.

The programs in the study taught medical students, residents, doctoral students, sleep fellows, and postdoctoral fellows. Though many faculty

---

BOX 9-2
Areas Addressed in Semistructured Interviews

1. A description of the program's revenue stream(s)
   a. Tests, including polysomnograms
   b. Treatment protocols
   c. Clinical consults
   d. Other services

2. Approximate operating budget for:
   a. Number of staff
      i.   Administrative
      ii. Technical support
      III. Practitioners
   b. Number of beds allocated to sleep
   c. Equipment maintenance and upgrades
   d. Training and continuing education
   e. Basic and clinical research
   f. The amount and source of discretionary funds controlled by the sleep center director

3. What percentage of the center's revenue goes to its parent department or division?

4. What percentage of the center's revenue goes to other departments through cost-sharing agreements?

5. What percentage of the center's operating budget does your sleep center receive from its parent department or division?

6. What are the challenges in working under the current system—does this create any barriers in care or service?

7. Are changes in the infrastructure needed? If so, why and what?

---

taught these medical students, there was not a formal mechanism for offsetting the expense through tuition revenue sharing. This is a more substantial problem in administrative structures in which the academic hospital is a separate legal entity from the university. Although there is generally a formal revenue sharing arrangement between the university and the hospital, there is seldom a similar arrangement between the university and the medical faculty.

Direct observations of programs being profiled here are consistent with findings of other studies that "teaching moments" increase the time spent for each clinical encounter by 20 to 30 percent. All programs examined for this study participated in fellowship training. Funding, with the exception

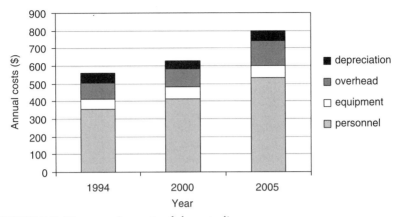

FIGURE 9-3 Direct service costs of sleep studies.

of direct NIH training grant support, was done without transparency and with minimal recognition of the expenses involved.

For research, there is a broad range of costs involved, depending on whether the research is basic or applied. This analysis focused only on direct costs and did not take into account start-up costs or shared or under-utilization of space or personnel costs.

Revenue Streams

There are three major clinical revenue steams: sleep studies—technical and professional components (the latter being for interpretation) and clinical encounters, teaching revenue streams (student tuition fees, graduate medical education [GME] funding, and NIH training grants), and one research revenue stream (grant funding both from federal and nonfederal sources).

Sleep studies generate the largest net revenue but mostly in the technical component. Clinical interpretations of sleep studies exhibited positive but lower margins. Clinical encounters were, at best, a breakeven proposition. This reflects general reimbursement patterns and the relatively higher overhead in academic practice by comparison to private practice settings. The relative efficiency of office practice varied considerably based on the organizational structure, but even under the best structure there was little evidence of net revenue beyond salary support for this part of the activity.

Interpretation of sleep studies does offer moderate net revenues even in the least efficient of the organizational structures. Direct costs are minimal, and federal and commercial insurance payments are predictable and above direct costs. Net revenue can support program development for both clinical and teaching purposes. Whether a given sleep program can access the net revenue for development depends on the organizational structure and financial arrangements between the sleep program and its parent organization(s).

By far the greatest net revenue comes from sleep diagnostic procedures. However, compared with other outpatient procedures (e.g., endoscopy and surgery) and many inpatient procedures, the net revenue from sleep studies may represent a type of "opportunity cost," insofar as they are not as profitable as other procedures. The net revenue is sufficient, however, to support clinical, teaching, and research program development. Even so, whether a sleep laboratory is a potential source of programmatic reinvestment is very much affected by the entity that owns the laboratory. In a hospital setting, the sleep laboratory margins compete for space and personnel with other services that generate much higher net margins. The difficulty in acquiring sleep laboratory space and sharing in the revenue has resulted in many academic programs outsourcing sleep laboratory studies to private contractors. Revenue sharing plans, such as those at Emory University and the University of Pennsylvania, with private contractors can support clinical teaching.

Three sources of revenue for teaching include capture of student tuition, federal GME funding, and NIH training grants. However, none of the sleep programs profiled here received student tuition revenue despite the substantial time spent teaching students. This generally reflects funds flow in most academic centers and is therefore not specific to sleep programs. Training grants support the education of fellows during their research training. Support of the fellows' clinical education is derived from a variety of sources and therefore differs from one institution to another.

Federal and nonfederal research grants support the direct costs of research, but the indirect cost recovery, even when distributed, does not completely cover the overhead costs of doing research. Institutional supplements generally close the gap.

Findings About the Role of Organizational Structure

There are two major parameters defining the effect of organizational structure on academic sleep centers. The first is the relationships among the university, school of medicine, university hospital, and faculty practice group. The second is the relationship between the sleep program and the rest of the faculty practice groups.

Macrostructure

The relationships among the university, university hospital, and faculty group have a major bearing on transparency in career development, resource sharing, and program development. For a fortunate few, these organizational units exist within the same legal entity. For most, they are disaggregated, with many having the hospital as a separate legal entity. In others, the faculty practice group, hospital, and school of medicine are all separate legal entities. Under the disaggregated organizational structures, all the complications and barriers exist to multidisciplinary collaboration in clinical, teaching, and research activities. Even more relevant to the purpose of this report, the ability to reinvest net revenues generated by the various sleep programs' revenue streams is dependent on individual initiative, personal relationships, and historical fiscal arrangements.

Microstructure

The relationship between the sleep program and the rest of the faculty practice group controls program development. In a few instances, the program is a formally recognized administrative structure (either as a separate division or as a formal "center"). A formally recognized program enhances the likelihood of revenue and resource sharing, faculty recruitment and development, decisions about how to reinvest revenue, and the ability to respond to local conditions. All too often, however, the sleep program is informally recognized. Net revenues are folded back into the department—with no advantage to the sleep program. The sleep program often has little control over faculty selection and evaluation, risk of multiple sleep services being offered by competing departments, and significant barriers to cross-discipline teaching activities and credit. This, in turn, limits the program's capacity to attract new faculty of high quality. Consequently, most programs have relied on the charisma, determination, persistence, and persuasiveness of their program leader. However, successful sleep programs do not need to be established in separate administrative structures. Many large, successful programs with strong leadership are housed within long-established medical departments or divisions.

The degree of transparency (or lack thereof) in administrative policy and procedures governing cost and revenue allocation and the weighting of teaching and research activities relative to clinical income at both the individual faculty member and program level varied considerably. The integrated model demonstrated the greatest transparency, greatest growth, and least concern about how to reinvest in the program.

Summary of Fiscal and Organizational Analysis

Sleep programs can generate higher revenues than costs. The net revenues (i.e., profits) can be used for reinvestment to sustain and build the program. Programs studied here have three sources of revenues: grants, clinical revenues, and teaching revenue. The technical revenue for sleep studies is the most profitable type of clinical revenue. It often is more profitable when contracted out to a private management firm with lower cost structures and more efficient operations. Contracting out also brings an added dividend: it gives the sleep program a dedicated source of revenue over which it may exert greater control. Training's financial benefits or disadvantages cannot be calculated, largely because none of the programs profiled here captured those costs.

The ability to control reinvestment in the sleep program is largely governed by the administrative structure within which the program is located. The ideal structure for controlling reinvestment exists when the program is a formal division within a medical school or the health science center—and when the medical school operates under the same administration as does the university hospital and faculty group. However, the committee recognizes that establishment of independent sleep departments is not possible in the vast majority of medical centers. Many successful sleep programs are divisions or centers in an existing medical department (e.g., internal medicine, neurology, or psychiatry). Therefore, facilitating growth of sleep programs can best occur by following the key principles previously set forth and the organization guidelines that will be discussed in the following section.

If the emphasis of the sleep program is on clinical services and clinical teaching, then the greatest reinvestment opportunities occur when the program is recognized as a formal clinical center, especially one that contracts out for sleep studies. If research is its greatest priority, then the greatest opportunities for program reinvestment occur when the sleep program is its own center administering its own grant activity.

Sleep programs have come into existence because of the vision and dedication of their leaders. Constructing a new enterprise requires that type of leadership, but sustaining and enhancing a program requires more: it requires a self-supporting organizational structure with transparent goals, rules of participation, and the capability to control reinvestment opportunities.

ACCREDITATION AND CERTIFICATION ARE ESSENTIAL TO QUALITY CARE

Although somnology and sleep medicine is a relatively new field, it is coming of age during this transformative period in medicine as a whole. Sleep medicine needs to be committed to the same high standards and evolving system of care influencing other fields of medicine, starting with the basics—accreditation and certification. The American Academy of Sleep Medicine (AASM) has standards for sleep centers, which include standards dealing with three broad functions: (1) accreditation of sleep centers and laboratories; (2) accreditation of sleep fellowship training programs;

and (3) certification of specialists in sleep medicine. Two of the AASM's functions recently have been assumed, at its request, by national certifying organizations (Table 9-1). The transition to these national certifying bodies is still in progress.

Accreditation of Sleep Centers or Laboratories

In 2005, the AASM accredited a total of 900 sleep centers and laboratories. There are two types of accreditation. One type, which accounts for the vast majority of accreditations (832 of 900), is a *sleep disorders center*. The centers are described as having a "comprehensive or full-service sleep disorders program" (American Academy of Sleep Medicine, 2006b). The other type of accreditation is for a more limited *laboratory for sleep-related breathing disorders only*.

The committee identified several problems with respect to quality of care. The foremost problem is that only 30 percent of sleep centers nationwide are accredited (Tachibana et al., 2005). Considering that an estimated 1 million polysomnograms were performed in 2001, it is likely that approximately 700,000 of them were not performed in accredited centers. Although there is no systematic evidence of poor quality of care in unaccredited centers, there is no assurance of quality care either. Because many of the serious health outcomes of sleep disorders may not manifest until years later, it would be difficult to link those outcomes with quality problems at the time of testing. Further, the fact that a majority of programs are not accredited taints the credibility of the field, preventing it from achieving the legitimacy that it has long sought.

TABLE 9-1 Evolution in Accrediting and Certifying Organizations in Somnology and Sleep Medicine

	Past Accrediting or Certifying Organization	Current Accrediting or Certifying Organization	Number Accredited or Certified in 2005
Sleep Centers or Laboratories	American Academy of Sleep Medicine	American Academy of Sleep Medicine	894 (832 centers, 62 labs)
Sleep Fellowship Training Programs	American Academy of Sleep Medicine	Accreditation Council for Graduate Medical Education	50 AASM 24 ACGME
Board Certification in Sleep Medicine	American Board of Sleep Medicine	American Board of Medical Specialties[a]	3,250

[a]The American Board of Medical Specialties will begin certification in 2007.

Finally, the absence of accreditation impedes sleep centers moving toward better care for patients (by embracing both diagnosis and treatment, rather than diagnosis alone). The overview to the standards indicates that accredited centers provide a comprehensive approach to patient care (AASM, 2006a). But this broad mission is not reflected in the actual criteria for accreditation. Accrediting criteria emphasize personnel, patient acceptance, facilities, and technical staff. The criteria lack specific emphasis on long-term disease management and improved outcomes provided by patient care. The committee heard testimony that many patients who are evaluated and diagnosed at centers are not systematically tracked in terms of follow-up care—either for treatment or for monitoring adherence with treatment. This testimony is consistent with research revealing that compliance with CPAP is poor (Kribbs et al., 1993; Reeves-Hoche et al., 1994). The committee could not find studies that directly address the extent to which diagnosed patients are not receiving treatment and follow-up care. The committee believes, however, that the accreditation procedure represents a unique opportunity to ensure that sleep centers are primarily focused on improving patient outcomes rather than diagnosis.

Accreditation of Fellowship Training Programs in Sleep Medicine

Starting in the mid-1990s, the AASM began to accredit sleep fellowship training programs. These are 1-year programs for medical doctors, which may be taken after completion of a residency (e.g., internal medicine, neurology, otolaryngology, psychiatry, or pediatrics or fellowships such as pulmonary medicine). In 2003, the ACGME approved AASM's application for transferring its fellowship training program to ACGME. AASM had actively sought approval in order to further elevate the standards for training and education. The newly established ACGME accreditation program began in June 2004. Accreditation criteria cover such areas as curriculum, qualifications of faculty, fellow competencies, scholarly activities, duty hours, and evaluation. By 2011, eligibility for board certification in sleep medicine will require attending an ACGME-accredited fellowship program in sleep medicine. Currently there are 24 ACGME-accredited fellowship programs and approximately 50 AASM accredited programs.

Certification of Specialists in Sleep Medicine

Since its inception, the AASM (or its predecessor organization) certified specialists by a specialty examination. By 1991, the AASM formed an independent body to serve that function, the American Board of Sleep Medicine. Certified professionals are known as diplomates in sleep medicine. The number of diplomates rose from 21 in the late 1970s to 3250 in 2005.

One of the board's major goals was realized in 2005, when it was accorded recognition as a bona fide subspecialty by the American Board of Medical Specialties. The timetable calls for a 6-year transition period. By 2011, board certification in sleep medicine will become available under the auspices of the American Boards of Internal Medicine, Pediatrics, Otolaryngology, and Psychiatry and Neurology. However, as discussed in Chapter 5, not all clinicians will be eligible to sit for the exam. The ACGME only permits accreditation of medical doctors; thus nurses, dentists, and doctorally prepared sleep specialists (e.g., psychologists and behavioral health specialists) in other fields will require alternative means of credentialing. It is possible that this may continue to be performed through the American Board of Sleep Medicine. Alternatively, other appropriate professional organizations may wish develop their own standards.

Health Insurance Role in Improving Quality

Health insurance, whether private or public (e.g., Medicare or Medicaid), is a driving force in health care delivery. Health insurance coverage drives the types of services that are offered and the incentives under which physicians operate. Health insurance coverage also influences who has access to services and how consumers select and use them (Hillman, 1991; Miller and Luft, 1994).

Health insurance coverage also influences the quality of care, often in unintentional ways. For example, fee-for-service health insurance may promote *overuse* of services—ones may not be necessary or that may expose patients to greater harm than benefit. Conversely, managed care may promote potential *underuse* of services from which patients might benefit (IOM, 2001). A major recommendation of the IOM report, *Crossing the Quality Chasm*, was to use health insurance as a means to ensure development of programs in quality improvement. Payment policies, the report recommended, should be used to reward higher quality of care.

The concept of using payment methods to reward better quality of care already has taken hold in many areas of medicine. It also is occurring in sleep medicine. In several regions, private health insurers require as a condition of reimbursement that sleep studies be conducted in accredited laboratories or centers (AASM, 2006a).

NEXT STEPS

Continued clinical advances and growth of the field depends on the appropriate emphasis and organization of academic sleep programs. These structures require special attention, not only to diagnosis, but also to long-term patient care that recognizes the need for chronic disease management and strategies. The committee recommends a three-tier structure that ensures all academic health centers have at least a minimum set of organizational components that ensure adequate interdisciplinary clinical care, with subsequent tiers also emphasizing training and research components. Further, to ensure improved care and scientific advances, the committee recommends accreditation standards be updated to include patient care criteria.

Proposed Organizational Guidelines for Interdisciplinary Sleep Programs

As suggested throughout this chapter and the entire report, the current organizational structures at many academic health centers are not sufficient to ensure continued advances in clinical care and research. Consequently, the committee recommends that each health center strive to put in place an interdisciplinary sleep program. However, the committee recognizes that each of the 125 academic health centers has a different organizational structure and resources. Consequently, a three-tier model for interdisciplinary sleep programs is recommended, progressing from programs that emphasize clinical care and education, to programs with a considerable research capacity, advanced training, and public education (Table 9-2). The first tier

TABLE 9-2 Guidelines for Interdisciplinary Type I, II, and III Academic Sleep Programs

Attribute	Type I (clinical)	Type II (clinical, training, research)	Type III (regionalized comprehensive centers)
Structure and Composition			
Clinical specialties represented:[a]			
Internal medicine and relevant subspecialties	x	x	x
Neurology	x	x	x
Psychiatry and subdisciplines	x	x	x
Otolaryngology	x	x	x
Pediatrics and subspecialties (as necessary may be separate program)	x	x	x
Nursing	x	x	x
Psychology		x	x
Dentistry			x
Medical director certification in sleep medicine (American Board of Medical Specialties or American Board of Sleep Medicine)[b]	x	x	x
Consultant services from specialties not represented	x	x	x

TABLE 9-2 continued

Attribute	Type I (clinical)	Type II (clinical, training, research)	Type III (regionalized comprehensive centers)
Sleep specialists provide consultant services	x	x	x
Single accredited clinical sleep center	x	x	x
Comprehensive program for diagnosis and treatment of individuals	x	x	x
Training Program			
Training program for health care professionals and/or researchers	x	x	x
Medical school training and education	x	x	x
Education for residents in primary care	x	x	x
Residents in neurology, psychiatry, otolaryngology, and fellows in pulmonary medicine rotate through sleep program		x	x
Accredited fellowship program for physicians		x	x
Research training for clinical fellows		x	x
NIH-sponsored training grants for graduate and postgraduate researchers		x	x
Research Program			
Research areas of emphasis:[c]			
Neuroscience		x	x
Epidemiology/public health		x	x
Pharmacology			x
Basic *or* clinical research program		x	
Basic *and* clinical research program			x
Member of proposed national somnology and sleep medicine research and clinical network	x[d]	x	x
Regional coordinator for:			
Core facilities for basic research			x
Multisite clinical trials			x
Core facilities for clinical research			x
Mentoring of sleep fellows			x
Public education			x
Data coordinating site			x

[a]This list is not meant to be exclusive or exhaustive and should be modified as relevant specialties and training programs emerge.

[b]Currently this is American Board of Sleep Medicine. It is anticipated that in 2007 the examination would be supplanted by the American Board of Medical Specialties.

[c]This list is not meant to be exclusive or exhaustive. Other research areas could be involved (e.g., genetics, systems neurobiology, and bioengineering).

[d]Type I programs would be responsible for generating and submitting data to the national data registry established by the proposed national somnology and sleep medicine research and clinical network.

represents a comprehensive program that emphasizes diagnosis and patient care. Type II and III interdisciplinary programs require a progressively larger commitment to clinical care, research, and training.

It is the belief of the committee that, if these components and guiding principles are followed, interdisciplinary sleep programs can thrive, whether as a freestanding department or as a program within an existing department, division, or unit. There is the danger that establishing stand-alone centers will result in the formation of additional barriers. Therefore, academic sleep programs must be organized to limit the formation of silos and facilitate interdisciplinary care and research. In most academic health centers, faculty participating in a sleep program will likely continue to have their primary appointment in departments, programs, or centers. To ensure interdisciplinary research and care, as well as prevent the formation of additional silos, faculty appointed in sleep programs are encouraged to maintain a connection with both the sleep program and their primary appointment.

Many academic health centers have in place the components to establish these types of programs. However, organizing and coordinating the components to reach the committee's vision is not an inconsequential task. Not all academic health centers are currently positioned to create interdisciplinary sleep programs. The committee recognizes that there must be incentives to facilitate this transition. To achieve this lofty goal will take great effort by the leaders of sleep programs and support and commitment from academic leadership. Establishing Type II and Type III interdisciplinary programs will require additional support from the NIH. As discussed in Chapter 8, the increased availability of training grants and program project grants will also help aid the establishment of these programs. However, simply increasing the funding available for these activities may not be effective. It is important to also establish comprehensive interdisciplinary sleep programs that will provide an environment conducive for interdisciplinary sleep-related research, training, and career development. Finally, comprehensive patient care will also be facilitated through the creation of accreditation standards for interdisciplinary academic programs in Somnology and Sleep Medicine that cover the diagnosis, treatment, and long-term follow-up of individuals with sleep disorders. As discussed previously in this chapter, the AASM has a demonstrated track record and the expertise to develop these criteria, which could be expanded to include the overall management of sleep disorders.

The need to establish novel structures for Somnology and Sleep Medicine within academic health centers is in line with current changes occurring in many other areas of science and medicine. The organization of basic science departments in academic health centers has been in a continuing state of transition in recent years, according to new data analysis from the American Association of Medical Colleges (AAMC). Medical schools are restructuring their basic science departments by consolidating the number of traditional departments and adding new departments to reflect scientific complexity and opportunity, as well as the changing nature of interdisciplinary biomedical research. The number of traditional discipline-based departments decreased from 2000 to 2004, but the overall number of departments has remained steady (Bunton 2006; Mallon et al., 2003). The creation of viable interdisciplinary sleep programs by the medical school leadership should benefit from ongoing experimentation in parallel areas.

Recommendation 9.1: New and existing sleep programs in academic health centers should meet the criteria of a Type I, II, or III interdisciplinary sleep program.

New and existing sleep programs should at a minimum conform to the criteria of a Type I clinical interdisciplinary sleep program. Academic medical centers with a commitment to interdisciplinary training are encouraged to train sleep scientists and fellows in sleep medicine, which would require at least a Type II training and research interdisciplinary sleep program. Research-intensive medical centers should aspire to become Type III regional interdisciplinary sleep programs and coordinators of the National Somnology and Sleep Medicine Research Network. The American Academy of Sleep Medicine should develop accreditation criteria for sleep programs specific to academic health centers.

Type I Clinical Interdisciplinary Sleep Program

The Type I Clinical Interdisciplinary Sleep Program, which if not already in existence, is achievable by the majority of centers nationwide and focuses on clinical care specialties. It further highlights the importance of increased awareness among health care professionals by requiring educational programs for medical students and residents in primary care. This minimum commitment to training is so important because of the sheer commonality of sleep disorders in primary care. Optimally, each academic health center should have a single Type I Clinical Interdisciplinary Sleep Program accredited center that emphasizes a comprehensive diagnosis and treatment program and includes representation from internal medicine and its relevant subspecialties, such as pulmonary medicine, neurology, psychiatry, otolaryngology, pediatrics, and nursing. Often pediatrics and its relevant subspecialties—especially in large, freestanding children's hospitals—may be better served by a separate program. Further, this list of participating specialties is not meant to be exclusive or exhaustive but should be modified as relevant specialties and training programs emerge. Although it is important that generalists and the key specialists are capable of treating individuals with sleep disorders, programs should also ensure that patients are referred to relevant specialists as needed. The medical director of each program should be certified in sleep medicine, and it should be a goal of each program that all physicians also be certified.

Type II Training and Research Interdisciplinary Sleep Program

A Type II Training and Research Interdisciplinary Sleep Program includes the characteristics of a Type I program but in addition is designed to provide optimal education, training, and research in somnology and sleep medicine. Nurses and psychologists should be included in the programs. Further, a Type II program should have an accredited fellowship program for all eligible physician rotations through the sleep program for all pulmonology, neurology, otolaryngology, and psychiatry residents. In addition, as described in Chapter 8, a Type II program would serve as an active member of the proposed National Somnology and Sleep Medicine Research and Clinical Network through at least an active basic or clinical research program. Research areas of emphasis should include, but not be limited to, science in the biological basis of sleep and population-based research on sleep patterns and problems.

Type III Regional Interdisciplinary Sleep Program

A Type III Regional Interdisciplinary Sleep Program includes the characteristics of Type I and II programs; however, in addition, a Type III program is designed to serve as a center for public health education, training for clinical care and research, basic research, patient-oriented research, translational research, and clinical care. As described in Chapter 8 the committee envisions that this type of program would act as a regional coordinator for the proposed National Somnology and Sleep Medicine Research and Clinical Network for education, training, mentoring, clinical care, research, clinical research studies, and large-scale population genetics studies. The committee does not recommend a specific number of Type III programs but recognizes that only a minimum number of programs currently have the necessary resources. However, as the field grows, more programs should develop the resources necessary to become a Type III program. Establishing these programs will not only require a significant investment from academic programs, but also, as described in Chapter 8, a long-term commitment by the NIH.

Chronic Care Accreditation Standards

As described earlier in this chapter, sleep disorders are chronic conditions with complex treatments. However, despite the importance of early recognition and treatment, the primary focus of most existing sleep centers is on diagnosis rather than on comprehensive management of sleep loss and sleep disorders as chronic conditions. This narrow focus may largely be the unintended result of compliance with criteria for accreditation of sleep laboratories, which emphasize diagnostic standards and reimbursement, for diagnostic testing. Clinical accreditation standards should be updated to address patient care needs.

Chronic disease management models, such as those used to provide optimal care for individuals with diabetes, asthma, congestive heart failure, and depression, have been proven to be effective at providing better-integrated care (Tsai et al., 2005). Therefore, the committee recommends that accreditation criteria for all sleep centers, embedded in either academic health centers or private sleep laboratories, be expanded to emphasize treatment, long-term patient care, and management strategies. Although sleep laboratories may face a financial burden implementing the changes, the committee believes this is the most effective way to ensure optimal patient care. Such criteria should be subject to further analysis and a demonstration that chronic care is a worthwhile investment. If such studies demonstrate a benefit, this may then change reimbursement patterns.

Recommendation 9.2: Sleep laboratories should be part of accredited sleep centers, the latter to include long-term strategies for patient care and chronic disease management.

All private and academic sleep laboratories should be under the auspices of accredited sleep centers and include adequate mechanisms to ensure long-term patient care and chronic disease management. Accreditation criteria should expand beyond a primary focus on diagnostic testing to emphasize treatment, long-term patient care, and chronic disease management strategies.

REFERENCES

AASM (American Academy of Sleep Medicine). 2006a. *Standards for Accreditation of Sleep Disorders Centers*. [Online]. Available: http://www.aasmnet.org/PDF/CenterStandards.pdf [accessed January 3, 2006].

AASM. 2006b. *Accreditation Standards*. [Online]. Available: http://www.aasmnet.org/center Lab.aspx [accessed January 18, 2006].

Allison PJ, Nicolau B, Edgar L, Archer J, Black M, Hier M. 2004. Teaching head and neck cancer patients coping strategies: Results of a feasibility study. *Oral Oncology* 40(5):538–544.

Baker TL, Guilleminault C, Nino-Murcia G, Dement WC. 1986. Comparative polysomnographic study of narcolepsy and idiopathic central nervous system hypersomnia. *Sleep*
9(1 pt 2):232–242.
Benca RM. 2005. Diagnosis and treatment of chronic insomnia: A review. *Psychiatry Services*
56(3):332–343.
Bodenheimer T, Wagner EH, Grumbach K. 2002. Improving primary care for patients with
chronic illness. *Journal of the American Medical Association* 288(14):1775–1779.
Bunton SA. 2006. Recent trends in basic science department reorganizations. *American Association of Medical Colleges Analysis in Brief* 6(1)1–21.
Cherniack NS. 2005. Sleep apnea and insomnia: Sleep apnea plus or sleep apnea minus. *Respiration* 72(5):458–459.
Chung KF. 2005. Insomnia subtypes and their relationships to daytime sleepiness in patients
with obstructive sleep apnea. *Respiration* 72(5):460–465.
Chung SA, Jairam S, Hussain MR, Shapiro CM. 2001. Knowledge of sleep apnea in a sample
grouping of primary care physicians. *Sleep and Breathing* 5(3):115–121.
Davidson JR, Waisberg JL, Brundage MD, MacLean AW. 2001. Nonpharmacologic group
treatment of insomnia: A preliminary study with cancer survivors. *Psycho-Oncology*
10(5):389-397.
Ehrenberg RG, Epifantseva J. 2001. Has the growth of science crowded out other things at
universities? *Heldref Publications/Gale Group* 26:46–52.
Ehrenberg RG, Rizzo MJ, Jakubson GH. 2003. *Who Bears the Growing Cost of Science at
Universities?* [Online] Available: http://www.nber.org/papers/w9627 [accessed December 15, 2005] (unpublished work).
Epstein DR, Bootzin RR. 2002. Insomnia. *The Nursing Clinics of North America*
37(4):611–631.
Hendricks JC, Finn SM, Panckeri KA, Chavkin J, Williams JA, Sehgal A, Pack AI. 2000. Rest
in *Drosophila* is a sleep-like state. *Neuron* 25(1):129–138.
Hillman AL. 1991. Managing the physician: Rules versus incentives. *Health Affairs (Millwood)*
10(4):138–146.
IOM (Institute of Medicine). 2000. *To Err Is Human: Building a Safer Health System.* Washington, DC: National Academy Press.
IOM. 2001. *Crossing the Quality Chasm: A New Health System for the 21st Century.* Washington, DC: National Academy Press.
Kapur V, Strohl KP, Redline S, Iber C, O'Connor G, Nieto J. 2002. Underdiagnosis of sleep
apnea syndrome in U.S. communities. *Sleep and Breathing* 6(2):49–54.
Kribbs NB, Pack AI, Kline LR, Smith PL, Schwartz AR, Schubert NM, Redline S, Henry JN,
Getsy JE, Dinges DF. 1993. Objective measurement of patterns of nasal CPAP use by
patients with obstructive sleep apnea. *American Review of Respiratory Diseases* 147(4):
887–895.
Lach S, Schankerman M. 2001. Organizational structure as a determinant of academic patent
and licensing behavior: An exploratory study of Duke, Johns Hopkins, and Pennsylvania
State Universities. *Journal of Technology Transfer* 26(1):21–35.
Lach S, Schankerman M. 2003. *Incentives and Invention in Universities.* [Online] Available:
http://www.nber.org/papers/w9727 [accessed December 15, 2005] (unpublished work).
Lee K, Cho M, Miaskowski C, Dodd M. 2004a. Impaired sleep and rhythms in persons with
cancer. *Sleep Medicine Reviews* 8(3):199–212.
Lee KA, Landis C, Chasens ER, Dowling G, Merritt S, Parker KP, Redeker N, Richards KC,
Rogers AE, Shaver JF, Umlauf MG, Weaver TE. 2004b. Sleep and chronobiology: Rec-
ommendations for nursing education. *Nursing Outlook* 52(3):126–133.
Likar LL, Panciera TM, Erickson AD, Rounds S. 1997. Group education sessions and compli-
ance with nasal CPAP therapy. *Chest* 111(5):1273–1277.

Luszki MB. 1958. *Interdisciplinary Team Research Methods and Problems*. Vol. 3. Research Training Series Edition. New York: New York University Press.

Mallon WT, Biebuyck JF, Jones RF 2003. The reorganization of basic science departments in U.S. medical schools, 1980–1999. *Academic Medicine* 78(3):302–306.

Miaskowski, C. 2004. Gender differences in pain, fatigue, and depression in patients with cancer. *Journal of the National Cancer Institute* (32):139–143.

Miaskowski C, Lee KA. 1999. Pain, fatigue, and sleep disturbances in oncology outpatients receiving radiation therapy for bone metastasis: A pilot study. *Journal of Pain and Symptom Management* 17(5):320–332.

Miller RH, Luft HS. 1994. Managed care plan performance since 1980. A literature analysis. *Journal of the American Medical Association* 271(19):1512–1519.

Mock V, Pickett M, Ropka ME, Muscari Lin E, Stewart KJ, Rhodes VA, McDaniel R, Grimm PM, Krumm S, McCorkle R. 2001. Fatigue and quality of life outcomes of exercise during cancer treatment. *Cancer Practice* 9(3):119–127.

National Academy of Sciences. 2004. *Facilitating Interdisciplinary Research*. Washington, DC: The National Academies Press.

NHLBI (National Heart, Lung, and Blood Institute). 2003. *National Sleep Disorders Research Plan, 2003*. Bethesda, MD: National Insitutes of Health.

Nieto FJ, Young TB, Lind BK, Shahar E, Samet JM, Redline S, D'Agostino RB, Newman AB, Lebowitz MD, Pickering TG. 2000. Association of sleep-disordered breathing, sleep apnea, and hypertension in a large community-based study. Sleep Heart Health Study. *Journal of the American Medical Association* 283(14):1829–1836.

Parker KP, Kimble LP, Dunbar SB, Clark PC. 2005. Symptom interactions as mechanisms underlying symptom pairs and clusters. *Journal of Nursing Scholarship* 37(3): 209–215.

Punjabi NM, Shahar E, Redline S, Gottlieb DJ, Givelber R, Resnick HE, Sleep Heart Health Study Investigators. 2004. Sleep-disordered breathing, glucose intolerance, and insulin resistance: The Sleep Heart Health Study. *American Journal of Epidemiology* 160(6):521–530.

Rechtschaffen A, Bergmann BM, Everson CA, Kushida CA, Gilliland MA. 1989. Sleep deprivation in the rat: X. Integration and discussion of the findings. *Sleep* 12(1):68–87.

Reeves-Hoche MK, Meck R, Zwillich CW. 1994. Nasal CPAP: An objective evaluation of patient compliance. *American Journal of Respiratory and Critical Care Medicine* 149(1): 149–154.

Reuveni H, Tarasiuk A, Wainstock T, Ziv A, Elhayany A, Tal A. 2004. Awareness level of obstructive sleep apnea syndrome during routine unstructured interviews of a standardized patient by primary care physicians. *Sleep* 27(8):1518–1525.

Richards K, Nagel C, Markie M, Elwell J, Barone C. 2003. Use of complementary and alternative therapies to promote sleep in critically ill patients. *Critical Care Nursing Clinics of North America* 15(3):329–340.

Shahar E, Whitney CW, Redline S, Lee ET, Newman AB, Javier Nieto F, O'Connor GT, Boland LL, Schwartz JE, Samet JM. 2001. Sleep-disordered breathing and cardiovascular disease: Cross-sectional results of the Sleep Heart Health Study. *American Journal of Respiratory and Critical Care Medicine* 163(1):19–25.

Shaw PJ, Cirelli C, Greenspan RJ, Tononi G. 2000. Correlates of sleep and waking in *Drosophila melanogaster*. *Science* 287(5459):1834–1837.

Singh M, Drake C, Roehrs T, Koshorek G, Roth T. 2005. The prevalence of SOREMPs in the general population. *Sleep* 28(abstract suppl):A221.

Spiegel K, Tasali E, Penev P, Van Cauter E. 2004. Brief communication: Sleep curtailment in healthy young men is associated with decreased leptin levels, elevated ghrelin levels, and increased hunger and appetite. *Annals of Internal Medicine* 141(11):846–850.

Sullivan CE, Issa FG, Berthon-Jones M, Eves L. 1981. Reversal of obstructive sleep apnoea by continuous positive airway pressure applied through the nares. *Lancet* 1(8225):862–865.

Tachibana N, Ayas TA, White DP. 2005. A quantitative assessment of sleep laboratory activity in the United States. *Journal of Clinical Sleep Medicine* 1(1):23–26.

Taheri S, Lin L, Austin D, Young T, Mignot E. 2004. Short sleep duration is associated with reduced leptin, elevated ghrelin, and increased body mass index. *PLoS Medicine* 1:210–217.

Tsai AC, Morton SC, Mangione CM, Keeler EB. 2005. A meta-analysis of interventions to improve care for chronic illnesses. *American Journal of Managed Care* 11(8):478–488.

Weaver TE, Laizner AM, Evans LK, Maislin G, Chugh DK, Lyon K, Smith PL, Schwartz AR, Redline S, Pack AI, Dinges DF. 1997. An instrument to measure functional status outcomes for disorders of excessive sleepiness. *Sleep* 20(10):835–843.

Young T, Evans L, Finn L, Palta M. 1997. Estimation of the clinically diagnosed proportion of sleep apnea syndrome in middle-aged men and women. *Sleep* 20(9):705–706.

A

Study Process

The committee reviewed and considered a broad array of information in its work on issues involving sleep disorder research. Information sources included the primary scientific literature, books and scientific reviews, and presentations from researchers, as well as representatives from federal agencies and academic, professional, and nonprofit organizations.

LITERATURE REVIEW

Extensive bibliographic searches were conducted, resulting in a reference database of more than 2,000 entries. Searches of the primary biomedical bibliographic databases, MEDLINE and EMBASE,[1] were supplemented with searches of Dissertation Abstracts Online, LexisNexis, and THOMAS (a federal legislative database). The Dissertation Abstracts database provided information on the current level of Ph.D. thesis production in the field of sleep disorders.[2]

---

[1]Excerpta Medica.

[2]Institute of Medicine staff searched the Dissertation Abstracts database using the search terms *sleep, sleep disorders, sleep apnea, dream, insomnia, hibernation, periodic limb movement, restless legs syndrome, circadian rhythm, narcolepsy,* and *sudden infant death syndrome.* The question mark is used to search for terms with multiple endings. For example, the search term *sleep disord?* resulted in hits that included *sleep disorder* and *sleep disorders.*

GRANT ANALYSIS

To identify information on funding mechanisms and trends from the National Institutes of Health (NIH), Institute of Medicine (IOM) staff queried the Computer Retrieval of Information on Scientific Projects (CRISP) database. This database collects information on the number of federally funded biomedical research projects. Data from the CRISP database were used to assess the number of fellowships (F grants), career grants (K grants), research grants (e.g., R01 grants), project grants (P grants), training (T grants), cooperative agreements (U grants), and Small Business Innovation Research and Small Business Technology Transfer awards funded by the NIH. To discern the number of NIH grants directed toward sleep-related research, IOM staff used appropriate keywords (which appeared in a 9,000-word thesaurus) for various sleep disorders, including: *insomnia, periodic limb movement disorder, restless legs syndrome, circadian rhythm, sudden infant death syndrome, sleep disorder, narcolepsy, sleep apnea, sleep, hibernation,* and *dream.* To limit the number of grants that were not relevant to somnology or sleep disorders the committee included only grants in which the keywords appeared in the thesaurus terms and not the abstract. Additional information on general funding trends at NIH was located in published documents and was provided by NIH staff.

PUBLIC WORKSHOPS

The committee held five meetings over the course of the study to address the study charge, review the data collected, and develop the report. Three of those meetings included public workshops: April 11–12, 2005; June 29–30, 2005; and September 15–16, 2005.

The first workshop (Box A-1) included three sessions that covered the public health significance of sleep deprivation and disorders, sleep deprivation and society, sleep apnea, and the impact of sleep deprivation and disorders on specific populations.

The committee held the second public workshop (Box A-2) in Washington, D.C. In that workshop the committee heard from 17 speakers who had expertise in surveillance and monitoring programs and technologies, model interdisciplinary programs, and training and education in sleep research.

The third meeting took place at the Jonsson Conference Center in Woods Hole, Massachusetts. The public workshop (Box A-3) consisted of two sessions that included a review of results from a survey and commissioned paper on sleep and a discussion with Dr. Charles Czeisler, director of Harvard Medical School's Division of Sleep Medicine and president-elect of the Sleep Research Society.

BOX A-1

Institute of Medicine
Committee on Sleep Medicine and Research

April 11–12, 2005

Monday April 11, 2005
Session I: Sponsors' Perspective, Panel Discussion with Committee

10:15   **National Sleep Foundation**
Richard Gelula, Executive Director

National Institutes of Health
Stuart Quan, Chair, NIH Sleep Disorders Research
Advisory Board
Carl Hunt, Director, National Center on Sleep Disorders
Research, National Heart, Lung, and Blood Institute
Merrill Mitler, Program Director, Extramural Research
Program, National Institute of Neurological Disorders
and Stroke

Sleep Research Society
Charles Czeisler, President-Elect
Jerry Barrett, Executive Director

American Academy of Sleep Medicine
Michael Sateia, President
Lawrence Epstein, President-Elect
Jerry Barrett, Executive Director
Jennifer Markkanen, Assistant Executive Director

Tuesday, April 12, 2005
Session I: Public Health Significance of Sleep Deprivation and Disorders

8:25   **Welcome and Introductions**
Harvey Colten, Chair

8:30   **Impact of Insomnia and Periodic Leg Movements**
Thomas Roth, Henry Ford Health System of Detroit

9:00   **Overview of the Public Health Significance of Sleep Deprivation and Disorders**
Terry Young, University of Wisconsin

continued

BOX A-1 continued

9:30   **Sleep Duration: Neurobehavioral, Physiological, and Epidemiological Issues**
David Dinges, University of Pennsylvania School of Medicine

Session II: Sleep Deprivation and Society

10:15   **Accidents Caused by Sleep Deprivation and Disorders**
Allan Pack, University of Pennsylvania Medical Center

10:45   **Metabolic Consequences of Sleep Deprivation**
Daniel Gottlieb, Boston University School of Medicine

Session III: Sleep Apnea

11:15   **Effect of Apnea on Cardiovascular Disease and Metabolic Functions**
Susan Redline, Case Western Reserve University School of Medicine

11:45   Discussion of Morning Session

Session IV: Impact of Sleep Deprivation and Disorders on Specific Populations

1:00   **Snoring in Children: Sound the Alarm!**
David Gozal, University of Louisville

1:30   **Sleep Loss and Women's Health**
Kathy Lee, University of California, San Francisco

2:00   **Sleep Disturbance in Geriatrics**
Donald Bliwise, Emory University

2:30   Discussion of Afternoon Session

BOX A-2

Institute of Medicine
Committee on Sleep Medicine and Research

June 29–30, 2005

June 29, 2005

11:15   **Lee Goldman**
         University of California, San Francisco, Department of
         Medicine

Surveillance Programs and Technologies

1:00   **Welcome and Introductions**
         Harvey Colten, Chair
         Paul Eggers, NIDDK, Co-Project Officer, United States
         Renal Data System
         Ed Sondik, Director, National Center for Health Statistics

2:15   **Open Discussion**

2:45   **Roger Rosa**
         Senior Scientist, National Institute for Occupational Safety
         and Health

3:15   **Eugene J. Lengerich**
         Co-Chair, Pennsylvania Cancer Control Consortium

3:45   **Andrea Califano**
         Co-Director, Center for Computational Biochemistry and
         Biosystems, Bioworks and the NCI caCORE platform

4:15   Open Discussion

June 30, 2005
Organizational Impediments

8:30   **David Lewis**
         President and Chief Executive Officer, SleepMed, Inc.

9:00   **Michael Martin**
         Director of the Division of Physiology and Pathology in the
         Center for Scientific Review, NIH

                                                          continued

BOX A-2 continued

9:30   **William Dement**
           Director, Sleep Research Center, Stanford University
           School of Medicine

10:15   **David White**
           Director, Sleep Disorders Program, Brigham and Women's
           Hospital

10:45   General Discussion

Model Interdisciplinary Programs

12:30   **Kathleen C. Buckwalter**
           , Codirector University of Iowa Center on Aging

1:00   **Story Landis**
           Director, NINDS, Co-chair NIH Pain Consortium

1:30   **Hal Moses**
           Founding Director of the Vanderbilt-Ingram Cancer
           Center

2:00   **David J. Kupfer**
           Chair, Department of Psychiatry, University of Pittsburgh
           School of Medicine

2:30   **Steven Wolinsky**
           Division Chief of Infectious Diseases
           Northwestern University

3:00   General Discussion

Training and Education

3:30   **Judith Owens**
           Brown University Medical School, AASM MED Sleep
           Program

4:00   **Daniel Buysse**
           Department of Psychiatry, UPMC Sleep Medicine Center
           and Sleep Medicine Fellowship Training Program

4:30   **Roger Bulger**
           President, Association of Academic Health Centers

5:00   General Discussion

BOX A-3

Institute of Medicine
Committee on Sleep Medicine and Research

September 15–16, 2005

September 15, 2005
12:45 **Results from AASM Academic Health Centers Survey**
Michael Sateia, Section of Sleep Medicine Chief,
Dartmouth University
Past President, American Academy of Sleep Medicine

1:30 **Preliminary Findings of Commissioned Paper**
John Fontanesi, Center for Management Science in
Public Health, University of California, San Diego

September 16, 2005
10:15 **Discussion with Charles Czeisler**
Director, Division of Sleep Medicine, Harvard Medical School
President-Elect, Sleep Research Society

B

Acronyms

AASM	American Academy of Sleep Medicine
ABSM	American Board of Sleep Medicine
ACGME	Accreditation Council for Graduate Medical Education
ADHD	attention-deficit hyperactivity disorder
ADSM	Academy of Dental Sleep Medicine
AHI	apnea-hypopnea index
AMA	American Medical Association
APSS	annual meeting of sleep professional societies
ASAA	American Sleep Apnea Association
ATS	American Thoracic Society
BEARS	B = bedtime issues, E = excessive daytime sleepiness, A = night awakenings, R = regularity and duration of sleep, S = snoring
BMI	body mass index
CDC	Centers for Disease Control and Prevention
CNS	central nervous system
CPAP	continuous positive airway pressure
CRISP	Computer Retrieval of Information on Scientific Projects
CRP	C-reactive protein
CSA	central sleep apnea
CSF	cerebrospinal fluid

DCI	Diseases and Conditions Index
DNA	deoxyribonucleic acid
EEG	electroencephalogram
GABA	gamma-aminobutyric acid
HCRT	hypocretin
HLA	human leukocyte antigen
HPA	hypothalamic-pituitary axis
IRG	integrated review groups
L-DOPA	levo-dopa
MEPS	Medical Expenditure Panel Survey
MRI	magnetic resonance imaging
mRNA	messenger ribonucleic acid
MS	multiple sclerosis
MSLT	multiple sleep latency test
NAMCS	National Ambulatory Medical Care Survey
NCHS	National Center for Health Statistics
NCMRR	National Center for Medical Rehabilitation Research
NCSDR	National Center for Sleep Disorders Research
NEHIS	National Employer Health Insurance Survey
NHAMCS	National Hospital Ambulatory Medical Care Survey
NHANES	National Health and Nutrition Examination Survey
NHDS	National Hospital Discharge Survey
NHHCS	National Home and Hospice Care Survey
NHIS	National Health Interview Survey
NHLBI	National Heart, Lung, and Blood Institute
NHPI	National Health Provider Inventory
NIH	National Institutes of Health
NIMH	National Institute of Mental Health
NNHS	National Nursing Home Survey
NREM	nonrapid eye movement
NSAS	National Survey of Ambulatory Surgery
NSF	National Sleep Foundation
NTSB	National Transportation Safety Board

OSA	obstructive sleep apnea
PA	program announcement
PLMI	periodic limb movement index
PSG	polysomnography
REM	rapid eye movement
RFA	request for application
RLS	restless legs syndrome
RNA	ribonucleic acid
SAA	sleep academic award
SBIR	Small Business Innovative Research
SCN	suprachiasmatic nucleus
SCOR	specialized center of research
SDB	sleep-disordered breathing
SIDS	sudden infant death syndrome
SOREMP	sleep onset REM period
SRS	Sleep Research Society
SWS	slow-wave sleep
WASO	wake time after sleep onset
YRBSS	Youth Risk Behavior Surveillance System

C

Glossary of Major Terms

Acoustic reflectometry A technique that allows for noninvasive measurement of human airways to quantify anatomical obstruction of the upper airway.

Actigraph A movement detector coupled with software that uses movement patterns to diagnose sleep disorders.

Adenoid An enlarged mass of lymphoid tissue at the back of the nasopharynx that, when enlarged, can obstruct the nasal and ear passages, forcing respiration through the mouth and inducing nasality, postnasal discharge, and dullness of facial expression.

Adenotonsillectomy The surgical removal of tonsils and adenoids.

African trypanosomiasis A category of disease caused by infection with the *Trypanosoma brucei (Tb)* parasite and resulting in sleeping sickness.

Antihypertensive A class of drugs that are used to reduce high blood pressure.

Antipsychotic A powerful tranquilizer typically used to treat psychosis.

Apnea Transient stop of respiration due to either normal or abnormal causes.

Apnea-hypopnea index The total number of episodes of apnea and hypopnea per hour of sleep. A value of 5 or greater is abnormal and may be associated with excessive daytime sleepiness.

Atonia Lack of physiological muscle tone.

Attention-deficit/hyperactivity disorder (ADHD) A syndrome of disordered learning and disruptive behavior, with no known cause, and characterized by one or all of the following symptoms: inattentiveness,

335

hyperactivity, and impulsive behavior. Also known as attention deficit disorder (ADD).

Autoimmune   Referring to or caused by autoantibodies or white blood cells that attack molecules, cells, or tissues of the organism producing them.

BEARS   A 5-step pediatric sleep screening form to identify sleep problems (B = bedtime issues, E = excessive daytime sleepiness, A = night awakenings, R = regularity and duration of sleep, S = snoring).

Body mass index (BMI)   A measure of body fat that is the ratio of the weight of the body in kilograms to the square of its height in meters.

Carotid body   A small body of vascular tissue that is able to sense changes in the partial pressures of oxygen and carbon dioxide in the blood and to mediate reflex changes in respiration.

Cataplexy   A symptom of narcolepsy, characterized by a sudden loss of muscle control with retention of clear consciousness in response to a strong emotional stimulus.

Catecholamine   An amine (such as norepinephrine or dopamine), derived from tyrosine, that functions as a neurotransmitter, hormone, or both.

Central sleep apnea   Cessation of breathing during sleep that is caused a disturbance in the brain's respiratory center.

Cerebral cortex   The surface layer of the brain's gray matter, which coordinates sensory and motor information.

Cerebrospinal fluid (CSF)   A liquid that is secreted from the blood into the internal cavities in each cerebral hemisphere of the brain and circulates through the cavities to the spaces formed between the brain or spinal cord and the surrounding membranes; serves chiefly to maintain uniform pressure within the brain and spinal cord.

Chemoreflex   A physiological reflex initiated in a chemoreceptor or in response to a chemical stimulus.

CHQ-PF50   A parent report measure of children's physical, emotional, and social functional status and well-being.

Chronobiology   The science of biological rhythms.

Circadian rhythms   24-hour periods or cycles of biological activity or function.

Cognitive therapy   Psychotherapeutic method aimed at changing faulty beliefs and attitudes about sleep, insomnia, and the next-day consequences. Other cognitive strategies are used to control intrusive thoughts at bedtime and prevent excessive monitoring of the daytime consequences of insomnia.

Confusional arousal   One type of disorder of arousal associated with NREM sleep. Individuals display mental confusion or confusional behavior during or following arousal, typically from slow-wave sleep.

Corticosteroids   Any of various adrenal-cortex steroids used medically, especially as anti-inflammatory agents.

Dementia   A condition characterized by the progressive development of multiple cognitive deficits, such as memory impairment, difficulty in speech comprehension and production, and inability to plan and initiate complex behavior.

Dialysis   A category of medical procedures to remove wastes or toxins from the blood and adjust fluid and electrolyte imbalances.

Diurnal   Occurring in the daytime.

Dysesthesia   The impairment of tactile sensitivity.

Electroencephalograph (EEG)   Machine used to monitor and categorize sleep stages by measuring changes in brain wave activity.

Electro-oculogram   A record of the standing voltage between the front and back of the eye that is correlated with eyeball movement (as in REM sleep) and obtained by electrodes suitably placed on the skin near the eye.

Electrophysiology   The study of the electrical activity related to physiological function of living tissue.

Epilepsy   A category of disorders characterized by abnormal electrical activity in the brain and featuring symptoms such as sudden brief episodes of altered or diminished consciousness, involuntary movements, or convulsions.

Epworth sleepiness scale   A series of questions used to determine whether an individual is sleepy or not.

Excessive daytime sleepiness   Background of constant sleepiness with sleep attacks leading to unintended napping during the day; a characteristic symptom of narcolepsy.

Exploding head syndrome   Characterized by a sudden, loud noise or explosion in the head, this is an imagined, painless noise.

F30 fellowship   Individual Predoctoral National Research Service Award for M.D./Ph.D. degrees. Fellowship award that provides combined medical school and predoctoral Ph.D. support for a maximum of 6 years.

F31 fellowship   Predoctoral Individual National Research Service Award. Fellowship award that provides up to 5 years of support for research training leading to the Ph.D. or equivalent research.

F32 fellowship   Postdoctoral Individual National Research Service Award. Fellowship award that provides postdoctoral research training to broaden scientific background.

F33 fellowship   National Research Service Award for Senior Fellow. Fellowship award that provides opportunities for experienced scientists to broaden scientific background.

Gene   A DNA sequence that encodes a protein.

Gene loci   The term used to describe the locations of genes on a chromosome.

Generalized anxiety disorder   An anxiety disorder characterized by chronic excessive anxiety and worry that is difficult to control, and it consequently impairs daily functioning and causes stress. Primary symptoms include: restlessness, irritability, poor concentration, and sleep disturbances.

Hemodialysis   The removal and purification of blood from an artery, followed by the addition of vital substances and reintroduction into the circulatory system through a vein.

Hypersomnia   Periods of normal duration of sleep and waking are interspersed with excessive periods of sleep.

Hypersomnolence   Excessive drowsiness.

Hypertension   Abnormally high arterial blood pressure that typically results in a thickening and inelasticity of arterial walls and left heart ventricle hypertrophy. A risk factor for various pathological conditions or events such as heart attack, heart failure, stroke, end-stage renal disease, or retinal hemorrhage.

Hypnagogic   Relating to or occurring in the drowsiness stage that immediately precedes the onset of sleep.

Hypnagogic hallucinations   A characteristic symptom of narcolepsy that is marked by frightening dreamlike REM sleep experiences when falling asleep.

Hypnopompic   Referring to the semiconsciousness period that precedes waking.

Hypnopompic hallucinations   A characteristic symptom of narcolepsy that is marked by frightening dreamlike REM sleep experiences when waking up from sleep.

Hypnotic   An agent that induces sleep.

Hypocretin-1   One of a pair of highly excititory neuropeptide hormones (the other being hypocretin-2) that are biosynthesized in the hypothalamus and are involved in the cause of narcolepsy-cataplexy. Also known as orexin-A.

Hypopnea   Extremely shallow or abnormally slow respiration.

Hypoxia   Impaired oxygenation of the tissues of the body.

Insomnia   A prolonged and usually abnormal inability to obtain adequate sleep that may result in sleepiness, fatigue, difficulty concentrating, and irritability.

Interleukin   Compounds of low molecular weight that chiefly function in immune system regulation and cell-mediated immunity.

K award   Career development awards offered by the NIH to assist new investigators at stages beyond postdoctoral training in order to become independent scientists. Support for the awards is limited to one 3- to 5-year term and is usually restricted to one mentored career award per individual.

K01 award   Mentored Research Scientist Development Award. Provides salary and fringe benefits for awardees for career development experience.

K02 award   Independent Scientist Award. Provides up to 5 years of salary and fringe benefit support for newly independent scientists.

K05 award   Senior Scientist Award. Provides salary and fringe benefit support for outstanding scientists to enhance skills in their research field.

K07 award   Academic Career Award. Provides up to 5 years of funding to develop or improve curricula changes that emphasize development and leadership skills of scientists.

K08 award   Mentored Clinical Scientist Development Award. Provides salary and fringe benefit support for the development of clinician research scientists.

K12 award   Mentored Clinical Scientist Development Program Award. Provides support to an educational institution for career development experiences for clinicians leading to research independence.

K23 award   Mentored Patient-Oriented Research Career Development Award. Provides salary and fringe benefit support for the development of patient-oriented research scientists.

K24 award   Midcareer Investigator Award in Patient-Oriented Research. Provides salary and fringe benefit support to allow protected time for patient-oriented research and time to act as mentors for beginning clinical investigators.

K25 award   Mentored Quantitative Research Career Development Award. Provides salary and fringe benefit support for career development for scientists with quantitative and engineering backgrounds to foster interdisciplinary collaboration in biomedical research.

K-complex   Negative sharp waves followed immediately by slower positive component; sleep spindles may ride on K-complexes. May occur in response to sound or spontaneously but may be distinguished from background activity on the EEG.

Kleine-Levin syndrome   Characterized by recurrent episodes of dramatic hypersomnia lasting from 2 days to several weeks. These episodes are associated with behavioral and cognitive abnormalities, binge eating or hypersexuality, and alternate with long asymptomatic periods that last months to years.

Leptin   A peptide hormone produced by fat cells and involved in the regulation of body weight by acting on the hypothalamus to suppress appetite and burn fat stored in connective tissue.

Magnetic resonance imaging (MRI)   A type of diagnostic imaging technique that relies on the interactions of magnetic fields and radiofrequency radiation with body tissues.

Melatonin   A vertebrate hormone that has been linked to circadian rhythm regulation, is derived from serotonin, and is secreted by the pineal gland especially in response to darkness.

Multiple Sleep Latency Test (MSLT)   A test that objectively quantifies daytime sleepiness.

Myoclonic epilepsy   Epilepsy characterized by myoclonic seizures, which involve brief and involuntary contractions of a muscle.

Narcolepsy   A chronic neurological condition marked by transient attacks of deep sleep, with symptoms of cataplexy, hypnagogic hallucinations, sleep disruption, and sleep paralysis.

Nares   The pair of openings of the nose.

Nightmare disorder   Recurrent nightmares that are coherent dream sequences and manifest as disturbing mental experiences, generally occurring during REM sleep.

Night terrors   One type of disorder of arousal associated with NREM sleep. Typically initiated by a loud scream associated with panic, followed by intense motor activity, which can result in injury.

Nocturnal groaning   Characterized by disruptive groaning that occurs during expiration, particularly during the second half of night. Also known as catathrenia.

Non-rapid eye movement sleep (NREM)   A state of deep, usually dreamless, sleep that occurs regularly during a normal period of sleep with intervening periods of REM sleep and is characterized by delta waves and a low level of autonomic physiological activity—called also non-REM sleep or slow-wave sleep.

Obstructive sleep apnea (OSA)   Obstructive sleep apnea is caused by recurrent interruption of breathing during sleep due to upper airway obstruction caused by sleep-related loss of upper airway muscle tone or anatomical obstruction of the upper airway. Also called obstructive sleep apnea syndrome.

P01 grant   Federally supported research program project grant that is sponsored by the National Institutes of Health and that funds as many as three separate, multidisciplinary research projects that are based on a central research theme. Funding is limited to about $1 million each year in direct costs.

P20 grant Federally supported research program project grant that is sponsored by the National Institutes of Health and that funds exploratory grants. Provides support for the development of new or interdisciplinary programs or the expansion of existing resources.

P30 grant Federally supported center core grant that is sponsored by the National Institutes of Health and that provides funds to develop an infrastructure that supports centralized research, facilities, and resources. Core grants provide resources to investigators to help them achieve a higher level of productivity. Awards are limited to 5 years and about $500,000 in direct costs per year.

P50 grant Federally supported specialized center grant that is sponsored by the National Institutes of Health and that provides funds for multi-investigator, multidisciplinary research. Funding is limited to about $1 million each year in direct costs.

Parasomnia Unpleasant or undesirable behaviors or experiences that occur during entry into sleep, during sleep, or during arousals from sleep.

Pharyngeal Relating to or located in the pharynx area.

Polysomnogram A sleep test that continuously acquires physiological data obtained during sleep, including brain wave activity, eye movements, muscle activity (chin and legs), heart rate, body position, and respiratory variables, including oxygen saturation.

Polysomnography Use of a polygraph to record multiple physiological variables during sleep.

Prader-Willi syndrome A genetic disorder marked by mental retardation, below average height, hypotonia, abnormally small hands and feet, gonadal incompetence, and excessive appetite resulting in extreme obesity.

R01 award Federal research project grant that supports specific health-based research for 1 to 5 years. It can be investigator initiated or submitted in response to a request for application or program announcement.

R03 award Federal grant that supports small research projects for a limited period of time and with limited resources. Grants are awarded for up to 2 years with direct costs limited to $50,000 per year.

R13 award Federal grant that supports conference grants. Provides support for a symposium, seminar, workshop, or other formal conference assembled to exchange and disseminate information or to explore a subject, problem, or field of knowledge.

R21 award Federally supported exploratory or developmental research grant that supports the early development of an innovative project. Grants are awarded for up to 2 years, with total direct costs not to exceed $275,000 for the length of the project.

R25 award Federal grant that supports education project grants. Provides support to develop a program in education, information, training, technical assistance, or evaluation.

Rapid eye movement (REM) Rapid and simultaneous movement of both eyes, and associated with REM sleep.

Rapid eye movement sleep A state of sleep that is experienced in several cycles during a normal period of sleep and is marked by increased forebrain and midbrain neuronal activity and by reduced muscle tone. Humans experience dreams, rapid eye movements, and vascular congestion of the sex organs during REM sleep.

Rapid eye movement sleep behavior disorder A complex set of behaviors, including mild to harmful body movements associated with dreams and nightmares and loss of muscle atonia.

Restless legs syndrome (RLS) A neurological condition characterized by an irresistible urge to move that occurs or worsens at rest and is relieved by activity. It is also sometimes characterized by worsening in the evening and night.

Sleep apnea A condition marked by transient cessation of breathing during sleep, as a result of either airway obstruction or a disturbance in the brain's respiratory center. Especially associated with excessive daytime sleepiness.

Sleep drunkenness Difficulty waking up and being foggy for long periods of time after wake onset. Also known as sleep inertia.

Sleep hygiene Describes the practice of maintaining proper sleep health.

Sleep medicine A branch of clinical medicine devoted to the diagnosis and treatment of individuals suffering from chronic sleep loss or sleep disorders.

Sleep paralysis Muscle paralysis akin to REM sleep atonia while awake, when falling asleep, or waking up.

Sleep-related dissociative disorder A dissociative episode that can occur in the period from wakefulness to sleep or from awakening from stages 1 or 2 or from REM sleep.

Sleep-related eating disorder Marked by repeated episodes of involuntary eating and drinking during arousals from sleep.

Sleep-related hallucination Hallucinatory images that occur at sleep onset or on awakening from sleep.

Sleep restriction therapy A method to curtail time in bed to the actual sleep time, thereby creating mild sleep deprivation, which results in more consolidated and more efficient sleep.

Sleep spindle Waxing and waning electrical brain activity at 7 to 14 Hz, grouped in sequences that last 1 to 2 seconds and recur periodically with a slow rhythm of 0.1 to 0.4 Hz. Typically appear during sleep stage 2.

Sleepwalking One type of disorder of arousal associated with NREM sleep. Involves a series of behaviors initiated during arousals from slow-wave sleep that culminate in walking around in an altered state of consciousness.

Slow-wave sleep (SWS) Term used to describe sleep stages 3 and 4 together due to characteristic slow waves.

Somnology The branch of science devoted to the study of the physiology of sleep, the behavioral dimensions of sleep, and the consequences of sleep loss and sleep disorders on an individual's and the general population's health, performance, safety, and quality of life.

Somnolence Drowsiness.

Spasticity A state of increased muscular tone in which abnormal stretch reflexes intensify muscle resistance to passive movements.

Stage 1 sleep First stage of NREM sleep characterized by low-voltage, mixed frequency waves on the EEG; small eye movements; and tonic muscles.

Stage 2 sleep Second stage of NREM sleep characterized by low-voltage, mixed frequency waves on the EEG, sleep spindles, and K-complexes; occasional small eye movements near sleep onset; and tonic muscles.

Stage 3 sleep Third stage of NREM sleep characterized by high-voltage, slow-wave activity on EEG; no eye movements; and tonic muscles.

Stage 4 sleep Fourth stage of NREM sleep characterized by high-voltage, slow-wave activity on EEG; no eye movements; and tonic muscles.

Sudden Infant Death Syndrome (SIDS) The death of an apparently healthy infant usually before 1 year of age that is of unknown cause and occurs especially during sleep.

Suprachiasmatic nucleus (SCN) Either of a pair of neuron clusters in the hypothalamus that receive visual information from the retina via the optic nerve and that regulate the body's circadian rhythms.

T32 training grant National Research Service Award Institutional Research Training Grants. Provides support to institutions to develop or enhance research training opportunities for predoctoral and postdoctoral students.

T34 training grant National Research Service Award Institutional Undergraduate Research Training Grant. Provides support to institutions to promote undergraduate research training to underrepresented groups in the biomedical and behavioral sciences.

T35 training grant   Short-Term Institutional Research Training Grant. Provides support to institutions for predoctoral and postdoctoral training focused on biomedical and behavioral research.

Type 2 diabetes mellitus   Diabetes that develops especially in adults and especially in obese individuals. Marked by high blood sugar that is a consequence of impaired insulin utilization and a physiological inability to compensate with increased insulin production. Also called adult-onset diabetes, late-onset diabetes.

U Cooperative Agreements   Provided to support any part of the full range of research and development activities composing a multidisciplinary attack on a specific disease entity or biomedical problem area.

D

Congressional Language Establishing the National Center on Sleep Disorders Research, § 285b–7

The following is the congressional language that was part of the 1993 National Institutes of Health (NIH) Revitalization Act, which created the National Center on Sleep Disorders Research. The NIH Revitalization Act became law (*P.L. 103-43*) on June 10, 1993.

a) **Establishment** Not later than 1 year after June 10, 1993, the Director of the Institute shall establish the National Center on Sleep Disorders Research (in this section referred to as the "Center"). The Center shall be headed by a director, who shall be appointed by the Director of the Institute.

b) **Purpose** The general purpose of the Center is—
   1. the conduct and support of research, training, health information dissemination, and other activities with respect to sleep disorders, including biological and circadian rhythm research, basic understanding of sleep, chronobiological and other sleep related research; and
   2. to coordinate the activities of the Center with similar activities of other Federal agencies, including the other agencies of the National Institutes of Health, and similar activities of other public entities and nonprofit entities.

c) **Sleep Disorders Research Advisory Board**
   1. The Director of the National Institutes of Health shall establish a board to be known as the Sleep Disorders Research Advisory Board (in this section referred to as the "Advisory Board").

2. The Advisory Board shall advise, assist, consult with, and make recommendations to the Director of the National Institutes of Health, through the Director of the Institute, and the Director of the Center concerning matters relating to the scientific activities carried out by and through the Center and the policies respecting such activities, including recommendations with respect to the plan required in subsection (c)[1] of this section.

3.

     A. The Director of the National Institutes of Health shall appoint to the Advisory Board 12 appropriately qualified representatives of the public who are not officers or employees of the Federal Government. Of such members, eight shall be representatives of health and scientific disciplines with respect to sleep disorders and four shall be individuals representing the interests of individuals with or undergoing treatment for sleep disorders.

     B. The following officials shall serve as ex officio members of the Advisory Board:

         i. The Director of the National Institutes of Health.

         ii. The Director of the Center.

         iii. The Director of the National Heart, Lung, and Blood Institute.

         iv. The Director of the National Institute of Mental Health.

         v. The Director of the National Institute on Aging.

         vi. The Director of the National Institute of Child Health and Human Development.

         vii. The Director of the National Institute of Neurological Disorders and Stroke.

         viii. The Assistant Secretary for Health.

         ix. The Assistant Secretary of Defense (Health Affairs).

         x. The Chief Medical Director of the Veterans' Administration.

4. The members of the Advisory Board shall, from among the members of the Advisory Board, designate an individual to serve as the chair of the Advisory Board.

5. Except as inconsistent with, or inapplicable to, this section, the provisions of section 284a of this title shall apply to the advisory board established under this section in the same manner as such provisions apply to any advisory council established under such section.

---

[1]So in original. Probably should be subsection "(d)".

d) **Development of comprehensive research plan; revision**
   1. After consultation with the Director of the Center and the advisory board established under subsection (c) of this section, the Director of the National Institutes of Health shall develop a comprehensive plan for the conduct and support of sleep disorders research.
   2. The plan developed under paragraph (1) shall identify priorities with respect to such research and shall provide for the coordination of such research conducted or supported by the agencies of the National Institutes of Health.
   3. The Director of the National Institutes of Health (after consultation with the Director of the Center and the advisory board[2] established under subsection (c) of this section) shall revise the plan developed under paragraph (1) as appropriate.
e) **Collection and dissemination of information** The Director of the Center, in cooperation with the Centers for Disease Control and Prevention, is authorized to coordinate activities with the Department of Transportation, the Department of Defense, the Department of Education, the Department of Labor, and the Department of Commerce to collect data, conduct studies, and disseminate public information concerning the impact of sleep disorders and sleep deprivation.

---

[2]So in original. Probably should be capitalized.

E

Sleep Disorders Research Advisory Board Membership

Name	Affiliation	Year of Term Expiration
Scientific and Health		
Wayne E. Crill, MD	Professor and chair, Department of Physiology and Biophysics, School of Medicine, University of Washington	1996
Debra J. Meyers, MD	Private Physician Pulmonary Associates	1996
Thomas Roth, PhD	**Director, Sleep Disorders and Research Center, Henry Ford Hospital**	**1996**
J. Christian Gillin, MD	Professor, Department of Psychiatry/UCSD/ VAMC	1997
Allan Pack, MB, ChB, PhD	Director of Medicine Center on Sleep and Respiratory Neurobiology, Hospital of the University of Pennsylvania	1997
Barbara A. Phillips, MD, MSPH	Professor, Division of Pulmonary and Critical Care; Medicine Director, Sleep Apnea Laboratory, University of Kentucky and Good Samaritan Hospitals	1997
James K. Walsh, PhD	Director, Sleep Medical Center St. Luke's MSPH	1997
Sudhansu Chokroverty, MD	Professor and associate chair of neurology; chief of neurophysiology, Department of Neurology, St. Vincent's Hospital & Medical Center	1998
Martha U. Gillette, PhD	Professor, Department of Cell and Structure Biology, University of Illinois	1999

Name	Affiliation	Year of Term Expiration
Fred W. Turek, PhD	Director, Center for Circadian Biology & Medicine; professor and chair, Department of Neurobiology and Physiology, Northwestern University	2000
Richard P. Millman, MD	Director, Sleep Disorders Center Rhode Island Hospital	2001
Michael Rosbash, PhD	Howard Hughes Medical Institute, Department of Biology, Brandeis University	2001
David P. White, MD	Director, Sleep Disorders Program, Division of Endocrinology, Brigham and Women's Hospital	2001
Carol Landis, DNSc, RN	Department of Biology, Behavioral Nursing and Health Systems, University of Washington Seattle	2002
Emmanuel Mignot, MD, PhD	Director, Center for Narcolepsy, Stanford University School of Medicine	2002
Gene Block, PhD	Vice president and provost, University of Virginia	2004
Mary Carskadon, PhD	Professor, Department of Psychiatry and Human Behavior, Brown University School of Medicine	2004
Stuart F. Quan, MD	Chief Pulmonary and Critical Care Medicine Section Director, Sleep Disorders Center Professor of Medicine, University of Arizona	2005
Clifford Saper, MD, PhD	Professor and chair, Department of Neurology and Program in Neuroscience, Harvard Medical School	2005
Kathryn A. Lee, RN, PhD, FAAN	Professor, family health care nursing, School of Nursing, University of California, San Francisco	2006
Rafael Pelayo, MD	Assistant professor, Department of Psychiatry and Behavioral Sciences, Stanford University	2006
Susan Redline, MD, MPH	Chief, Division of Clinical Epidemiology, Department of Pediatrics, Rainbow Babies and Children's Hospital Professor of pediatrics, medicine, epidemiology, and biostatistics, Case School of Medicine	2006
Michael J. Sateia, MD	Professor of psychiatry; Director, Section of Sleep Medicine, Dartmouth University	2006
Gina Poe, PhD	Assistant professor, Department of Anesthesiology, University of Michigan Medical Center	2007
Michael H. Smolensky, PhD	Professor of environmental sciences, University of Texas-Houston	2008

continued

Name	Affiliation	Year of Term Expiration
Howard P. Roffwarg, MD	Professor of psychiatry and human behavior; Director, Division of Sleep Medicine, co-director, Animal Sleep Neurophysiology Laboratory, University of Mississippi Medical Center	2009
Phyllis C. Zee, MD, PhD	Professor of neurology, neurobiology, and physiology; director, Sleep Disorders Center, Northwestern University	2009
Public and Patient Advocates		
Carol C. Westbrook		1996
Carla G. Kidd		1998
Victoria P. Haulcy, MPH		1999
Morris L. Lyons		2000
Carol Upchurch Walker		2000
Carol Bell Anderson		2002
James Everett, Jr., MD		2002
Sandra McGinnis		2003
Dara Spearman		2003
Phillip Williams		2004
Sara Caddick, PhD		2005
Lorraine Wearley, PhD		2007
Sheila C. Connolly, RN		2007
M. Elizabeth Johns		2008
Julianne Hill		2009

NOTE: Members in bold indicate a former or the current chair of the NCSDR Advisory Board. Each term is 4 years in length.

F

National Institutes of Health
Sleep-Related Initiatives:
1994–2004

TABLE F-1 Sleep Initiatives (RFAs) Sponsored by the National Institutes of Health, 1994–2004

Title	Primary Purpose	Participating Institutes/Centers	Funding Activity	Year
SCOR in Neurobiology of Sleep & Sleep Apnea: RFA-HL-96-014	Establish specialized centers of research (SCORs) programs to foster translational research.	NHLBI	P50	1996
Molecular Biology and Genetics of Sleep and Sleep Disorders: RFA-HL-96-015	Advance the understanding of the molecular and genetic basis of sleep and sleep disorders.	NHLBI, NIMH, NICHD	R01	1996
Sleep Academic Award: HL-97-015; HL-96-021	Develop and/or improve the quality of medical curricula for the prevention, management, and control of sleep disorders.	NHLBI	K07	1996, 1997
Obstructive Sleep Apnea in Children: HL-98-004	Define abnormalities in airway structure and function responsible for obstructive sleep apnea in children, and identify physiological and clinical measures associated with increased morbidity.	NHLBI, NIDR, NICHD	R01	1997
Phenotypic Characterization of Sleep in Mice: RFA-HL-99-001	Develop improved molecular, cellular, and systems approaches to investigate sleep and circadian phenotypes in mice.	NHLBI, NIMH, NIA, NINDS	R01	1998
Nocturnal Asthma, Chronobiology, and Sleep: RFA-HL-99-011	Establish the mechanisms that underlie the chronobiology of nocturnal exacerbations of asthma and airway inflammation, as well as the role played by sleep and sleep disturbances.	NHLBI	R01	1999
Implementation of the National Occupational Research Agenda: RFA-OH-99-002	Develop knowledge that can be used in preventing occupational diseases and injuries and to better understand their underlying pathophysiology.	NIOSH, NCI, NHLBI, NIA, NIDCD, NIEHS	R01, R18	1999
Data Coordinating Center for Sleep Heart Health Study: RFA-HL-99-014	Establish a new data coordinating center for the Sleep Heart Health Study.	NHLBI	U01	1999
Research on Alcohol and Sleep: RFA-AA-00-005	Stimulate research on alcohol and sleep in areas that may improve understanding of the etiology and treatment of alcoholism.	NIAAA	R01, R21	2000

Title / RFA Number	Purpose	Institutes	Type	Year
Oxygen Sensing During Intermittent Hypoxia: RFA-HL-00-004	Improve understanding of how intermittent hypoxia contributes to the pathophysiology of cardiopulmonary, vascular, hematological, and sleep disorders.	NHLBI	R01	2000
Ancillary Studies in Conjunction with SHOW Trial: RFA-DK-00-017	Develop basic, clinical, and behavioral ancillary research studies of the Study of Health Outcomes of Weight-Loss (SHOW) clinical trial.	NIDDK, NHLBI, NINR, NIAMS, NIDCR	R01	2000
Interrelationships Between Sleep and Heart, Lung, and Blood Diseases: RFA-HL-01-009	Elucidate characteristics of sleep physiology, sleep disorders, and pathophysiological mechanisms mediating the interrelationship between sleep disturbance and heart, lung, and blood diseases.	NHLBI, NIDA	R01	2001
Sleep and Sleep Disorders in Children: RFA-HL-01-006	Improve the understanding of fundamental biological mechanisms through which sleep deprivation and sleep disorders affect the cardiopulmonary, hematological, immunological, mental, and behavioral health of children.	NHLBI, NIMH, NINR, NICHD	R01	2001
Role of Sleep and Sleep Disordered Breathing in the Metabolic Syndrome: RFA-HL-03-008	Elucidate the relationship of sleep deprivation and sleep-disordered breathing to characteristics of the metabolic syndrome including obesity, high blood pressure, dyslipidemia, insulin resistance, and vascular inflammation.	NHLBI, NIA	R01	2002
Inter-relationships of Sleep, Fatigue, and HIV/AIDS: RFA-HL-04-010	Elucidate the etiology of sleep disturbances and fatigue associated with human immunodeficiency virus infection and acquired immunodeficiency disease syndrome.	NHLBI, NIMH	R01	2003

NOTE: Primary purpose of each PA and RFA are adapted from language in NIH announcements. NCCAM = National Center for Complementary and Alternative Medicine; NCI = National Cancer Institute; NCSDR = National Center on Sleep Disorders Research; NHLBI = National Heart, Lung, and Blood Institute; NIA = National Institute on Aging; NIAAA = National Institute on Alcohol Abuse and Alcoholism; NIAID = National Institute of Allergy and Infectious Diseases; NIAMS = National Institute of Arthritis and Musculoskeletal and Skin Diseases; NICHD = National Institute of Child Health and Human Development; NIDA = National Institute on Drug Abuse; NIDCD = National Institute on Deafness and Other Communication Disorders; NIDCR = National Institute of Dental and Craniofacial Research; NIDDK = National Institute of Diabetes and Digestive and Kidney Diseases; NIDR = National Institute of Dental Research; NIEHS = National Institute of Environmental Health Sciences; ; NIH= National Institutes of Health; NIMH = National Institute of Mental Health; NINDS = National Institute of Neurological Disorders and Stroke; NINR = National Institute of Nursing Research; NIOSH = National Institute for Occupational Safety and Health; PA = program announcement; RFA = request for application.

SOURCE: National Heart, Lung, and Blood Institute, 2003; *National Sleep Disorders Research Plan*, 2003. Bethesda, MD: NIH.

TABLE F-2 Sleep Initiatives (PAs) Sponsored by the National Institutes of Health, 1994–2004

Title	Primary Purpose	Participating Institutes/Centers	Funding Activity	Year
Basic and Clinical Research on Sleep & Wakefulness: PA-95-014	Enhance sleep research in the following areas: neuroscience and behavioral science; molecular and cellular mechanisms of sleep and circadian rhythms across the life span; development of sleep from fetal life through infancy; role of dreaming in humans; etiological factors and pathophysiology of transient or persistent insomnia; and the treatment of sleep disorders.	NIA, NIAAA, NICHD, NIDA, NHLBI, NIMH, NINDS, NINR	R01, R03, R29, P01	1994
Innovative Approaches to Developing New Technologies: PA-97-014	Support research to identify, create, and develop innovative technologies and to provide these technologies for biomedical research.	NCRR	R21	1996
Research on Musculoskeletal Fitness and Sports Medicine: PA-97-025	Study a broad range of basic and clinical topics related to musculoskeletal fitness, exercise physiology, and sports medicine.	NIAMS, NICHD, NINR	R01, R03, R29, K01, K02, K08, P01	1997
Institutional National Research Service Award in Sleep Research: PA-97-064	Ensure that scientists, highly trained in sleep research, are available in adequate numbers to address important gaps in our biomedical and biological understanding of sleep, including those outlined in the NIH director's Sleep Disorders Research Plan.	NHLBI, NIA, NIAAA, NICHD, NIDA, NIMH, NINDS, NINR	T32	1997
Bioengineering Research Grants: PAR-99-009	Support basic bioengineering research whose outcomes are likely to advance health or health-related research within the mission of the NIH.	NCI, NCRR, NEI, NHGRI, NHLBI, NIA, NIAAA, NIAID, NIAMS, NICHD, NIDA, NIDCD, NIMH, NINDS, NINR, NLM	R01	1998

Human Brain Project (Neuroinformatics): PAR-99-138	Encourage and support investigator-initiated, neuroinformatics research that will lead to new digital and electronic tools for all domains of neuroscience research.	NIMH, NIDA, NSF, NIA, NICHD, NIDCD, NLM, NASA, FIC, DOE, NIAAA, NHLBI, NIDCR, NCI, NINDS	R01, P01, P20	1999
Occupational Safety and Health Research: PA-99-143	Develop knowledge that can be used in preventing occupational diseases and injuries, and better understand their underlying pathophysiology.	NIOSH, NCI, NHLBI, NIA, NIAAA, NIAID, NIAMS, NIDCD, NIEHS	R01	1999
Restless Legs Syndrome and Periodic Limb Movement Disorder: PA-01-086	Develop an understanding of the pathogenesis of RLS and PLMD that will lead to new forms of treatment.	NINDS, NHLBI, NIA, NIMH	R01	2001
Research on Sleep and Sleep Disorders: PA-05-046	Advance biomedical knowledge related to sleep or sleep disorders; improve understanding of the neurobiology or functions of sleep over the life span; enhance timely diagnosis and effective treatment for individuals affected by sleep-related disorders; or implement and evaluate innovative community-based public health education and intervention programs.	NHLBI, NCSDR, NIA, NIAAA, NIAMS, NCI, NICHD, NCCAM, NIDA, NIMH, NINDS, NINR, ORWH	R01, R21	2004

NOTE: Primary purpose of each PA and RFA are adapted from language in NIH announcements. DOE = Department of Energy; FIC = Fogarty International Center; NASA = National Aeronautics and Space Administration; NCCAM = National Center for Complementary and Alternative Medicine; NCI = National Cancer Institute; NCRR = National Center for Research Resources; NCSDR = National Center on Sleep Disorders Research; NEI = National Eye Institute; NHGRI = National Human Genome Research Institute; NHLBI = National Heart, Lung, and Blood Institute; NIA = National Institute on Aging; NIAAA = National Institute on Alcohol Abuse and Alcoholism; NIAID = National Institute of Allergy and Infectious Diseases; NIAMS = National Institute of Arthritis and Musculoskeletal and Skin Diseases; NICHD = National Institute of Child Health and Human Development; NIDA = National Institute on Drug Abuse; NIDCD = National Institute on Deafness and Other Communication Disorders; NIDCR = National Institute of Dental and Craniofacial Research; NIEHS = National Institute for Environmental Health Sciences; NIH= National Institutes of Health; NIMH = National Institute of Mental Health; NINDS = National Institute of Neurological Disorders and Stroke; NINR = National Institute of Nursing Research; NIOSH = National Institute for Occupational Safety and Health; NLM = National Library of Medicine; NSF = National Sleep Foundation; ORWH = Office of Research on Women's Health; PA = program announcement; RFA = request for application.

SOURCES: National Heart Lung and Blood Institute, 2003; *National Sleep Disorders Research Plan*, 2003. Bethesda, MD: NIH.

G

National Institutes of Health
Support of Sleep-Related R01 Grants

The following information is a summary of extramural sleep research grants at the National Institutes of Health (NIH).

Institute of Medicine staff searched the Computer Retrieval of Information on Scientific Projects (CRISP) database for key-terms relevant to sleep. These terms include *insomnia, periodic limb movement disorder, restless legs syndrome, circadian rhythm, sudden infant death syndrome, sleep disorder, narcolepsy, sleep apnea, sleep, hibernation,* and *dream.* Abstracts were reviewed and only those grants with these terms listed in both the thesaurus and abstract, and not the abstract alone, were considered in the counts. The numbers for each grant reflect individual, unduplicated counts for a given year (Table G-1 and Figure G-1). All institutes were searched. Note that every abstract from 1995 and 2004 was analyzed to determine its relevance to somnology and somnopathy (see Table 6-3). This resulted in even fewer grants being relevant to the field. This analysis was not performed on grants awarded from 1996 to 2003; therefore these numbers may be slightly inflated.

TABLE G-1 Sleep-Related R01 Grants, 1995–2004

Fiscal Year	1995	1996	1997	1998	1999	2000	2001	2002	2003	2004
Number of Awards	116	79	243	259	244	332	369	402	420	331
Number of New Awards	37	24	68	71	43	86	118	101	113	82

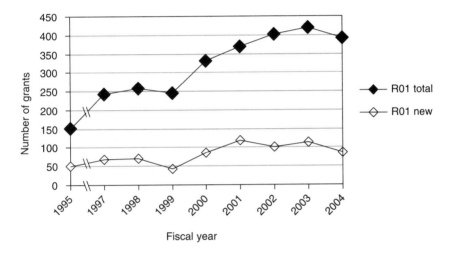

FIGURE G-1 Sleep-Related R01 Grants, 1995 to 2004.

There are 12 institutes that are members of the Trans-NIH Sleep Research Coordinating Committee. Table G-2 shows the annual NIH support of sleep-related research for various institutes. However, analysis of NIH support of sleep-related R01 grants shows that two of the largest supporters of sleep grants, the National Institute of General Medical Sciences and the National Eye Institute, are not members of the Trans-NIH Sleep Research Coordinating Committee.

TABLE G-2 Annual NIH Institute Support of Sleep-Related Research

	NIMH	NHLBI	NINDS	NIA	NIGMS	NINR	NEI	NIDA	NIAAA
1995	35	20	29	16	2	9	8	4	7
1996	26	15	14	11	0	6	0	1	1
1997	56	46	41	30	7	12	11	8	10
1998	57	47	49	32	10	10	10	11	8
1999	53	48	57	29	9	10	11	10	11
2000	72	84	59	33	10	16	14	11	9
2001	87	80	53	35	16	15	15	14	12
2002	105	93	50	40	17	15	16	17	11
2003	101	104	53	36	21	22	16	12	13
2004	88	102	49	31	22	19	15	13	12

ABBREVIATIONS: NCCAM = National Center for Complementary and Alternative Medicine; NCI = National Cancer Institute; NEI = National Eye Institute; NHLBI = National Heart, Lung, and Blood Institute; NIA = National Institute on Aging; NIAAA = National Institute on Alcohol Abuse and Alcoholism; NIAID = National Institute of Allergy and Infectious Diseases; NIAMS = National Institute of Arthritis and Musculoskeletal and Skin Diseases; NICHD = National Institute of Child Health and Human Development; NIDA = National Institute on Drug Abuse; NIDCD = National Institute on Deafness and Other Communication Disorders; NIDCR = National Institute of Dental and Craniofacial Research; NIDDK = National Institute of Diabetes and Digestive and Kidney Diseases; NIGMS = National Institute of General Medical Sciences; NIH = National Institutes of Health; NIMH = National Institute of Mental Health; NINDS = National Institute of Neurological Disorders and Stroke; NINR = National Institute of Nursing Research; NIOSH = National Institute for Occupational Safety and Health.

NIDDK	NICHD	NCI	NIAMS	NIDCD	NIOSH	NCCAM	NIAID	NIDCR	FIC
2	17	0	2	0	1	0	2	0	0
1	6	0	0	0	0	0	1	0	0
8	15	2	2	0	1	0	2	0	0
8	11	2	3	0	0	0	1	1	0
2	15	3	3	0	4	0	0	1	
29	17	3	7	3	3	2	0	1	0
14	17	4	7	4	3	3	0	0	0
16	16	5	5	4	2	3	0	0	0
15	13	6	6	3	3	4	1	0	0
11	10	7	5	4	3	3	1	0	1

H

Summary of NIH Support of Sleep-Related Career Development Awards

The following information is a summary of extramural sleep research grants at the National Institutes of Health. Institute of Medicine staff searched the Computer Retrieval of Information on Scientific Projects (CRISP) database for key-terms relevant to sleep. These terms include *insomnia, periodic limb movement disorder, restless legs syndrome, circadian rhythm, sudden infant death syndrome, sleep disorder, narcolepsy, sleep apnea, sleep, hibernation,* and *dream.* Abstracts were reviewed and only those grants with these terms listed in both the thesaurus and abstract, and not the abstract alone, were considered in the counts. The numbers for each grant reflect individual, unduplicated counts for a given year. All institutes were searched.

Grant	Title	Description	Number of Awards (New Awards)		
			1995	2000	2004
K01	Mentored Research Scientist Development Award	Provides salary and fringe benefits for awardees for career development experience	1 (1)	9 (3)	6 (1)
K02	Independent Scientist Award	Provides up to 5 yeasrs of salary and fringe benefit support for newly independent scientists	10 (1)	8 (1)	3 (1)

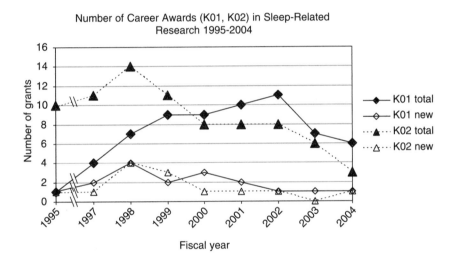

Number of Career Awards (K01, K02) in Sleep-Related
Research 1995-2004

Grant	Title	Description	Number of Awards (New Awards)		
			1995	2000	2004
K05	Senior Scientist Award	Provides salary and fringe benefit support for outstanding scientists to enhance skills in their research field	6 (2)	5 (0)	1 (0)
K07	Academic	Provides up to 5 years of funding to develop or improve curricula changes that emphasize development and leadership skills of scientists	1 (0)	20 (0)	3 (3)

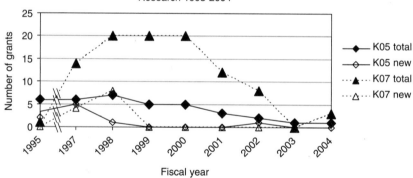

Number of Career Awards (K05, K07) in Sleep-Related Research 1995-2004

Grant	Title	Description	Number of Awards (New Awards)		
			1995	2000	2004
K08	Mentored Clinical Scientist Development Award	Provides salary and fringe benefit support for the development of clinician research scientists	8 (1)	12 (1)	8 (1)
K12	Mentored Clinical Scientist Development Program Award	Provides support to an educational institution for career development experiences for clinicians leading to research independence	0	0	0
K23	Mentored Patient-Oriented Research Career Development Award	Provides salary and fringe benefit support for the development of patient-oriented research scientists	0 (0)	10 (6)	28 (8)

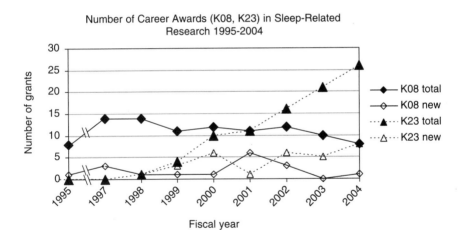

Number of Career Awards (K08, K23) in Sleep-Related Research 1995-2004

Grant	Title	Description	Number of Awards (New Awards)		
			1995	2000	2004
K24	Midcareer Investigator Award in Patient-Oriented Research	Provides salary and fringe benefit support to allow protected time for patient-oriented research and time to act as mentors for beginning clinical investigators	0 (0)	5 (1)	8 (3)
K25	Mentored Quantitative Research Career Development Award	Provides salary and fringe benefit support for career development for scientists with quantitative and engineering backgrounds to foster interdisciplinary collaboration in biomedical research	0 (0)	0 (0)	1 (0)

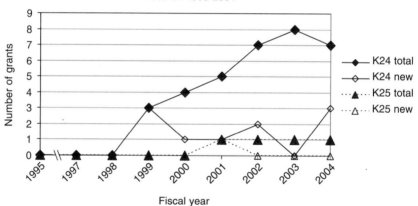

Number of Career Awards (K24, K25) in Sleep-Related Research 1995-2004

Summary of NIH Institute Support of K Awards

Of the 314 career development awards that were funded during the 5 years between 2000 and 2004, the National Heart, Lung, and Blood Institute (NHLBI) sponsored 94 (29 percent). Thirty-two of all the NHLBI-sponsored training grants were K07 grants awarded in 2000 and 2001. K07 grants are designed to provide 5 years of funding to develop or improve curricula changes that emphasize development and leadership skills of scientists.

K01: Mentored Research Scientist Development Award

	Number of Awards (New Awards)						
	NIMH	NCCAM	NINR	NIA	NIDDK	NCRR	Total
2000	4 (1)	1 (1)	2 (1)	1 (0)	1 (0)	0 (0)	9 (3)
2001	4 (0)	1 (0)	2 (1)	1 (0)	1 (0)	1 (1)	10 (2)
2002	6 (1)	1 (0)	2 (0)	1 (0)	0 (0)	1 (0)	11 (1)
2003	3 (0)	1 (0)	1 (0)	1 (1)	0 (0)	1 (0)	7 (1)
2004	2 (0)	1 (0)	0 (0)	1 (0)	1 (1)	1 (0)	6 (1)

K02: Independent Scientist Award

	Number of Awards (New Awards)			
	NIMH	NINDS	NICHD	Total
2000	6 (1)	2 (0)	0 (0)	8 (1)
2001	6 (1)	2 (0)	0 (0)	8 (1)
2002	7 (1)	1 (0)	0 (0)	8 (1)
2003	5 (0)	1 (0)	0 (0)	6 (0)
2004	2 (0)	0 (0)	1 (1)	3 (1)

K05: Senior Scientist

	Number of Awards (New Awards)	
	NIMH	Total
2000	5 (0)	5 (0)
2001	3 (0)	3 (0)
2002	2 (1)	2 (1)
2003	1 (0)	1 (0)
2004	1 (0)	1 (0)

K07: Academic Career Award

	Number of Awards (New Awards)	
	NHLBI	Total
2000	20 (0)	20 (0)
2001	12 (0)	12 (0)
2002	8 (0)	8 (0)
2003	0 (0)	0 (0)
2004	3 (3)	3 (3)

K08: Mentored Clinical Scientist Development Award

	NIMH	NINDS	NHLBI	NICHD	NCI	AHRQ	NEI	NIGMS	Total
	Number of Awards (New Awards)								
2000	4 (1)	4 (0)	1 (0)	1 (0)	1 (0)	0 (0)	1 (0)	0 (0)	12 (1)
2001	5 (2)	3 (2)	0 (0)	1 (1)	0 (0)	0 (0)	1 (0)	1 (1)	11 (6)
2002	4 (0)	3 (1)	1 (1)	1 (0)	0 (0)	1 (1)	1 (0)	1 (0)	12 (3)
2003	4 (0)	1 (0)	1 (0)	1 (0)	0 (0)	1 (0)	1 (0)	1 (0)	10 (0)
2004	3 (0)	1 (1)	1 (0)	1 (0)	0 (0)	1 (0)	0 (0)	1 (0)	8 (1)

K23: Mentored Patient-Oriented Research Career Development Award

	NIMH	NIA	NIDDK	NCRR	NINDS	NHLBI	NICHD	Total
	Number of Awards (New Awards)							
2000	1 (1)	2 (1)	0 (0)	2 (2)	0 (0)	5 (2)	0 (0)	10 (6)
2001	1 (0)	2 (0)	0 (0)	2 (0)	0 (0)	6 (1)	0 (1)	11 (2)
2002	3 (2)	1 (0)	1 (1)	3 (1)	0 (0)	7 (1)	1 (0)	16 (5)
2003	4 (1)	1 (0)	1 (0)	4 (1)	0 (0)	9 (2)	2 (1)	21 (5)
2004	7 (2)	2 (1)	2 (1)	5 (1)	1 (1)	7 (2)	2 (0)	26 (8)

K24: Midcareer Investigator Award in Patient-Oriented Research

	NIMH	NIAAA	NIA	NCRR	NHLBI	NICHD	Total
	Number of Awards (New Awards)						
2000	1 (0)	1 (0)	1 (1)	0 (0)	1 (0)	0 (0)	4 (1)
2001	1 (0)	0 (0)	1 (0)	0 (0)	1 (0)	1 (1)	4 (1)
2002	2 (1)	1 (0)	1 (0)	0 (0)	2 (1)	1 (0)	7 (2)
2003	3 (0)	1 (0)	1 (0)	0 (0)	2 (0)	1 (0)	8 (0)
2004	1 (0)	0 (0)	1 (0)	1 (1)	3 (2)	1 (0)	7 (3)

K25: Mentored Quantitative Research

	Number of Awards (New Awards)	
	NHLBI	Total
2000	0 (0)	0 (0)
2001	0 (1)	0 (1)
2002	1 (0)	1 (0)
2003	1 (0)	1 (0)
2004	1 (0)	1 (0)

ABBREVIATIONS: AHRQ = Agency for Healthcare Research and Quality; NCCAM = National Center for Complementary and Alternative Medicine; NCI = National Cancer Institute; NCRR = National Center for Research Resources; NEI = National Eye Institute; NHLBI = National Heart, Lung, and Blood Institute; NIA = National Institute on Aging; NIAAA = National Institute on Alcohol Abuse and Alcoholism; NICHD = National Institute of Child Health and Human Development; NIDDK = National Institute of Diabetes and Digestive and Kidney Diseases; NIGMS = National Institute of General Medical Sciences; NIMH = National Institute of Mental Health; NINDS = National Institute of Neurological Disorders and Stroke; NINR = National Institute of Nursing Research.

I

Summary of NIH Support of Sleep-Related R13, R25, P, F, T, and U Grants

The following information is a summary of extramural sleep research grants at the National Institutes of Health. Institute of Medicine staff searched the Computer Retrieval of Information on Scientific Projects (CRISP) database for key terms relevant to sleep. These terms include *insomnia, periodic limb movement disorder, restless legs syndrome, circadian rhythm, sudden infant death syndrome, sleep disorder, narcolepsy, sleep apnea, sleep, hibernation, and dream.* Abstracts were reviewed and only those grants with these terms listed in both the thesaurus terms and abstract, not the abstract alone, were considered in the counts. The numbers for each grant reflect individual, unduplicated counts for a given year. All institutes were searched. Note that no sleep-related U grants were funded between 1994 and 2004.

Grant	Title	Description	Number of Awards (New Awards)		
			1995	2000	2004
R13	Conference Grant	Provides support for a symposium, seminar, workshop, or other formal conference assembled to exchange and disseminate information or to explore a subject, problem, or field of knowledge	0	0	2
R25	Education Project Grant	Provides support to develop a program in education, information, training, technical assistance, or evaluation	0 (0)	4 (1)	1 (0)

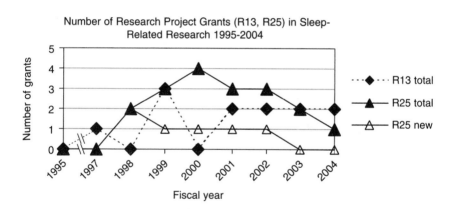

Number of Research Project Grants (R13, R25) in Sleep-Related Research 1995-2004

Grant	Title	Description	Number of Awards (New Awards)		
			1995	2000	2004
P01	Research Program Project	Provides support for an integrated, multiproject research program involving a number of independent investigators who share knowledge and common resources	5 (1)	17 (5)	11 (6)
P20	Exploratory Grant	Provides support for the development of new or interdisciplinary programs or the expansion of existing resources	0 (0)	1 (0)	2 (2)
P30	Center Core Grant	Provides support for shared resources and facilities to a program providing a multi-disciplinary approach with existing research funds	0 (0)	6 (3)	4 (2)
P50	Specialized Center Grant	Provides support to assemble "critical masses" of basic and clinical scientists to work together collaboratively	6 (3)	10 (3)	7 (5)

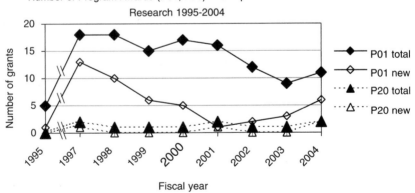

Number of Program Awards (P01, P20) in Sleep-Related Research 1995-2004

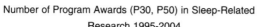

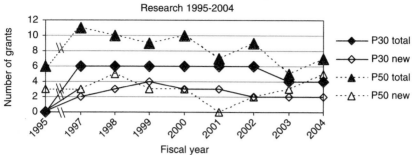

Fiscal year

			Number of Awards (New Awards)		
Grant	Title	Description	1995	2000	2004
F30	Individual Predoctoral National Research Service Award for M.D./Ph.D. Fellowship	Fellowship award that provides combined medical school and predoctoral Ph.D. support for a maximum of 6 years	1 (1)	3 (0)	3 (1)
F31	Predoctoral Individual National Research Service Award	Fellowship award that provides up to 5 years of support for research training leading to the Ph.D. or equivalent research	3 (0)	8 (0)	28 (14)
F32	Postdoctoral Individual National Research Service Award	Fellowship award that provides postdoctoral research training to broaden scientific background	5 (3)	13 (3)	25 (13)
F33	National Research	Fellowship award that provides opportunities for experienced scientists to broaden scientific background	0	0	0

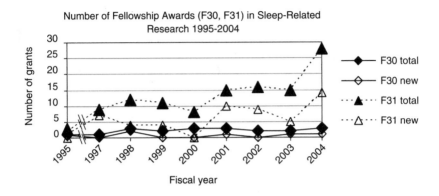

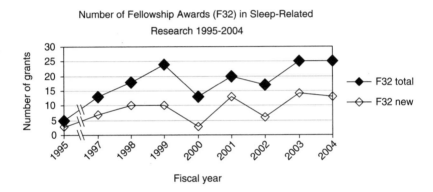

Grant	Title	Description	Number of Awards (New Awards)		
			1995	2000	2004
T32	National Research Service Award Institutional Research Training	Provides support to institutions to develop or enhance research training opportunities for predoctoral and postdoctoral students	3 (0)	11 (1)	16 (2)
T34	National Research Service Award—Institutional Undergraduate Research Training	Provides support to institutions to promote undergraduate research training to underrepresented groups in the biomedical and behavioral sciences	0	0	0
T35	Short-Term Institutional Research Training	Provides support to institutions for predoctoral and postdoctoral training focused on biomedical and behavioral research	0 (0)	0 (0)	7 (4)

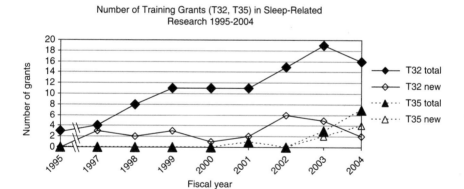

Number of Training Grants (T32, T35) in Sleep-Related
Research 1995-2004

J

Summary of Investment in Sleep-Related Projects at the Top 30 NIH-Funded Institutions

The following is a summary of the amount the top 30 National Institutes of Health (NIH)-funded institutions, ranked according to the total number of awards each institution received from the NIH in 2004. Institute of Medicine staff searched the Computer Retrieval of Information on Scientific Projects (CRISP) database for key-terms relevant to sleep. These terms include *insomnia, periodic limb movement disorder, restless legs syndrome, circadian rhythm, sudden infant death syndrome, sleep disorder, narcolepsy, sleep apnea, sleep, hibernation, and dream.* Abstracts were reviewed and only those grants with these terms listed in both the thesaurus terms and abstract, not the abstract alone, were considered in the counts. The committee then examined each institute's grant portfolio to determine the number of sleep-related awards it received.

TABLE J-1 Sleep-Related Research at the Top 30 NIH-Funded Institutions

Rank by Number of Total Grants	Rank by Number of Sleep Grants	Institution	Number of Awards Received
1	6	Johns Hopkins University	1,304
2	1	University of Pennsylvania	1,176
3	12	University of Washington	1,031
4	11	University of California, San Francisco	977
5	5	University of Michigan	945
6	2	University of Pittsburgh	938
7	3	University of California, Los Angeles	890
8	13	Washington University	885
9	17	Yale University	852
10	17	University of North Carolina-Chapel Hill	777
11	13	Duke University	759
12	NA[b]	Columbia University	747
13	9	Stanford University	739
14	13	Harvard University (Medical School)	723
15	18	Massachusetts General Hospital	672
16	10	Case Western Reserve University	670
17	19	University of California, San Diego	663
18	10	University of Wisconsin, Madison	653
19	10	Vanderbilt University	642
20	15	University of Minnesota	606
21	8	Emory University	580
22	19	Baylor College of Medicine	559
23	17	University of Alabama at Birmingham	553
24	2	Brigham and Women's Hospital	535
25	NA[b]	Cornell University	490
26	16	University of Colorado Denver/HSC Aurora	486
27	8	Oregon Health & Science University	473
28	11	Scripps Research Institute	465
29	12	Northwestern University	451
30	13	University of Virginia	450
Total			21,691

NOTES: To isolate only qualifying sleep-specific grants in the Total Number of Sleep Grants column, grants were obtained by searching the NIH CRISP database for key terms relevant to sleep. These terms include *insomnia, periodic limb movement disorder, restless legs syndrome, circadian rhythm, sudden infant death syndrome, sleep disorder, narcolepsy, sleep apnea, sleep, hibernation,* and *dream.* Abstracts were reviewed, and only those grants with these terms listed in the thesaurus were considered in the counts. The number for each institution reflects individual, unduplicated counts for a given year.

[a]The totals for P Awards are for "parent grants" and do not include subprojects.
[b]Columbia and Cornell Universities both received zero sleep awards in 2004.

Number of Sleep Awards	Sleep-Related Awards				
	Number of Career Development Awards	Number of Program Awards[a]	Number of Fellowship Awards	Number of Training Awards	Number of Research Project Awards
16	3	0	2	2	9
27	7	2	2	3	13
9	1	1	1	1	5
9	1	0	3	0	5
16	0	1	0	2	13
21	4	2	2	2	11
19	2	2	1	0	14
7	0	0	2	0	5
3	0	0	0	0	3
3	0	0	1	0	2
7	0	0	0	0	7
0	0	0	0	0	0
11	0	1	0	1	9
7	1	0	1	0	5
2	1	0	1	0	0
10	3	0	0	0	7
19	2	1	2	1	13
10	0	0	1	1	8
10	1	0	0	0	9
6	1	0	0	0	5
12	0	0	3	0	9
1	0	1	0	0	0
3	0	0	0	0	3
22	6	2	3	1	10
0	0	0	0	0	0
4	0	0	0	0	4
12	2	0	0	0	10
9	0	0	3	0	6
8	0	0	2	1	5
7	1	0	1	0	5
290					

K

Biographical Sketches of
Committee Members and Staff

Harvey R. Colten, M.D., (IOM) (*Chair*), recently retired as vice president and senior associate dean for Academic Affairs at Columbia University Medical Center. He was the chief medical officer, iMetrikus, Inc., and a clinical professor of pediatrics at the University of California, San Francisco, between 2000 and 2002. Previously, he served as dean of the medical school and vice president for medical affairs at Northwestern University from 1997 to 1999 and was the Harriet B. Spoehrer Professor and chair of the Department of Pediatrics at Washington University School of Medicine in St. Louis, Missouri, from 1986 to 1997. Dr. Colten earned a B.A. degree at Cornell in 1959, an M.D. from Western Reserve University in 1963, and an M.A. (honorary) from Harvard in 1978. Following his clinical training in 1965, he was an investigator at the National Institutes of Health until 1970. In 1970, he was appointed to the faculty at the Harvard Medical School, where he was named professor of pediatrics in 1979 and chief of the Division of Cell Biology, Pulmonary Medicine, and director of the Cystic Fibrosis Program at Children's Hospital Medical Center in Boston. Dr. Colten's research interests include the regulation of acute phase gene expression and genetic deficiencies of proteins that play a major role in pulmonary diseases, autoimmunity, and inflammation, on which he has published more than 270 original articles, book chapters and invited reviews. He is a member of Alpha Omega Alpha and a recipient of other honors, including a Special Faculty Research Award from Western Reserve University, the E. Mead Johnson Award for Pediatric Research, a MERIT Award from the National Institutes of Health (NIH), Distinguished Service Award from the American Association of Immunologists, and honorary membership in the Hungarian

Society of Immunology. He has been listed in Who's Who in America since 1982. Dr. Colten has been on editorial boards and advisory committees of several leading scientific and medical journals. He served on and was vice chairman of the Council of the Institute of Medicine and has served on multiple committees including the Committee on Drug Use in Food Animals, Committee on Palliative and End-of-Life Care for Children and Their Families, and the Committee for Review and Assessment of the NIH's Strategic Plan to Reduce and Ultimately Eliminate Health Disparities.

Francois M. Abboud, M.D., (IOM), is currently the Edith King Pearson Chair in Cardiovascular Research; professor of medicine, physiology, and biophysics; director, University of Iowa Cardiovascular Research Center; and associate vice president for research at the University of Iowa. He was chair of the Department of Internal Medicine from 1976 through 2002. His research is focused on integrative neurobiology of cardiovascular regulation, including the molecular determinants of sensory signaling and autonomic control. Human studies have focused on the integrated control of sympathetic activity in physiological and pathological states (e.g., sleep apnea and hypertension). He has received a number of awards, including ASPET Award for Experimental Therapeutics, American Society for Pharmacology and Experimental Therapeutics, the Wiggers Award of the American Physiological Society, the Research Achievement Award and the Gold Heart Award from the American Heart Association, and the CIBA award and medal for hypertension research of the Council for High Blood Pressure Research. He was editor-in-chief of *Circulation Research*, has served on the advisory council of the National Heart, Lung, and Blood Institute (1995–1999), is former president of the American Heart Association and the Association of American Physicians, and is currently associate editor of the journal *Physiology in Medicine*.

Gene D. Block, Ph.D., is the Thomas Jefferson Professor of Biology and the vice president and provost of the University of Virginia. Dr. Block's area of expertise is in circadian biology; he has studied the neurophysiological basis of circadian rhythms in mammals and in invertebrate models. He was founding director of the National Science Foundation's Science and Technology Center in Biological Timing. He also served as the University of Virginia's vice president for research and is past president of the Society for Research on Biological Rhythms. He received his A.B. degree from Stanford University and his Ph.D. degree from the University of Oregon.

Thomas F. Boat, M.D., (IOM), is director of the Children's Hospital Research Foundation and the professor and chair of the Department of Pediatrics at the University of Cincinnati. Dr. Boat has served as a member and chair of the Biochemistry II Study Section of the National Institutes of Health and as a council member of the National Heart, Lung, and Blood Institute. He chairs the Research Development Program Advisory Committee for the National Cystic Fibrosis Association and is a member of their Medical Advisory Committee. Dr. Boat is a recipient of the St. Geme Award from the Federation of Pediatric Organizations as well as former chair of the American Board of Pediatrics, president of the Association of Medical School Pediatric Department Chairs, and past president of the American Pediatric Society. His areas of expertise include pathophysiology of lung disease in children, subspecialty pediatric education, improvement of health services for children, and academic health center management.

Iris F. Litt, M.D., (IOM), is the Marron and Mary Elizabeth Kendrick Professor of Pediatrics and national director of the Robert Wood Johnson Clinical Scholars Program at the Stanford University School of Medicine. Dr. Litt's research focus is on the health problems of adolescent women, with particular emphasis on the interaction of psychosocial phenomena with biological features of the second decade of life. She previously participated in multiple Institute of Medicine (IOM) committees including the Committee on Lesbian Health Research Priorities, the Committee on Youth Development, and the Forum on Adolescence, and was workshop participant on Sleep Needs, Patterns, and Difficulties of Adolescents. She has been a member of the IOM since 1995; she served as editor of the *Journal of Adolescent Health* from 1990 to 2005 and was the former director for the Division of Adolescent Medicine at Stanford University from 1976 to 2005.

Emmanuel Mignot, M.D., Ph.D., (IOM), is professor of psychiatry and behavioral sciences and director of the Center for Narcolepsy at Stanford University, as well as a Howard Hughes Medical Institute investigator. Dr. Mignot has experience in clinical and basic research in the area of sleep disorders medicine. He is board certified in sleep disorders medicine. Dr. Mignot has extensive experience in basic and clinical research of sleep disorders, most particularly with narcolepsy. He is currently on the Board of Scientific Councilors of the National Institute of Mental Health and serves on the editorial board of scientific journals in the field of sleep disorders research. Dr. Mignot is a past chair of the National Center on Sleep Disorders Research Advisory Board of the National Institutes of Health, former president of the Sleep Research Society, and former board member of the National Sleep Foundation. Dr. Mignot received both his M.D. and Ph.D. degrees from Paris University in 1984 and 1986, respectively.

Robert H. Miller, M.D., M.B.A., is the executive director of the American Board of Otolaryngology. Previously, he was professor and chair of

Otolaryngology-Head and Neck Surgery and vice chancellor at Tulane University Medical Center, dean of the University of Nevada School of Medicine, and was a Robert Wood Johnson Health Policy Fellow. His research interests have focused on the medical workforce and health policy. He received his M.D. degree in 1973 from Tulane University, did a residency in otolaryngology, performed head and neck surgery at UCLA, and received his M.B.A. degree from Tulane in 1996.

F. Javier Nieto, M.D., Ph.D., is the Helfaer Professor of Public Health, and professor and chair of the Department of Population Health Sciences at the University of Wisconsin School of Medicine and Public Health in Madison. His areas of research interest include cardiovascular disease epidemiology, markers of subclinical atherosclerosis, emerging risk factors for cardiovascular disease, and health consequences of sleep disorders and psychosocial stress. He is a board member of the American College of Epidemiology; a member of the American Society of Epidemiology; a fellow of the American Heart Association's Council on Epidemiology and Prevention; and he is affiliated with the American Public Health Association, Society for Epidemiologic Research, Spanish Epidemiologic Society, and Spanish Society of Public Health and Health Services Administration. He received his M.D. degree from University of Valencia in 1978, his M.P.H. from University of Havana, Cuba, and his Ph.D. in epidemiology from the Johns Hopkins School of Public Health in 1991.

Allan I. Pack, M.D., Ph.D., is professor of medicine and director of the Center for Sleep and Respiratory Neurobiology and chief of the Division of Sleep Medicine at the University of Pennsylvania. Dr. Pack's current major research focus is sleep and its disorders, particularly sleep apnea. In 1988, Dr. Pack was awarded one of three specialized centers of research (SCOR) in cardiopulmonary disorders during sleep from the National Institutes of Health; in 1998, he received a second SCOR in neurobiology of sleep and sleep apnea. Dr. Pack is the author of over 190 original papers and chapters and has edited three books. He has received a number of awards, including the Nathaniel Kleitman Award and the William C. Dement Academic Achievement Award from the American Academy of Sleep Medicine. He received his M.B.ChB. degree in 1968 and his Ph.D. in 1976, both from the University of Glasgow.

Kathy P. Parker, Ph.D., R.N., F.A.A.N., is the Edith F. Honeycutt Professor at the Nell Hodgson Woodruff School of Nursing and professor of neurology at Emory University. In 2001, she established the Center for Research on Symptoms, Symptom Interactions, and Health Outcomes, one of nine exploratory nursing research centers funding by the National Institute of

Nursing Research. She has more than 20 years of clinical experience in nursing and is one of five nurses in the country certified in Clinical Sleep Disorders by the American Board of Sleep Medicine. She is a fellow in the American Academy of Sleep Medicine and the American Academy of Nursing. Dr. Parker's program of research focuses on sleep-wake disturbances in hemodialysis patients and the effects of pain and opioids on sleep in cancer patients.

Samuel J. Potolicchio, M.D., is professor of neurology at the George Washington University Medical Center. Dr. Potolicchio's research interests are in sleep and convulsive disorders, particularly epilepsy, and in other neurological disorders. He also treats patients with peripheral neuropathies, sleep disturbances, mental confusion, impaired memory, and memory loss. Dr. Potolicchio has served as a member on previous Institute of Medicine Committees on the Gulf War and health.

Susan Redline, M.D., M.P.H., is professor of pediatrics, medicine, epidemiology and biostatistics at Case Western Reserve University School of Medicine and is the chief of the Division of Clinical Epidemiology in the Department of Pediatrics at Rainbow Babies & Children's Hospital. Her research interest focuses on the epidemiology of chronic diseases with an emphasis on sleep apnea, and on pulmonary and cardiovascular diseases. She directs the Case Sleep and Epidemiology Research Center, which serves as a national sleep reading center for numerous large-scale sleep epidemiological studies. Dr. Redline also directs the University Hospitals of Cleveland Sleep Disorders Center. She is an associate editor of *Sleep* and a current member of Scientific Advisory Committee of the American Thoracic Society and a member of the National Center on Sleep Disorders Research Advisory Board of the National Institutes of Health.

Charles F. Reynolds III, M.D., is a University of Pittsburgh, School of Medicine Endowed Professor of Geriatric Psychiatry, and senior associate dean of the University of Pittsburgh, School of Medicine. He directs the National Institute of Mental Health (NIMH)-sponsored Advanced Center for Interventions and Services Research in Late-Life Mood Disorders and the John A. Hartford Center of Excellence in Geriatric Psychiatry at the Western Psychiatric Institute and Clinic. Dr. Reynolds' primary research interests focus on mood and sleep disorders of later life, the prevention and treatment of those disorders, suicide prevention, and the dissemination of evidence-based practice to general medical settings. Dr. Reynolds is the past recipient of a MERIT Award and a Senior Scientist Award from the NIMH; he has led the field in studies of maintenance treatment of mood disorders in old age. He currently serves on the National Mental Health Advisory

Council and has previously served on the Institute of Medicine Committee on the Pathophysiology and Prevention of Adolescent and Adult Suicide. Dr. Reynolds is immediate past president of the American College of Psychiatrists. He graduated from the Yale University School of Medicine in 1973 and from the University of Virginia in 1969.

Clifford B. Saper, M.D., Ph.D., is James Jackson Putnam Professor of Neurology and Neuroscience at Harvard Medical School and chair of the Department of Neurology at Beth Israel Deaconess Medical Center. Previously, he was an assistant, then associate, professor in the Departments of Neurology and Anatomy and Neurobiology at the Washington University School of Medicine and associate professor and then the William D. Mabie Professor of Neurology and Neuroscience at the University of Chicago, where he chaired the graduate program in neuroscience. Dr. Saper's research interests focus on identifying neuronal circuitry involved in regulating integrated functions maintained by the hypothalamus, including wake-sleep cycles, body temperature, and feeding, and determining the homologous circuitry in human brains and examining how it may be disrupted in specific neurological and psychiatric disorders. Currently, he is editor-in-chief of the *Journal of Comparative Neurology* and serves on the editorial boards of *Neurology, Physiological Genomics, Sleep,* and *Neuroimmunomodulation.* Dr. Saper formerly was a member of the National Center on Sleep Disorders Research Advisory Board of the National Institutes of Health and previously served on the National Research Council's Howard Higher Medical Institute (HHMI) Predoctoral Fellowships Panel on Neurosciences and Physiology.

IOM STAFF

Bruce M. Altevogt, Ph.D., is a senior program officer in the Board on Health Sciences Policy at the Institute of Medicine (IOM). He received his doctoral thesis from Harvard University's Program in Neuroscience. While at Harvard Dr. Altevogt studied how the glial cells in the central and peripheral nervous system form a network of cells through intracellular communication, which is critical for maintaining myelin. After receiving his Ph.D., Dr. Altevogt was a policy fellow with the Christine Mirzayan Science & Technology Policy Graduate Fellowship Program at the National Academies. He has over 10 years of research experience. In addition to Dr. Altevogt's work at Harvard, he also performed neuroscience research at the National Institutes of Health and the University of Virginia. He received his B.A. degree from the University of Virginia in Charlottesville, where he majored in biology and minored in south Asian studies. Since joining the Board on Health Sciences Policy, he was a program officer on the IOM study *Spinal Cord*

Injury: Progress, Promise, and Priorities and is serving as the director of the Forum on Neuroscience and Nervous System Disorders and Stem Cell Research Advisory Committee.

Andrew Pope, Ph.D., is director of the Board on Health Sciences Policy at the Institute of Medicine. With a doctoral degree in physiology and biochemistry, his primary interests focus on environmental and occupational influences on human health. Dr. Pope's previous research activities focused on the neuroendocrine and reproductive effects of various environmental substances in food-producing animals. During his tenure at the National Academies and since 1989 at the Institute of Medicine, Dr. Pope has directed numerous studies; topics include injury control, disability prevention, biological markers, neurotoxicology, indoor allergens, and the enhancement of environmental and occupational health content in medical and nursing school curricula. Most recently, Dr. Pope directed studies on National Institutes of Health priority-setting processes, organ procurement and transplantation policy, and the role of science and technology in countering terrorism.

Miriam Davis, Ph.D., is an independent medical writer and consultant. She is a frequent contributor to reports of the Institute of Medicine and United States Surgeon General. After receiving her doctorate in neurobiology from Princeton University, she gained nearly 10 years of health policy experience at the Assistant Secretary for Health's office in the Department of Health and Human Services. She later became Director of Policy for the National Institutes of Health's National Institute of Environmental Health Sciences. For the past 10 years, she has been a medical writer and consultant on high-profile reports and publications and has coauthored review articles in *Science, Journal of the American Medical Association,* and *Neurology.* She holds an adjunct faculty post at the George Washington University School of Public Health and Health Services.

Sarah L. Hanson is a research associate in the Board on Health Sciences Policy at the Institute of Medicine. Ms. Hanson is working for the Committee on Sleep Medicine and Research. Prior to joining the Institute of Medicine, she served as research and program assistant at the National Research Center for Women & Families. Ms. Hanson has a B.A. degree from the University of Kansas with a double major in political science and international studies.

Lora K. Taylor is a senior project assistant for the Board on Health Sciences Policy working on the Sleep Medicine and Research project. She has 14 years of experience working in the academy and prior to joining the Institute of Medicine, she served as the administrative associate for the Report

Review Committee and the Division on Life Sciences' Ocean Studies Board. Ms. Taylor has a B.A. degree from Georgetown University with a double major in psychology and fine arts.

Eleanore Edson, Ph.D., a Christine Mirzayan Science & Technology Policy Graduate Fellow in the Board on Health Sciences Policy. Dr. Edson successfully defended her Ph.D. thesis in neurobiology at Harvard University in August 2005 and holds a B.S. degree in biology from Stanford University. Between college and graduate school, she studied abroad at the Glasgow School of Art on a Rotary International Scholars Fellowship.

Amy Haas is the administrative assistant for the Board on Health Sciences Policy. She previously served as a senior project assistant for the Clinical Research Roundtable. Prior to joining the Institute of Medicine, she worked as a project manager for a medical education and publishing firm in Washington, DC. She graduated from Whitman College in Walla Walla, Washington with a B.A. degree in biology.

Catharyn T. Liverman, M.L.S., is a senior program officer at the Institute of Medicine (IOM). In her 12 years at the IOM, she has worked on studies addressing a range of topics, primarily focused on public health and science policy. Most recently she was the study director for the IOM committee that produced the report *Preventing Childhood Obesity: Health in the Balance.* Other recent studies include *Testosterone and Aging: Clinical Research Directions, Gulf War and Health,* and *Reducing the Burden of Injury.* Her background is in medical library science, with previous positions at the National Agricultural Library and the Naval War College Library. She received a B.A. degree from Wake Forest University and an M.L.S. degree from the University of Maryland.

Kathleen M. Patchan was a research associate at the Institute of Medicine (IOM). She served as a research associate on the *Sleep Medicine and Biology* study until July 2005. She worked on a study on health literacy and assisted with staffing IOM's Sarnat Award. She also worked on an IOM study that resulted in the report *Incorporating Research into Psychiatry Residency Training.* Previously, at the Congressional Research Service and the Center on Budget and Policy Priorities, she conducted research and wrote reports on Medicaid, the State Children's Health Insurance Program (SCHIP), and state-funded immigrant health care. She has also worked at the Institute for Health Policy Solutions, where she developed reports on SCHIP and employer-sponsored health insurance. Ms. Patchan graduated from the University of Maryland at College Park with a B.S. degree in cell and molecular biology and a B.A. degree in history.

Index

chronic disease management model, 28,
304, 321
consortia, 185, 187
constraints on, 26-28, 300-303
diagnosis-treatment linkages, 28, 303-
305
direct costs, 307-309
education and training, 304
examples of approaches, 299
grants, 318, 370
guiding principles, 11, 14-16, 305-306
health insurance coverage, 315
institutional reward system and, 301
key components, 303-306
knowledge base, 26, 296
leadership, 305
macrostructure, 310-311
microstructure, 311
network participation, 12-13, 282, 284,
305, 320
next steps, 315-321
obstacles, 27, 301-302
organizational structures, 13-14, 27-28,
310-311, 312, 316-320
and quality of care, 27
rationale for, 26-28, 294-300
recommendations, 14, 319, 321
research component, 304-305
revenue generation and fiscal
independence, 28, 305-310,
311-312
staffing, 298-300, 302-303, 307
transparent policies and procedures, 306,
311
Type I clinical program, 13, 15-16, 279,
284, 316, 317, 319-320
Type II training and research program,
13, 15-16, 200, 284, 316, 317, 318,
320
Type III regional program, 13-14, 15-16,
200, 284, 316, 317, 318, 320
International Classification of Sleep
Disorders, 56, 86, 104, 107, 262
Internet, 21, 58
Interventions. *See also* Treatment
effectiveness of, 150-151
Iron deficiency, 98, 262, 295-296
Irregular sleep schedules, 58
Irregular sleep-wake disorder, 107
Irritability, 79, 108, 184

J

Jet lag, 58, 107

K

K awards. *See* Career development in sleep
research
K complexes, 36, 38
Kleine-Levin syndrome, 84, 86, 87, 273,
340

L

Learning and vocabulary, sleep loss and,
140, 145, 146, 184, 264
Leptin, 60, 72, 267, 340
Lewy body disease, 92, 262, 296
Light-dark cycle, 39, 40, 43
Light exposure, 47, 76, 109, 110, 143

M

Magnetic resonance imaging, 186, 227, 340
Maintenance of Wakefulness Test (MWT),
227
Maternal and Child Health Bureau, 180
Median thalamic stroke, 85
Medical disorders and sleep. *See also*
individual disorders
cancer, 103, 105
grants for research, 270
infectious diseases, 102-104
pain, 100-101
treatment-related effects, 104-106
Medical education in somnology. *See also*
Professional training
accreditation and certification, 189, 190,
191-192, 196, 197-201, 202
barriers to curriculum implementation,
25, 188
evaluation of effectiveness of, 188, 189-
190
inadequacy of, 187-188
multidisciplinary learning environment,
189, 192, 193, 202
nurses as care managers, 190-191
overview, 187-191
residency training curricula, 191-192

and mood and behavior, 63
and mortality, 63-64
and obesity, 59-61
prevalence, 2, 20, 56, 57, 206
public health burden, 2, 56, 294
and quality of life, 48, 151-153
Sleep medicine. *See* Somnology and sleep
medicine research
Sleep monitoring. *See* Portable monitoring
and therapeutic devices
Sleep paralysis, 84, 87, 89, 90, 342
Sleep patterns
age and, 44-47, 142, 143
circadian rhythm disruption, 21
temporal distribution, 108
Sleep Research Society, 2, 22, 25, 29, 177,
235, 237, 249
Sleep Research Society Foundation, 177
Sleep restriction therapy, 77, 342
*Sleep, Sleep Disorders, and Biological
Rhythms*, 176
Sleep spindles, 36, 186, 342-343
Sleep terrors, 89, 90, 227, 343
Sleep-wake regulation
brain processes and structures, 40-41,
43, 76-77, 80, 85, 92, 94, 261
iatrogenic effects of medical therapies,
104-106
immune system and, 102
phylogenetic studies, 261-262
two-process model, 39-40
Sleepiness, excessive daytime. *See*
Hypersomnia
Sleeping sickness, 102-104, 335
Sleepwalking, 88, 89-90, 343
Slow-wave sleep
arousal disorders, 90
body temperature and, 43
characteristics, 36-37
defined, 343
depression and, 79
endocrine function, 39
infections and, 102
opioids and, 105
Small Business Innovation Research (SBIR)
grants, 222
Snoring, 65, 66, 70, 73, 74, 99, 145, 150,
221, 266
Socioeconomic status
and insomnia, 160
and narcolepsy, 162
and OSA, 161-162

Somnology and sleep medicine research. *See
also* Career development in sleep
research; Interdisciplinary sleep
programs
academic programs, 5, 235-236, 375-
377
adolescents, 186
advances since 2003, 260-267
animal studies, 261-262, 271, 274, 352
basic, 23, 25, 240, 259, 261-262, 270,
272, 279, 282, 354
Basics of Sleep Research guide, 177
bias in studies, 59, 70, 74
Centers of Excellence, 278-282, 283
challenges, 6, 22-26
circadian rhythm, 260-261, 270, 272
clinical, 270, 272, 274, 279, 282, 285-
286
collaborations, 28, 276, 277-278
coordination by NIH, 2, 3-5, 22-24,
186, 229, 240, 241, 244, 250, 254-
256, 257-258, 267, 268, 275-276,
277, 357
defining, 2 n.1, 20, 23, 250, 342, 343
fellowship training, 192-197, 198, 199,
200
grants from NIH, 4, 200, 235-236, 254,
255, 256, 277, 282, 296, 340-342,
351-359, 368-373, 375-377; *see also*
Analysis of NIH grants
growth of field, 4, 22, 25, 234-238, 296
historical background, 21-22
human studies, 271, 274
insomnia, 265
interdisciplinary approach, 3-4, 6, 242,
254, 278-282, 297-300
investigator shortages, 2, 5, 6, 25-26, 27,
234, 296
knowledge base, 296
minorities in, 236-237
molecular/genetic studies, 262, 263, 271,
273
national network, 7, 14, 179, 279, 282-
285, 320
neurobiology-related, 260-262, 352
next steps, 276-286
outlook for, 254, 267-268
pediatric sleep sciences, 265-266
phylogenetic approaches, 261-262
professional societies, 22, 235
recommendations, 4-5, 277, 283, 285-
286